The Mental Health of Children and Adolescents

The Mental Health of Children and Adolescents

An Area of Global Neglect

A report from the World Psychiatric Association Presidential Programme on Child Mental Health

Editors

Helmut Remschmidt
Head of the Department of Child and Adolescent Psychiatry, Philipps University, Marburg, Germany

Barry Nurcombe
Professor Emeritus of Child and Adolescent Psychiatry, The University of Queensland, Brisbane, Australia

Myron L. Belfer
Professor of Psychiatry, Department of Social Medicine, Harvard Medical School, Boston MA, USA

Norman Sartorius
President, Association for the Improvement of Mental Health Programmes, Geneva, Switzerland

Ahmed Okasha
Professor and Director of WHO Collaborating Center for Research and Training in Mental Health, Institute of Psychiatry, Ain Shams University, Cairo, Egypt

BICENTENNIAL 1807 WILEY 2007 BICENTENNIAL

John Wiley & Sons, Ltd

Telephone (+44) 1243 779777

Email (for orders and customer service enquiries): cs-books@wiley.co.uk
Visit our Home Page on www.wiley.com

Other Wiley Editorial Offices

John Wiley & Sons Inc., 111 River Street, Hoboken, NJ 07030, USA

Jossey-Bass, 989 Market Street, San Francisco, CA 94103-1741, USA

Wiley-VCH Verlag GmbH, Boschstr. 12, D-69469 Weinheim, Germany

John Wiley & Sons Australia Ltd, 42 McDougall Street, Milton, Queensland 4064, Australia

John Wiley & Sons (Asia) Pte Ltd, 2 Clementi Loop #02-01, Jin Xing Distripark, Singapore 129809

John Wiley & Sons Canada Ltd, 6045 Freemont Blvd, Mississauga, ONT, L5R 4J3, Canada

Wiley also publishes its books in a variety of electronic formats. Some content that appears in print may not be available in electronic books.

Anniversary Logo Design: Richard J. Pacifico

British Library Cataloguing in Publication Data

A catalogue record for this book is available from the British Library

ISBN 978-0-470-51245-6

Typeset in 10/12 pt Times by Thomson Digital
Printed and bound in Great Britain by Antony Rowe Ltd, Chippenham, Wiltshire
This book is printed on acid-free paper responsibly manufactured from sustainable forestry
in which at least two trees are planted for each one used for paper production.

Contents

Contributors

Alan Apter, Department of Psychiatry, Feinberg Child Study Center, Schneider Children's Medical Center of Israel, 14 Kaplan Street, Petah Tikva 49202, Israel

Valeriya Andreyuk, Center for Mental Health of Children and Adolescents, Nizhny Novgorod, Nesterovstr. 3-17, Chrenoprudsky 4, 603005, Russia

Mary Azzer, Department of Community Medicine, Alexandria University and the Egyptian Child Mental Health Association, 36 Moustafa Fahmi Street, Gleem, Alexandria, Egypt

José J. Bauermeister, Behavioral Sciences Research Institute, University of Puerto Rico, PO Box 365067, San Juan, Puerto Rico

Carlotta Belaise, Department of Psychiatry and Mental Health, University of Modena and Reggio Emilia, Italy

Myron L. Belfer, Department of Social Medicine, Harvard Medical School, 641 Huntington Avenue Boston, Massachusetts 02115, USA

Ernesto Caffo, Department of Psychiatry and Mental Health, University of Modena Cattedra di Neuropsichiatria, Infantile Vil del Pozzo 71, 1-40100 Modena, Italy

Júlia Obst Comassetto, Federal University of Rio Grande do Sul, Brazil

Tatjana Dmitrieva, Center for Mental Health of Children and Adolescents Nizhny Novgorod, Nesterovstr. 3-17, Chrenoprudsky 4, 603005, Russia

Amira Seif El Din, Department, of Community Medicine, Alexandria University and the Egyptian Child Mental Health Association, 36 Moustafa Fahmi Street, Gleem, Alexandria, Egypt

John Fayyad, Department of Psychiatry and Clinical Psychology, St. George Hospital University Medical Center, Faculty of Medicine, Balamand University, Institute for Development, Research, Advocacy and Applied Care, P.O.Box: 16-6378 Beirut – Ashrafeih 1100 – 2807, Lebanon

Martine F. Flament, University of Ottawa, Institute of Mental Health Research, Royal Ottawa Hospital, 1145 Carling Ave, Ottawa, Ontario K1Z 7K4, Canada

Anat Fleischman, Geha Psychiatric Hospital, P.O. Box 102 49100 Petah-Tiqva, Israel

Claudia Furino, University of Ottawa, Institute of Mental Health Research, Royal Ottawa Hospital, 1145 Carling Ave, Ottawa, Ontario KIZ 7K4, Canada

Renata Rocha Gonçalves, Instituto de Pesquisa: Centro de Estudos da Metrópole, Rua Morgado de Mateus, 615, 04015-902, São Paulo, Brazil

Ana Soledade Graeff-Martins, Department of Psychiatry, Federal University of Rio Grande do Sul, Hospital de Clinicas de Porto Alegre, Rua Ramiro Barcelos, 2350, Porto Alegre, Rio Grande do Sul, 90035-003, Brazil

Doa Habib, Egyptian Child Mental Health Association, Egypt

Richard Harrington, Deceased

Kimberly Hoagwood, Professor of Clinical Psychology in Psychiatry, Columbia University, New York State Office of Mental Health, 1051 Riverside Dr., #78, New York NY 10032, USA

Jack S. F. Hung, Director of Research on Child & Adolescent Services Kwai Chung Hospital, Kwai Chung Hospital Road, Hong Kong

Peter S. Jensen, Center for the Advancement of Children's Mental Health, Department of Child Psychiatry, Columbia University/NY State Psychiatric Institute, 1051 Riverside Drive Unit #78, New York, NY10032, USA

Kelly Kelleher, Columbus Children's Research Institute, The Ohio State University, 700 Children's Drive, Columbus OH 43205, USA

Christian Kieling, Department of Psychiatry, Federal University of Rio Grande do Sul, Rua Ramiro Barcelos 2350, Porto Alegre 90035-003, RS, Brazil

Paulo Knapp, Klinika Ginekologii, Akademia Medyczna w Bialymstoku, ul. M. Skłodowskiej - Curie 24a, 15-276 Białystok

Orit Krispin, Lehrstuhl fur Mikrobiologie, Universitat Erlangen-Nuremberg, Staudtstrasse 5, D-91058 Erlangen, Germany

Cathy MacLean, Royal Ottawa Health Care Group, 1145 Carling Avenue, Ottawa, Ontario K1Z 7K4, Canada

Laura Murray, Boston University School of Public Health, Center for International Health and Development, Applied Mental Health Research Group, 715 Albany Street, Talbot Building, Boston, Massachusetts 02118, USA

Hien Nguyen, University of Ottawa, Institute of Mental Health Research, Royal Ottawa Hospital, 1145 Carling Ave, Ottawa, Ontario KIZ 7K4, Canada

Barry Nurcombe, University of Queensland, 49 Highview Terrace, St. Lucia, Brisbane, Queensland 4067, Australia

Ahmed Okasha, WHO Collaborating Centre, Institute of Psychiatry, Ain Shams University, 3 Ahmed Boraei Street, From Shehab St, Mohandessin, 12411 Giza, Egypt

Sylvia Oswald, University Hospital Ulm, Department for Child and Adolescent Psychiatry/ Psychotherapy, Steinhoevelstr. 5, D-89075 Ulm, Germany

Helmut Remschmidt, Philipps University, Hans-Sachs-Str. 4-8, D-35033 Marburg, Germany

Luis Augusto Rohde, Rua Ramiro Barcelos, 2350, Hospital de Clinicas de Porto Alegre, Porto Alegre-RS, 90035/003, Brazil

Per-Anders Rydelius, Astrid Lindgren's Children's Hospital, Karolinska Hospital, SE-17176 Stockholm, Sweden

Norman Sartorius, 14 Chemin Colladon, University of Geneva, 1209 Geneva, Switzerland

Howard Schachter, The Provincial Center of Excellence for Child and Youth Mental Health, Children's Hospital of Eastern Ontario Research Institute, 401 Smyth Road, Ottawa, Ontario K1H 8L1, Canada

Cheryl So, Kwai Chung Hospital, Kwai Chung Hospital Road, Hong Kong

Sam Tyano, Geha Psychiatric Hospital, P.O. Box 102, 49100 Petah-Tiqva, Israel

Danuta Wasserman, National Institute for Psychosocial Medicine, Karolinska Institute, Head of the Department of Public Health Sciences, Granits vag 4, Solna, SE-171 77 Stockholm, Sweden

Andrey Zanozin, Center for Mental Health of Children and Adolescents, Nizhny Novgorod, Nesterovstr. 3-17, Chrenoprudsky 4, 603005, Russia

Advisory Board

Members of the Advisory Board to the WPA Presidential Programme on Child Mental Health:

Thomas M. Achenbach, USA
Abd-Ul-Amir K. Al-Ganimee, Iraq
Alan Apter, Israel
Florence Baingana, World Bank (USA)
Cornelio G. Banaag, Philippines
Edgard Belfort, Venezuela
Zeinab Bishry, Egypt
Jan Buitelaar, Netherlands
Dirk Deboutte, Belgium
Saida Douki, Tunisia
Sue Estroff, USA
John Fayyad, Lebanon
Elizabeth Fivaz, Switzerland
Carole Florman, USA
Sherry Glied, USA
Ian Goodyer, UK
Luis Diego Herrera, Costa Rica
Ashfaq Ishaq, USA
Philippe Jeammet, France
Malavika Kapur (Psychology), India
Alla Kholmogorova, Russia
Anne-Liis von Knorring, Sweden
Valery Krasnov, Russia
Stan Kutcher, Canada
Francois Ladame, Switzerland
Stella Maris Maldonado, Argentina
Savita Malhotra, India
Virginia L. Mason, USA
Tiberiu Mircea, Romania
Driss Moussaoui, Morocco
Frank Njenga, Kenya
Frank Oberklaid, Australia
Mahmoud Okasha, USA
Marie-Odile Perouse de Montclos, France
Dainius Puras, Lithuania
Shobini Rao (Pediatric Neurology), India
Franz Resch, Germany
Agnes Rupp, USA
Maha Sayed, Egypt
Stephen Scott, UK
Anatoly A. Severny, Russia
Mimoza Shahini, Serbia and Montenegro
Yury S. Shevchenko, Russia
Sadaaki Shirataki, Japan
Wei-Tsuen Soong, Taiwan
Suna Taneli, Turkey
Eric Taylor, UK
Martina Tomori, Slovenia
Frank Verhulst, Netherlands
Agnes Vetro, Hungary
Donata Vivanti (Parent association), Italy
Andreas Warnke, Germany
Jean-Victor P. Wittenberg, Canada
Kosuke Yamazaki, Japan
Victor Zaretsky, Russia

Preface

It is an honour and a pleasure to write a preface to this book describing some of the activities of the Presidential Programme on Child Mental Health of the World Psychiatric Association (WPA) conducted in the years 2002–2005, while one of us (AO) was president of the Association.

The programme was the first of its kind, a fact that should surprise. Although the majority of the world's population are children and adolescents, of whom a significant proportion suffer from mental and neurological disorders, there had never been any international programme that aimed to improve the care for children and adolescents who suffer from such disorders.

The WPA programme came into existence and became a success because of the contribution of many, the world over. Child psychiatrists, psychologists, social workers, teachers, and other professionals contributed their time and wisdom. Organizations of family members gave advice and got involved in the use of the products of the programme. The institutions involved in the programme gave their moral support and facilitated the participation of their staff in the activities of the programme. Eli Lilly and Company provided financial support in the form of an unrestricted educational grant. For all of them, the main reward is that the goals of the programme were achieved in full and in accordance with the plans that were drawn up: On our part, however, we also wish to acknowledge all these contributions without which the programme would not have been possible.

The book has three main parts. In the first, there is a description of the programme, and two reviews – one of the evidence regarding ways and means of raising awareness of child mental health programmes and another of the epidemiology of mental disorders in childhood. The second part describes the findings of a feasibility study conducted to establish whether knowledge and information condensed in training programmes concerned with treatment of mental disorders in childhood and adolescence can be effectively distributed using modern means of communication, such as teleconferences and written media. In the third part of the book, there are several reviews of knowledge concerning the prevention of mental disorders in childhood and adolescence and the description of three studies – in Brazil, Egypt, and Russia – carried out to establish whether school dropout can be prevented by specific mental health interventions. The reviews and case studies are examples taken from an array of materials produced in the course of the programme. Other materials are likely to be published in the future, possibly in the local languages. This will be a part of the programmes undertaken by the International Association of Child and Adolescent Psychiatry and Allied Professions (IACAPAP) to develop this area further, using the bases that were produced in the World Psychiatric Association's programme.

Child and adolescent mental health has been a neglected area of public health efforts for a long time. The WPA programme was a first, successful, and important step in the development of international collaboration in this area. It is our hope that other steps will follow, including an active involvement of professional and nonprofessional organizations, of governments, of the health industries, the educational and health systems of parent organizations, and all other stakeholders who can help to improve health and quality of life of the world's children and adolescents and to thus create a solid basis for a better world for all people tomorrow.

Ahmed Okasha and Norman Sartorius

Acknowledgments

This book is a product of the World Psychiatric Association's Presidential Programme on Child Mental Health carried out in collaboration with the World Health Organization and the International Association for Child and Adolescent Psychiatry and Allied Professions.

The programme was organized and managed by a Steering Committee chaired by Professor Ahmed Okasha and co-chaired by Professor Norman Sartorius. Its members were Helmut Remschmidt (Scientific Director and Chairperson of the Primary Prevention Task Force), Sam Tyano (Vice Director and Chairperson of the Awareness Task Force), Peter Jensen (Chairman of the Service Development Task Force), Tarek Okasha (Secretary of the Steering Committee), Barry Nurcombe, Myron L. Belfer (WHO representative to the Steering Committee), and John Heiligenstein.

The programme had three task forces:

Task force on Awareness: Ange Agoussou (Congo), Myron L. Belfer (USA), Michael Hong (Korea), Christina Hoven (USA), Du Ya Song (China), Danuta Wasserman (Sweden).

Task force on Service Development and Management: José Jorge Bauermeister (Puerto Rico), John Fayyad (Lebanon), Richard Harrington (UK), Kimberly Hoagwood (USA), S.F. Hung (China), Kelly Kelleher (USA).

Task force on Primary Prevention: Ernesto Caffo (Italy), John Cox (UK), Amira Seif El Din (Egypt), Tatjana Dmitrieva (Russia), Martine F. Flament (Canada), Luis Augusto Rohde (Brazil), Per-Anders Rydelius (Sweden).

The programme was supported by an unrestricted educational grant from the Eli Lilly and Company Foundation and by the institutions and individuals who participated in the programme.

CHAPTER 1

A Global Programme for Child and Adolescent Mental Health: A Challenge in the New Millennium

Myron L. Belfer
Harvard Medical School, Boston MA, USA
Helmut Remschmidt
Philipps University, Marburg, Germany
Barry Nurcombe
The University of Queensland, Brisbane, Australia
Ahmed Okasha
WHO Collaborating Center, Ain Shams University, Cairo, Egypt
Norman Sartorius
Association for the Improvement of Mental Health Programmes, Geneva, Switzerland

BACKGROUND

In 2003, during the presidency of Dr Ahmed Okasha, the World Psychiatric Association (WPA) initiated the Global Programme for Child and Adolescent Mental Health. The Programme was conducted in collaboration with the World Health Organization (WHO) and the International Association for Child and Adolescent Psychiatry and Allied Professions (IACAPAP). This unique initiative focused on three key areas: *Awareness*, *Prevention*, and *Treatment*. The respective task forces generated products that will have a continuing impact on advocacy, training, prevention, and services development. A special product of the collaboration was the WHO Child and Adolescent Mental Health Atlas which for the first time documents objectively the gaps in global services and training available, worldwide, for child and adolescent mental health (World Health Organization, 2005).

The Mental Health of Children and Adolescents: an area of global neglect. Edited by H. Remschmidt *et al.*

The WPA Presidential Global Programme on Child Mental Health was always mindful of the need to respect and support the rights of children, adolescents, and their families. Its overall objectives were as follows:

- To increase awareness by health decision makers, health professionals, and the general public of the magnitude and severity of problems related to mental disorders in childhood and adolescence, and the possibility of their resolution.
- To promote the primary prevention of mental disorders in childhood and adolescence and foster interventions that will contribute to healthy mental development.
- To offer support for the development of services for children and adolescents with mental disorders and promote the use of evidence-based methods of treatment.

The Global Programme was initiated by Prof. Ahmed Okasha, as President of the WPA, and coordinated by an International Steering Committee chaired by Prof. Okasha and Prof. Norman Sartorius. In the process of implementation, the Programme generated several worldwide initiatives, for example, field trials for the prevention of school dropout in Alexandria (Egypt), Nizhnij Novgorod (Russia), and Porto Alegre (Brazil). The results of the Global Programme were presented in 2005 at the World Congress of Psychiatry in Cairo.

As will be detailed in later chapters, the Global Programme began a process that stimulated the task forces to focus on particular areas. The process itself is of interest in that it demonstrated the need for priority setting in an area of health care that requires resource rationing. The Programme harnessed the collective wisdom of knowledgeable individuals worldwide.

The Awareness Task Force recognized the need to help constituencies to develop informed advocacy. Consequently, it produced as its primary offering a manual for implementing an awareness campaign. Rather than focusing on a nebulous prevention campaign, the Prevention Task Force identified a key area in which it would be possible to make a demonstrable impact. The preventive setting chosen was in schools, specifically in regard to school dropout, a problem that has broad implications for child mental health. Recognizing the need for training materials that could be used in the developing world, the Treatment Task Force produced two manuals and collateral documents concerning the treatment of externalizing and internalizing disorders. As a whole, through these activities, the Global Programme accomplished the goal of raising global awareness of child and adolescent mental health needs and how these might be addressed. This volume gives details of the overall Programme and its research activities, provides background documents, and directs readers to available resources. The volume itself is part of a continuing effort to enhance advocacy and disseminate information.

CHILD RIGHTS CONTEXT FOR THE GLOBAL PROGRAMME

Children and adolescents must be respected as human beings with clearly defined rights. *The United Nations (UN) Convention on the Rights of the Child* delineates the rights that should be accorded children and their families (United Nations Convention on the Rights of the Child). The Convention is applicable to children in all cultures and societies and has particular relevance for those living in conditions of adversity. Two additional documents should be mentioned in connection with the convention: *The Optional Protocol on the Involvement of Children in Armed Conflicts* and *The Optional Protocol on the Sale of Children, Child Prostitution, and Child Pornography.* All three documents provide comprehensive guidance to the human-rights entitlements of children, adolescents, and their families.

Children with mental health problems are entitled to benefit from the guarantees of the Convention; however, this is not the case in many parts of the world. The magnitude and impact of mental health problems have not yet been properly recognized by many governments and decision makers. The world has failed to address not only well-defined mental disorders, but also the mental health problems of children exploited for labor and sex, orphaned by AIDS, or forced to migrate for economic and political reasons (Foster, 2002). These problems are increasing. It is estimated that, in 26 African countries, the number of children orphaned for any reason will be more than double by 2010, 68% of them as a result of AIDS. Fourteen million children in 23 developing countries will lose one or both parents by 2010 (World Health Organization, 2003).

Other important child rights documents and conventions are the following: *The Declaration of Helsinki* (1984), revised in Tokyo (1995) and Edinburgh (2000), codifying the principles of ethical research in medicine; *The Bioethics Convention of the European Union*; *The Belmont Report* proposed by the US National Commission for the Protection of Human Subjects in Biomedical and Behavioral Research (1978); and *The Declaration of Madrid of the WPA* (2002), concerning the principles of ethical research with human beings.

THE BURDEN OF CHILD AND ADOLESCENT MENTAL DISORDER

A disproportionately large percentage of the "burden of disease" (World Health Organization, 2001) falls into the category of "neuropsychiatric conditions in children and adolescents" (see Figure 1.1). This estimate of disability-adjusted life years (DALYs) actually underrepresents the burden caused by disorders such as attention-deficit/hyperactivity disorder (ADHD), conduct disorder, learning disorder, mood disorder, pervasive developmental disorder, and mental retardation (Fayyad, Jahshan, and Karam, 2001). The WHO report *Caring for Children and Adolescents with Mental Disorders* (Foster, 2002) highlights the following facts: (a) up to 20% of children and adolescents worldwide suffer from disabling mental illness (World Health Organization, 2000); (b) suicide is the third leading cause of death among adolescents worldwide (World Health Organization, 2001); (c) major depressive disorder often begins in adolescence, across diverse countries, and is associated with substantial psychosocial impairment and risk of suicide (Weissman *et al.*, 1999); and (d) conduct disorder tends to persist into adolescence and adulthood and is associated with juvenile delinquency, adult crime, dissocial behavior, marital problems, poor parenting, unemployment, and poor physical health (Patterson, DeBaryshe, and Ramsey, 1989). Kessler *et al.* (2005) has found that approximately 50% of adult mental disorders begin before the age of 14 years.

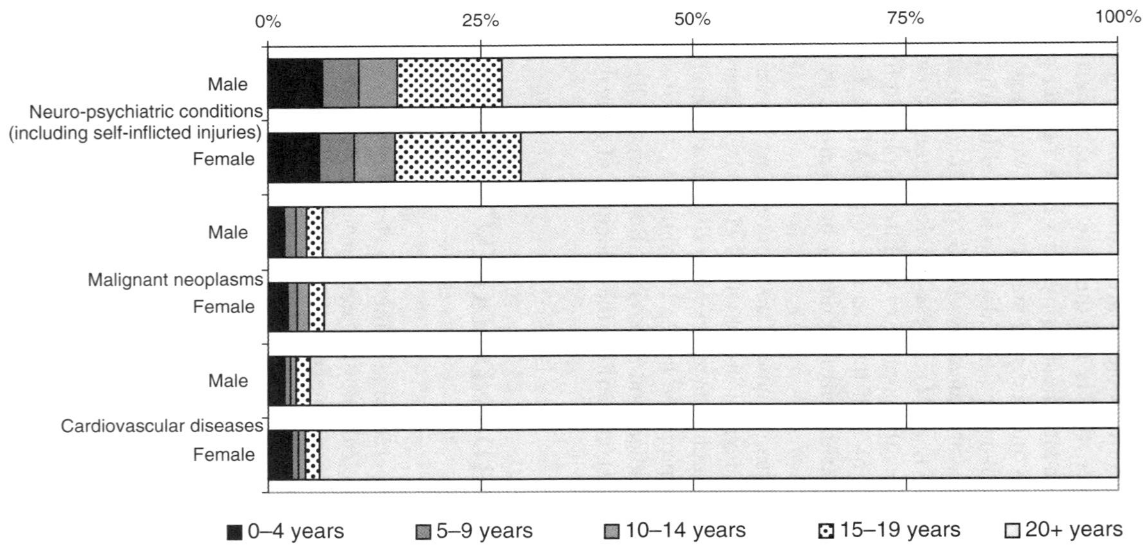

Figure 1.1 Disability-adjusted life years in the year 2000 attributable to specific causes by age and sex (World Health Organization, 2005)

The cost to society of the mental disorders of children can be calculated. Leibson *et al.* (2001) reported that, over a 9-year period, the median medical cost of a child with ADHD is 4306.00 USD compared to 1944.00 USD for a child without ADHD. These data suggest that mental health disorders in children represent a huge burden for children, families, and society; and that a human-rights framework is essential if children are to get effective, good quality care.

EPIDEMIOLOGY AS A BASIS FOR THE PLANNING OF SERVICES

Epidemiological data are important for the development of public policy and programmes to improve children's mental health. Epidemiological research answers the following questions (Leibson *et al.*, 2001): How many children in the community have mental health problems? How many children make use of mental health services? What is the distribution of mental health problems and services across age, sex, and ethnic group? Are there historical trends in the frequency of child mental health problems? What is the developmental course of mental health problems from childhood to adulthood? What etiological factors can be identified to inform the design of prevention and treatment programmes? How cost-effective are child mental health services? What are the outcomes for children who receive services? The answers to these questions provide a rational basis for service design and implementation.

The prevalence of child mental disorders worldwide appears quite similar. The 6-month prevalence rates for all mental disorders in the general population (boys and girls included) are 16.3% in 8-year-olds, 17.8% in 13-year-olds, 16% in 18-year-olds, and 18.4% in 25-year-olds. The most severe disorders vary in prevalence between 4.2% in 8-year-olds and 6.3% in 25-year-olds (Verhulst, 2004). Table 1.1 gives an overview of the prevalence of mental disorders in the general population, split into five groups, and classified according to developmental features and course of illness (Schmidt, 2006; Remschmidt and Schmidt, 2001).

These epidemiological data, based on studies in Europe and the United States, can be used for the planning of services in all regions of the world; however, it is crucial to supplement the data with local studies that reflect cultural dimensions of the presentation of disorders and the degree of impairment they convey.

THE CHILD AND ADOLESCENT MENTAL HEALTH ATLAS

The WHO Child and Adolescent Mental Health Atlas (World Health Organization, 2005) is one of the first systematic attempts to gather countrywide data on treatment resources available for children and adolescents with mental disorders. From key informants, the Atlas collected data on health policy and legislation, mental health financing, mental health services, human resources for care, data collection capacity, the care of special populations, and the use of medication.

The WHO Child and Adolescent Mental Health Atlas follows other Atlas projects such as those for general mental health services, neurological disorder, and epilepsy (World Health Organization, 2005). The findings related to children and adolescents are striking in comparison to the data obtained for adult mental health services (Table 1.2):

Table 1.1 Prevalence of mental disorders in children and adolescents based on population studies in Europe and the United States (Leibson *et al.*, 2001; Verhulst, 2004)

Early-onset disorders with lasting impairment		Developmentally dependent interaction disorders	
• Mental retardation	2%	• Feeding disorder (at age 2)	3%
• Autism	~0.5‰	• Physical abuse and neglect	~1.5%
• Atypical autism	1.1‰	• Sibling rivalry (in 8-year olds)	14%
• Receptive language disorder	2–3%		
• Expressive language disorder	3–4%		
• Dyslexia	4.5%		
Developmental disorders		*Early-onset adult-type disorders*	
• Disorders of motor development	1.5%	• Depressive episodes	2–4%
• Nocturnal enuresis in 9-year-olds	4.5%	• Agoraphobia	0.7–2.6%
• Encopresis in 7-year-olds	1.5%	• Panic disorders in adolescents	0.4–0.8%
• Oppositional defiant disorder	~6.0%	• Somatoform disorders	0.8–1.1%
		• Schizophrenia in adolescents	0.1–0.4%
		• Bipolar disorders in adolescents	<0.4%
		• Alcohol abuse in adolescents	~10%
		• Alcohol dependence in adolescents	4–6%
		• Personality disorders in 18-year olds	~1%
Disorders of age-specific onset			
• Mutism in 7-year-olds	0.8%		
• Stuttering	1.0%		
• Specific phobias	3.5%		
• Obsessive–compulsive disorder	1–3.5%		
• Anorexia nervosa	0.5–0.8%		

Table 1.2 Mental health services available for children and adolescents in most European countries

Outpatient Services
Child and adolescent psychiatrists in private practice
Psychoanalytical child and adolescent psychotherapists in private practice
Hospitals outpatient departments
Child psychiatric services in public health agencies
Child guidance clinics and family counseling services
Early intervention centers, social pediatric services

Day Patient Services
Day patient clinics
(two types: integrated into inpatient settings or independent)
Night clinic treatment facilities

Inpatient Services
Inpatient services at university hospitals
Inpatient services at state psychiatric hospitals
Inpatient services at general community hospitals or pediatric hospitals

Complementary Services
Rehabilitation services for special groups (e.g. children with severe head injury or epilepsy)
Different types of residential care setting
Residential groups for adolescents

- In less than one third of all countries, is it possible to identify an individual or a governmental entity with the sole responsibility for child mental health.
- In all but the wealthiest countries, public education regarding child mental health lags well behind that for other health problems.
- Worldwide the gap in meeting child and adolescent mental health needs is staggering. In most countries between one half and two thirds of all needs go unmet.
- School-based consultation services for child mental health do not operate regularly to the extent required in either developing or the developed countries. This gap leads to a failure to prevent school dropout and other significant consequences.
- Funding for child and adolescent mental health services is rarely identifiable in national health budgets. In low-income countries, services are often "paid out of pocket."
- While *The UN Convention on the Rights of the Child* is identified by most countries as a significant document, rarely are the child mental health provisions of the Convention exercised.
- The work of nongovernmental organizations in the provision of care is rarely connected to ongoing country-level programmes and too often lacks sustainability.
- In developing countries, the development and use of "self-help" or "practical help" programmes, not dependent on trained professionals, are more a myth than a reality.
- In 62% of the countries surveyed, there is no essential drug list for child psychotropic medication. In 53% of the countries, there are no specific controls in place for the prescription of medication to children.
- Although, worldwide, there is great interest in ADHD, in 47% of countries psychostimulants are either prohibited or not available for use.

CARING FOR CHILDREN WITH MENTAL DISORDERS: DIMENSIONS OF THE CHALLENGE

A system of care provides a range of services from least restrictive (community and family-based) to most restrictive (hospital-based). The concept of "system" does not dictate a particular theoretical orientation or the use of particular therapies. Implementation may lack uniformity depending on the particular setting. The geographic area covered by a "system" can be as small as a local community or as large as a country. In a system, it is assumed that there is some form of facilitated transfer of the patient between the components of the continuum of care. Facilitated transfer is difficult to ensure.

In Europe, systems of care have been very much connected to the development of child and adolescent psychiatry as a medical specialty (Blanz *et al.*, 2006). In recent decades, those working in the field have learned that interdisciplinary cooperation is an absolute necessity for scientific and clinical progress. In nearly all European countries, the number of child psychiatrists and other child mental health workers has increased dramatically over the past decades; however, in other areas of the world, mental health professionals are usually absent or in short supply. The situation in different countries is very heterogeneous with regard not only to the number of child psychiatrists, but also to the organization of departments and services, and the research, training, and continuing medical education that take place within them. In the planning and implementation of treatment, it is crucial to select appropriate components and integrate them as a coherent

Table 1.3 Salient results from the WHO Child Mental Health Atlas[a] (Belfer and Saxena, 2006)

	High income[b]	Low income[b]
National policy for CAMH	16/18	4/16
CAMH[c]	14/18	0/16
Epidemiological data	8/20	1/16
Annual health survey data about CAMH	12/20	3/16
Stigma as barrier to care	16/20	5/16
Financing of services:		
Consumer/family only	0/20	6/16
Tax-based/government	2/20	1/16
International grants	10/20	2/16
Nongovernmental organizations	4/20[†]	0/16
Social services	4/19	0/16
Medication available without cost to family	8/20	3/16

[†]Does not reflect emergency or disaster services.
[a]64 countries responded to the survey over a three-year period.
[b]World Bank country categories.
[c]CAMH = child and adolescent mental health.

treatment plan (Remschmidt, 2001). Table 1.4 summarizes the intervention possibilities for the major mental disorders encountered in children and adolescents.

Modern care for child and adolescent mental disorders reflects the following issues (Stroul and Friedman, 1986; Grimes, 2004). The main arena for service delivery is no longer inpatient, but rather in outpatient, day treatment, and complementary community services (Table 1.4).

Specialized services for particular disorders are provided by highly qualified personnel who implement pragmatic, effective, and efficient treatment programmes. Programmes should be evaluated. The private practice of child and adolescent psychiatry varies with country and local circumstances. However, the coordination of different services is too often inadequate, causing obstacles for patients and impeding the delivery of effective intervention. Increased

Table 1.4 Therapeutic interventions for priority mental disorders of children and adolescents (World Health Organization, 2005)

Disorder	Dynamic psychotherapy	Cognitive-behavioral therapy	Psychopharmaco-therapy	Family therapy	School intervention	Counseling	Specialized interventions	Other
Learning disorders			X		X	X		X
ADHD[a]		X	X[b]		X			
Tics		X	X	X				
Depression (and suicidal behaviors)	X	X	X*	X				
Psychoses			X	X	X		X	

[a]ADHD = Attention-deficit/hyperactivity disorder.
[b]Specific treatment depends on the age of the child or adolescent.

efforts are required to develop sustainable programmes. The worldwide absence of child and adolescent mental health policy requires correction (Shatkin and Belfer, 2004).

To address the lack of child and adolescent mental health policy, the WHO has developed *The Child and Adolescent Mental Health Policy Module* (World Health Organization, 2005b). This document is aimed at ministers of health and other policy developers. It provides precise guidance on policy development for child and adolescent mental health services. The module recognizes that, without a national policy, there is little likelihood of priority setting, financing, and accountability. The section of Child and Adolescent Psychiatry of the Union of European Medical Specialists (UEMS) has published guidelines for the design of training programmes in child and adolescent psychiatry. These guidelines have been implemented in several countries of the European Union and could serve as a universal model. They identify specific requirements and provide guidance on monitoring and quality assurance.

In developing countries, basic needs such as nutrition, water, and sanitation often overshadow mental health concerns. In many developing countries, up to half of the population are children (Rohde, Celia, and Berganza, 2004; Hong *et al.*, 2004; Robertson *et al.*, 2004). The difficult circumstances found in many countries violate the basic rights of children (Robertson, 2004) (e.g., armed conflict, the forced recruitment of children as soldiers, child abuse, prostitution, child-trafficking, homelessness, child labor, HIV/AIDS infection, a lack of provision for children's basic needs, and discrimination against minority children).

When present, systems of care in developing countries are either formal or informal (United Nations Children's Fund, 1990). Informal systems include those provided by families and their support network, natural healers, and faith-based organizations. Formal systems are provided either by the state or by an emerging private sector. In many countries, it is impossible to gather reliable data on services. A key problem for all developing countries is the provision of education and training programmes in child and adolescent mental health for doctors, psychologists, and other health and mental health workers.

THE ROLE OF INTERNATIONAL ORGANIZATIONS AND GLOBAL INITIATIVES

International organizations such as the WPA, the World Federation of Mental Health, WHO, the IACAPAP, the United Nations Educational, Scientific and Cultural Organization (UNESCO), and the United Nations Children's Fund (UNICEF) play an important role with regard to all aspects of child and adolescent mental health. The paramount goals and activities of these organizations are to raise public awareness of child mental health, facilitate the establishment of appropriate services in different parts of the world, establish training programmes for mental health workers in all parts of the world, fight for the rights of children, and ensure that *The UN Convention on the Rights of the Child* is observed in every country.

ADVOCACY

It is a constant challenge to develop and sustain programmes that support the care of children and adolescents with mental disorders. Advocacy seeks to keep the needs of these children on the agenda of nations and communities. The WPA Presidential Global Programme on Child Mental Health aims to promote the development of child and adolescent mental health services and policy and to facilitate prevention. At international, national, and local levels, parent advocacy is a force for the development and maintenance of programmes. It should be the aim of all international organizations devoted to mental health to facilitate broader advocacy for children and adolescents everywhere in the world. Beyond their guild interests, professional mental health organizations of all types have an important role to play in advocacy. The health, social service, juvenile justice, and education sectors also have key roles to play as advocates for child and adolescent mental health.

CONCLUSION

Child and adolescent psychiatry and child and adolescent mental health services have evolved in remarkable ways in the past few decades. Old myths, old treatments, and old policies are no longer to be tolerated. The new era provides an opportunity to develop and implement evidence-based interventions, modern training programmes, and imaginative policies. Advocacy for these initiatives is the responsibility of many. The WPA Global Programme is an example of the type of collaborative, focused effort needed to promote child and adolescent mental health worldwide. The reward will be healthier and happier children and adolescents in more productive and stable societies.

REFERENCES

Belfer, M. L. and Saxena, S. (2006) Child and adolescent mental health resources. Findings from the WHO Child Atlas Project. *Lancet*, **367**:551–52.

Blanz, B., Remschmidt, H., Schmidt, M., Warnke, A. (eds) (2006) *Psychische Störungen im Kindes- und Jugendalter*, Schattauer, Stuttgart.

Fayyad, J. A., Jahshan, C. S., and Karam, E. G. (2001) Systems development of child mental health services in developing countries. *Child Adolesc Psychiatr Clin North Am*, **10**, 745–63.

Foster, G. (2002) Supporting community efforts to assist orphans in Africa. *N Engl J Med*, **346**, 1907–10.

Grimes, K. E. (2004) Systems of care in North America, in *Facilitating Pathways: Care, Treatment and Prevention in Child and Adolescent Mental Health* (eds H. Remschmidt, M. Belfer, and I. Goodyer), Springer, Berlin, pp. 35–41.

Hong, K. M., Yamazaki, K., Banaag, C. G. *et al.* (2004) Systems of care in Asia, in Facilitating Pathways: Care, Treatment and Prevention in *Child and Adolescent Mental Health* (eds H. Remschmidt, M. Belfer, and I. Goodyer), Springer, Berlin, pp. 58–70.

Kessler, R. C., Berglund, P. M. B. A., Demler, O. *et al.* (2005) Lifetime prevalence and age-of-onset distributions of DSM-IV disorders in the National Co-morbidity Study Replication. *Arch Gen Psychiatry*, **62**, 593–602.

Leibson, C. L., Katusic, S. K., Barbaresi, W. J. *et al.* (2001) Use and costs of medical care for children and adolescents with and without attention-deficit-hyperactivity disorder. *JAMA*, **285**, 60–66.

Patterson, G. R., DeBaryshe, B. D., and Ramsey, E. (1989) A developmental perspective on antisocial behavior. *Am Psychol*, **44**, 329–35.

Remschmidt, H. (2001) Definition, classification, and principles of application, in *Psychotherapy with Children and Adolescents* (ed H. Remschmidt), Cambridge University Press, Cambridge, pp. 3–11.

Remschmidt, H., and Schmidt, M. H. (2001) Disorders in child and adolescent psychiatry, in *Contemporary Psychiatry*, Vol. 2 (F. Henn, N. Sartorius, H. Helmchen *et al.*) Springer, Berlin, pp. 60–116.

Robertson, B., Mandlhate, C., Seif El-Din, A. *et al.* Systems of care in Africa, in *Facilitating Pathways: Care, Treatment and Prevention in Child and Adolescent Mental Health* (eds H. Remschmidt, M. Belfer, and I. Goodyer), Springer, Berlin, pp. 71–88.

Rohde, L. A., Celia, S., and Berganza, C. (2004) Systems of care in South America, in *Facilitating Pathways: Care, Treatment and Prevention in Child and Adolescent Mental Health* (eds H. Remschmidt, M. Belfer, and I. Goodyer), Springer, Berlin, pp. 42–51.

Schmidt, M. H. (2006) Epidemiologie und Ätiologie psychischer Störungen im Kindes- und Jugendalter, in *Psychische Störungen im Kindes- und Jugendalter* (eds B. Blanz, H. Remschmidt, M. H. Schmidt) Schattauer, Stuttgart.

Shatkin, J. P. and Belfer, M. L. (2004) The global absence of child and adolescent mental health policy. *Child Adolesc Mental Health*, **9**, 104–08.

Stroul, B. and Friedman, R. (1986) A system-of-care for children and youths with severe emotional disturbance. Georgetown University Child Development Center, CASSP Technical Assistance Center, George Washington University, Washington.

United Nations Children's Fund. (1990) Children and development in the 1990s. United Nations, New York.

Verhulst, F. C. (2004) Epidemiology as a basis for the conception and planning of services, in *Facilitating Pathways: Care, Treatment and Prevention in Child and Adolescent Mental Health* (eds H. Remschmidt, M. Belfer, and I. Goodyer), Springer, Berlin, pp. 3–15.

Weissman, M. M., Wolk, S., Goldstein, R. B. *et al.* (1999) Depressed adolescents grown up. *JAMA*, **281**, 1707–13.

World Health Organization. (2000) World health report. World Health Organization, Geneva.

World Health Organization. (2001) World health report. World Health Organization, Geneva.

World Health Organization. (2003) Caring for children and adolescents with mental disorders. World Health Organization, Geneva.

World Health Organization (2005a) Child and adolescent country resources for mental health. World Health Organization.

World Health Organization. (2005b) Child and adolescent mental health policy. World Health Organization, Geneva, Switzerland.

CHAPTER 2

Public Awareness of Child and Adolescent Mental Health: A Review of the Literature

Sam Tyano and Anat Fleischman
Sackler School of Medicine, Tel-Aviv University, Israel

INTRODUCTION

Compared with adult psychiatry, child mental health is a growing but relatively new field. As childhood and adolescence are developmental phases, there has been vagueness in the diagnosis and treatment of young people and difficulty in drawing a distinct line between behavior that is part of normal development and that which is abnormal. Mental health, as a part of well-being, involves more than medical issues. It is strongly influenced by socioeconomic factors and has the potential to affect the strength and integrity of future society through family disruption, substance abuse, crime, violence, suicide, and lost productivity.

At the end of the twentieth century, the perception of childhood and children's mental health changed. *The United Nations Convention on the Rights of the Child* (UNCRC) (1989) formalized the rights of children and recognized "for the full and harmonious development of his or her personality the child should grow up in a family environment, in an atmosphere of happiness, love and understanding" (World Health Organization, 1989). Ratified by most countries in the world, the UNCRC is a landmark for children's mental health (Carlson, 2001). In 1999, the United States Health Administration called for the promotion of child mental health: "Mental health is a critical component of children's learning and general health. Fostering social and emotional health in children as a part of healthy child development must therefore be a national priority... Sadly, we have reached a point in the United States in which mental health/psychosocial problems, as well as risk-taking behaviors and preventable injuries, are resulting in more morbidity and mortality for children and adolescents than are physical illnesses and disorders" (US Department of

The Mental Health of Children and Adolescents: an area of global neglect. Edited by H. Remschmidt *et al.*

Health and Human Services, 1999). One of the main reasons for the focus on children's mental disorders is their high prevalence and the high burden they impose on society: "In advanced industrial societies such as the United Kingdom, the burden of disease is shifting from physical to mental health problems – emotional and behavioral problems currently being the major cause of disability in children." According to the Mental Health Foundation, "at any given time 20% of children and adolescents experience psychological problems" (Barlow and Underdown, 2005).

One of the aims of the United Kingdom's Health Administration White Paper *Our Healthier Nation* (1999) is to reduce suicide rates over the next 10 years by 17% (Department of Health, 1998). The British Green Paper *Every Child Matters* (2003) proposes an investment in preventive services such as home visitation, parenting training, and child and adolescent mental health services (Department for Education and Skills, 2003). *The WHO Report on Mental Health* (2001) reported that the prevalence of mental disorders among children ranges from 10 to 20% in different countries. Over 40% of countries have no mental health policy, and 90% have no mental health policy for children (World Health Organization, 2001). In the United States, one in ten young people suffers from mental illness severe enough to cause impairment, yet only about one in five of them receives the needed treatment (US Department of Health and Human Services, 1999). Similar prevalence levels have been reported in developing countries such as Nigeria, Arab Emirates, Sudan, Philippines, India, and Colombia (Fayyad, Jahshan, and Karam, 2001). However, a recent study has found that the prevalence of psychiatric disorder in Russian children is 70% higher than that observed in the United Kingdom (Goodman, Slobodskaya, and Knyazev, 2005). As the fall of communism left many Eastern European countries with shattered economies, more children are living in poverty. Approximately 150 million children were affected during this transition (Baingana, Bannon, and Thomas, 2005), obstructing access to education and health services, increasing suicide rates, alcohol abuse and parental abandonment, and leading to the placement of millions of children in institutions. War and ethnic cleansing have further exposed many children to psychological trauma (Lewis *et al.*, 2001).

CHILDREN'S UNMET MENTAL HEALTH NEEDS

The mental health needs of children around the world are seriously underserved. In the United States, 5–10% of children have made use of mental health services (Sturm, Ringel, and Andreyeva, 2003). About 50% of children aged 2–14 years involved with US welfare agencies have clinically significant emotional or behavioral problems, but only 25% of them receive specialized mental health care (Burns *et al.*, 2004). In the *Methods for the Epidemiology of Child and Adolescent Mental Disorders* (MECA) study (1989–1992), 17.1% of the population sampled reported that their need for mental health services was unmet, and only 25% of them actually accessed mental health services (Flisher *et al.*, 1997). In Europe, mental health services for children are less well developed than those for adults and are characterized by a paucity of specialized personnel, limited exposure of general practitioners and pediatricians to training in child psychiatry, and a scarcity of school psychological services and facilities for the treatment of children with conduct problems and mental retardation. The adequacy of child mental health services is correlated with national income level (Levav *et al.*, 2004). In the United Kingdom, only

23% of children with psychiatric disorder are in contact with a specialist (Ford, 2005); children in outpatient pediatric clinics are twice as likely to suffer from emotional and behavioral problems as those in control group, and only 25% of them receive help from a mental health specialist (Glazebrook *et al.*, 2003). In Canada, 14% of children aged 4–17 years have mental disorders but only 25% of them receive specialized treatment (Waddell *et al.*, 2005). In Australia, only 17% of children and adolescents with a mental disorder access specialized mental health services (Sawyer *et al.*, 2001). In a review of six large-scale studies in the United States, Canada, and the United Kingdom, specialized mental health service use by children with mental disorder was found to be not more then 16–27% (Waddell *et al.*, 2005). However, 40% of children with mental health problems in the United Kingdom and 59% of such children in Canada receive primary health care. In the United States, the education system is the sole provider of services for most children with mental health problems: 70–80% of children who receive mental health services do so in school (Burns *et al.*, 1995). In the United Kingdom, 50% of children receive special education services for mental disorders (Waddell *et al.*, 2002). In Australia, the providers most often accessed by children and adolescents with mental disorder are general practitioners and school counselors (Sawyer *et al.*, 2001).

Given the gap between prevalence and specialized health service utilization, researchers have studied the barriers to the use of services. In a review of help-seeking behavior in children and adolescents, Zwaanswijk *et al.* (2003) found two chief barriers to care: (1) lack of awareness by parents and children of mental health disorders and services; and (2) lack of understanding by general practitioners of mental health disorders. Help seeking by children is associated with comorbidity, severity, and the persistence of problems. If the child, in addition, has learning problems, the family is more likely to seek help. Help seeking by parents is related to the distress they experience rather than to the severity of the child's psychopathology. Help seeking is also related to parents' attitudes, beliefs, and level of education. Parental psychopathology is correlated with a greater recognition of child mental disorder but not with an increased use of services. Nevertheless, if parents are receiving mental health care, children are more likely to seek help. For children in foster care, physical and sexual abuse is related to increased service use, whereas neglect or the absence of a caregiver is related to less service use. Ethnic minority families are less likely to seek help, but this association disappears when socioeconomic status is controlled. The failure of general practitioners to recognize psychological problems is another barrier to specialized care. One of the reasons for low problem-recognition by general practitioners is the failure of parents and children to report mental health problems. However, problem recognition is greater in regard to boys, with increasing age and in single-parent families. Problem recognition is lower for children with whom the physician is not well acquainted, particularly if medical contact is episodic rather than extended (Zwaanswijk *et al.*, 2003).

PUBLIC KNOWLEDGE AND ATTITUDES

Public knowledge of and attitudes to adult mental illness have a significant effect on help seeking. To quote the WHO report of mental health, "the single most important barrier to overcome … is the stigma and associated discrimination toward persons suffering from mental and behavioral disorders" (World Health Organization, 2001). The public generally have disparaging attitudes toward the mentally ill. In Western countries, social rather than biological explanations of mental illness are favored, whereas non-Western cultures emphasize supernatural causes. In Western countries, mental health professionals and psychiatric treatments are not held in high regard. Psychiatric treatment, especially medication, is often regarded as harmful whereas nonpsychiatric treatments such as physical activity, diet, self-help books, or stress management are preferred. There is little discrimination between nonspecialized counseling and professional mental health treatment (Jorm, 2000).

Attitudes to child mental health are closely linked to the way mental disorders in children are perceived. Silk *et al.* (2000) have reviewed the historical trends that underlie current professional perceptions of childhood mental disorder. Until the end of the nineteenth century, it was thought that mental illness is not found in children. Children were regarded as "merely a miniature mirror image of the adult" (Rubinstein, 1948, p. 314), a viewpoint concurrent with the failure to accord human rights to children. It was only at the end of the nineteenth century that child welfare and labor laws and public education appeared. When child psychopathology was finally researched, the predominant foci were learning problems and delinquent behavior. At the beginning of the twentieth century, the concept of childhood mental disorder extended to "the problem child," who was regarded as normal apart from unwanted behavior, and who shed much of the stigma associated with seeking mental health care. The social changes that followed industrialization allowed many women to concentrate on child-rearing, increasing their concern for the care for children, and their inclination to seek help from professionals, a social change leading to "mother blaming." Recently, biological theories of mental disorder have emerged, further reducing the stigma of mental disorder. Today, psychopathology is regarded as "a mismatch between persons and their environments rather than an internal dysfunction" (Silk *et al.*, 2000). Nevertheless, while adult and child mental health literacy is flawed, old saws die hard (e.g., children grow out of their emotional difficulties; children misbehave to get attention; and children do not have mental problems, only bad parents).

The media can reinforce these fallacies. Butler and Hyler (2005) have discussed how child mental disorders and child psychiatry are portrayed in the cinema. Mental disorders are often depicted without any indication that they require help. Child psychiatrists are comic figures, "crazier" than their patients; or warm, dedicated professionals with endless amounts of time; or evildoers who wield incarceration, shock treatment, lobotomy, and medication for revenge or financial gain. Illness is caused by lack of parental support. The main treatment is a restoration of love. Although movies often support the importance of a therapeutic alliance, psychiatric diagnosis and treatment are trivialized as a simplistic form of blaming, rather than a bio-psychosocial enterprise, and parents are dissuaded from seeking help for fear of losing their children. The second myth (*There is nothing to psychiatry; anything can be considered treatment and anyone can be a psychiatrist.*) lauds the lone clinician who rebels against a cold psychiatric system in which science and medication are the enemy. This myth can give hope to patients and encourage a search for new treatments; however, it encourages opposition to empirically based treatment. The third myth (*If you do not do what we want, you will be locked up forever.*) refers to the perception of psychiatric treatment as punitive. Psychiatric hospitals are dirty, dark places peopled by hostile staff. The fourth myth (*Mental illness is a gift that psychiatrists take away.*) refers to the presentation of mental illness as an alternative and no less valid way of seeing the world; indeed, a way that may have special significance. The fifth myth (*Mental illness and evil overlap.*) appears in horror movies that depict psychiatric patients as possessed by demons, dismiss scientific explanations of mental illness, and perpetuate an image of the psychiatric patient as a violent madman (Butler and Hyler, 2005).

Mass media may have an adverse affect on children's mental health. The exposure of children to violent scenes and explicit sex in electronic media is often blamed in the popular press for youth violence. In a recent review of the use of media in the United States, Villani, Olson, and Jellinek (2005) discuss the effect of media exposure at different ages. The American Academy of Pediatrics advises against television watching before the age of two years (though special programmes can promote language learning). Children under eight years of age have difficulty in distinguishing fantasy from reality and are influenced more by visual than by verbal content. Commercials and shows with violent content should be monitored by adults. The media can enhance school readiness and serve as a source of information; however, exposure to violence can provoke aggression and risk-taking behavior (Villani, Olson, and Jellinek, 2005).

On the contrary, the media can promote knowledge and eradicate misconceptions. Recently, Olson and Kutner (2005) called on child and adolescent psychiatrists to use the media to enhance public awareness of mental illness and remove barriers to mental health care. Mass media can promote mental health (e.g., campaigns for cessation of alcohol and drug abuse, physical punishment, violence, and suicidal behavior) (World Health Organization, 2001). Such campaigns were used in the United Kingdom: The *You in Mind* BBC series was evaluated as a preventive programme. It had a beneficial impact on public understanding of mental illness but was less successful in promoting help seeking (Barker *et al.*, 1993). The *Defeat Depression* campaign that aimed to educate general practitioners and the general public succeeded in changing attitudes in the order of 5–10% (Paykel, Hart, and Priest, 1998). The *Changing Minds – Every Family in the Land* campaign attempted to counteract stigma against mental disorder. Both campaigns were launched by the Royal College of Psychiatrists (Crisp *et al.*, 2000). The *Like Minds, Like Mine* campaign initiated by the New Zealand Ministry of Health (1996) promulgated radio, television, and cinema advertisements concerning famous people who had mental illness in order to counter stigma (Vaughan and Hansen, 2004). In 1999, The World Psychiatric Association introduced an anti-stigma campaign *Open the Doors* to increase public awareness of and knowledge about schizophrenia (Thompson *et al.*, 2002). However, all these campaigns have addressed mental illness in adults. The *Positive Parenting Programme* (Triple-P) (Sanders, 2002) aims to prevent behavioral, emotional, and developmental problems in children. In the television component of Triple-P, parents watch a television series featuring coercive child-rearing and learn how to deal better with oppositional behavior. Before the intervention, 42.9% of the children whose parents watched the programme scored within the clinical range of the Eyberg Child Behavior Inventory. After the intervention, only 14.3% and at 6 months follow-up, and only 9.5% did so (Sanders, Montgomery, and Brechman-Toussaint, 2000).

MENTAL HEALTH PREVENTION AND PROMOTION

There is a growing awareness that hospital and outpatient mental health services alone are unable to meet all the mental health needs of children and adolescents. As school and primary health services are the two places where most children seek help, mental health services could be located conveniently with primary health care and community-based facilities (Sawyer *et al.*, 2001; Waddell *et al.*, 2002; Farmer, Dorsey, and Mustillo, 2004). Alperstein and Raman (2003) have proposed an aged-based framework of strategies to promote mental health (e.g., home visitation, parent training, and school-based intervention). Offord *et al.* (1998) reviewed interventions that could promote resilience and lower the prevalence of psychiatric disorder in children. The three types of programmes recommended are as follows: (1) *Universal health promotion (primary prevention)* (e.g., substance abuse prevention delivered to all grade 7 school children). These programmes do not stigmatize children but they are impersonal and expensive. They could have a cumulative effect; however, for individuals, the effect size is likely to be small, particularly for those at greatest risk. (2) *Targeted prevention (secondary prevention)* is delivered for selected children. These programmes involve personal care and are tailored for the individual. On the contrary, accurate tailoring may be difficult because the choice of screening method and the threshold selected for intervention may be unclear, and because different populations may differ in regard to the suitability of particular kinds of intervention. Children may risk stigmatization and an adverse programme effect (e.g., due to the grouping of at-risk youth with deviant peers). (3) *Indicated clinical intervention delivered by specialized mental health services (tertiary prevention)*. The treatment programmes offered by specialized services have proven effectiveness (at least in laboratory studies), are approved by the public, and provide individualized treatment. On the contrary, coverage may be inadequate because of inaccessibility, noncompliance (40–60% of families beginning treatment do not complete intervention), stigmatization, and expense.

No single level of prevention can lower the prevalence of psychiatric disorder; a combination of all three types is recommended (Offord *et al.*, 1998).

The relation between health, mental health, and socioeconomic status has long been apparent, Alperstein and Raman (2003) quote Rose (1992) as follows: "The primary determinants of disease are economic and social and therefore its remedies must also be economic and social. Medicine and politics cannot and should not be kept apart." One step toward decreasing social and economic inequity in health promotion is to deliver universal programmes to disadvantaged populations (Alperstein and Raman, 2003; Waddell *et al.*, 2005).

THE INTEGRATION OF PREVENTION WITH PRIMARY CARE

Bower *et al.* (2001) have reviewed three methods of integrating mental health into primary health care: (1) the use of primary health care professionals (with and without training); (2) the placement of mental health professionals in primary health settings; and (3) consultation-liaison. Training courses for primary health care professionals in short courses have generally not been effective. Specialized treatment training, especially in cognitive-behavior therapy, has produced some improvement in child health care utilization. The one study of consultation-liaison generated a decreased referral rate and more appropriate referrals (Bower *et al.*, 2001). In Egypt, a programme to improve school physicians' understanding of child mental disorder increased the rate of referrals to a psychiatric clinic (Attia *et al.*, 1991). General practitioners trained in the primary-care version of the Triple-P programme were more likely to use parent consultation skills and to be satisfied with the outcome (Sanders *et al.*, 2003). The Cambridge Health Alliance tested the feasibility of improving mental health diagnosis and treatment in a pediatric clinic. The pediatric symptom checklist (PSC) is a simple screening tool for behavioral problems that can be filled out by a parent in the waiting room (Stancin and Palermo, 1997; Jellinek *et al.*, 1999; Navon *et al.*, 2001). Parents completed the checklist in the waiting room, every child scoring in the clinical range was referred to an on-site social worker. The waiting time for treatment was shortened and psychiatric referral facilitated (Hacker, Weidner, and McBride, 2004).

HOME VISITATION (FROM DURING PREGNANCY TO TWO YEARS OF AGE)

Home visitation refers to the mode of delivery. It encompasses a variety of programmes that differ in content, time, and purpose. Such programmes can be universal or targeted and delivered by professionals or trained lay people (Bull *et al.*, 2004). Home visitation for parents is a form of universal general health care used in many countries and intended originally to lower infant mortality. In the United Kingdom, targeted programmes have been implemented, such as "Home-Start," "Sure Start," "First Parent Health Visitor," and "Community Mothers" (Barlow and Underdown, 2005). In the United States, home visitation was implemented as a targeted programme for families at risk (American Academy of Pediatrics, 1998). In a review of 177 prevention studies, Durlak and Wells (1997) found that intervention for primiparous mothers had a high effect size (0.87). In a meta-analysis of prevention programmes, Bull *et al.* (2004) found that home visitation has a beneficial effect on parenting, and improves the diagnosis and treatment of maternal depression and child behavioral problems. Effective programmes tend to be multi-focused, targeted, and of medium-to-long duration (Bull *et al.*, 2004). A 15-year follow-up randomized controlled trial (RCT) of a nurse – home-visitation programme – has been conducted in the United States. Visitation started before birth and lasted until the infant was 2 years old. Families at risk (mothers younger than 19, unmarried, or of low socioeconomic status) were actively recruited. The programme was found to have reduced the prevalence of child maltreatment and domestic violence (Eckenrode *et al.*, 2000). It also reduced the prevalence of serious antisocial behavior, particularly running away from home, arrests, convictions, and violations of probation. Adolescents whose mothers had been exposed to home visitation had fewer sex partners, smoked less, and drank less alcohol (Olds *et al.*, 1998). A 15-year follow-up study in Finland, of nurse – home visitation – found a reduction of psychiatric symptoms as measured by the child behavior checklist (CBCL), but no difference in effectiveness with low- and high-risk families (Aronen and Kurkela, 1996). Home visitation has been less effective when conducted by nonprofessionals (Barnet *et al.*, 2002; Olds *et al.*, 2002). The European Early Promotion Project that is taking place in urban populations in five countries is evaluating the effectiveness of home visitation by primary health professionals (health visitors in Greece and the United Kingdom, public health nurses in Finland, and community nurses in Yugoslavia and Cyprus). The study includes both entire populations and at-risk families. Visitation starts before birth and continues until the infant is 2 years old. The effectiveness of trained and nontrained visitors is being tested. After 2 years, a beneficial effect on mother–child interaction was observed in Finland and the United Kingdom (Puura *et al.*, 2005).

PARENT TRAINING (2–5 YEARS)

Parent training programmes are designed to educate parents and encourage them to build closer relationships with their children. These programmes usually involve weekly family or group sessions and are either behavioral or relationship-based in design. Despite their diversity, parenting programmes have proven effective for behavioral problems and are the treatment of choice for conduct disorder (Barlow and Underdown, 2005; Mabe, Turner, and Josephson, 2005). In a meta-analysis of 26 controlled studies, parent training yielded an effect size of 0.86 for child behavior improvement, and an effect size of 0.44 for parental adjustment (Serketich and Dumas, 1996). A further meta-analysis of eight random control trials of parenting intervention found that children subsequently spent less time in institutions (weighted mean differences, 56.34 days) and were less often rearrested (relative risk, 0.66) (Woolfenden, Williams, and Peat, 2002). A meta-analysis of five random controlled trials of group-based parenting for children under 3 years yielded a moderate effect size (0.55); but data about follow-up were insufficient (Barlow *et al.*, 2004). Parental training programmes delivered in universal settings had a moderate effect size for children with at-risk behavior and for those living in high-risk neighborhoods (with low socioeconomic conditions and divorced parents) (Spoth, Redmond, and Shin, 1998). Another review concluded that targeted and universal parenting programmes had a moderate effect size (Mabe, Turner, and Josephson, 2005). The Webster-Stratton parenting programme ameliorated conduct problems; for example, scores on the Goodman Conduct Problem and Eyberg Child Behavior Inventories were reduced at 6 months follow-up in children in the intervention group (Patterson *et al.*, 2002). On the contrary, Durlak and Wells (1997) found that parental training has a low effect size (0.16). The *Incredible Years* parent training programme, a targeted programme for low-income families, has produced improvement in child behavior, related to the level of parental participation and the initial severity of child behavior problems (Reid, Webster-Stratton, and Baydar, 2004). The Triple-P programme encompasses universal, targeted, and high-intensity targeted interventions at five levels and match the severity of the disorder. The first level of intervention includes a media-based information campaign addressed to all promote awareness of parenting and parental participation and parenting tip sheets and videotapes to all interested parents. This programme was originally developed in Australia and has now been exported with success to New Zealand, the United Kingdom, the United States, Canada, Germany, Switzerland, Hong Kong, and Singapore (Sanders, 2002). The programme has been found to have improved parental mental health and child behavior (Sanders, 1999).

SCHOOL-BASED PROGRAMMES (5–18 YEARS)

As a natural setting, the school may be an especially favorable site for preventive programmes. In school, children encounter adults other than their parents. Teachers and counselors are in a good position to identify children at risk of psychological problems. School-based programmes designed to address violence, substance abuse, adjustment, depression, school dropout, and delinquency have been evaluated. Durlak and Wells (1997) reviewed school-based prevention programmes. The effect size was only moderate (0.35). Problem-solving and affective education programmes were more effective in younger (2–7 years) than in older (7–11 years) children (0.93 and 0.70 versus 0.24 and 0.36, respectively). Behavioral programmes had a moderate effect size (0.49) (Durlak and Wells, 1997). In a review of school-based programmes, Hoagwood and Ervin (1997) concluded that cognitive-behavioral therapy was an effective preventive programme for substance abuse and depression. Social skills training was effective in preventing aggression and alcohol abuse and enhancing peer acceptance and locus of control. Teacher-consultation was effective in facilitating referral for special education (Hoagwood and Ervin, 1997). However, a meta-analysis of substance abuse prevention programmes showed low effectiveness; moreover, most studies were conducted in the United States and their effectiveness in other cultures is unknown (White and Pitts, 1998). Randomized control studies of cognitive-behavioral therapy for the prevention of depression and anxiety yielded improvement superior to controls; however, too few clinical psychologists are trained to deliver such therapy (Andrews and Wilkinson, 2002). A meta-analysis of programmes for aggressive behavior yielded a beneficial effect on aggressive behavior in all age groups, children at risk showing larger effect size. Most programmes were implemented and supervised by researchers as demonstrations, not as routine programmes that usually have smaller effect size (Wilson, Lipsey, and Derzon, 2003).

One universal prevention programme disseminated in the United States is the *Expanded School Mental Health*. This programme involves assessment, treatment, and prevention through a partnership between school and community mental health agencies. It is intended that all schools in the country implement the programme that has been associated with improved learning and behavior (Weist and Albus, 2004).

Botvin *et al.* (1995) have studied the effectiveness of a drug abuse prevention programme, *Life Skills training*. This programme involves 15 sessions in the seventh grade, 10 booster sessions in the eighth grade, and 8 booster sessions in the ninth grade. Information is provided about the consequences of drug abuse and social skills are provided to resist peer pressure. At 6-year follow-up, self-reported substance abuse was 44% less in the intervention group, and poly-drug abuse was 66% less (Botvin *et al.*, 1995).

The Australian *Gatehouse Project* aims to improve levels of emotional well-being and reduce substance abuse in school children. Substance abuse was decreased by 5–40% (Bond *et al.*, 2004). The United States *Incredible Years* is a teacher training programme aimed to help teachers provide praise and encouragement, manage inappropriate classroom behavior, and build a good relationship with students. After this intervention, children were less disobedient and aggressive, compared to controls. *Multi-systemic Therapy* (MST) is an indicated programme developed in the United States and operating in the United Kingdom, Canada, and Australia. MST is designed for chronic, violent, juvenile offenders, using multiple components of treatment (e.g., cognitive behavioral therapy and behavioral parent training). An intervention group has showed lower recidivism rates compared with controls (Kratochwill, Albers, and Shernoff, 2004). Another study indicated that the United States programme *Fast Track* involves social skills training, parent training, and teacher-based intervention for aggressive preschool and early elementary school children. By the end of the third grade, 37% of children in the intervention group were free of conduct problems compared with 27% in the control group (Rones and Hoagwood, 2000).

Other school-based programmes aim to increase knowledge of mental health and consequently help seeking. An educational programme for secondary school students increased knowledge and dceeased the stigma associated with mental illness in the United Kingdom

(Pinfold *et al.*, 2003), Pakistan (Rahman *et al.*, 1998), and Canada (Lauria-Horner, Kutcher, and Brooks, 2004).

In a meta-analysis of prevention studies, Nation *et al.* (2003) concluded that effective preventive programmes have the following characteristics: (1) multi-component intervention (aimed at family, school, and peer group); (2) active social-skill teaching; (3) early intervention, sufficient duration, the matching of intensity to individual risk, and booster sessions; (4) a basis in either etiological or intervention theory; and (5) the promotion of strong parent–child or adult–child relationships (Nation *et al.* 2003).

CONCLUSION

The twentieth century has seen great progress in children's mental health. An awareness that childhood is a special developmental stage and that development can be influenced by environmental factors has encouraged many governments and international organizations to step in when natural caregivers cannot function effectively. The classification of children's mental disorders and randomized control treatment trails have demonstrated that treatment can improve children's mental health. However, 10–20% of children and adolescents suffer from a mental disorder at any time, and of them only about 25% receive professional help (World Health Organization, 2001; Burns *et al.*, 2004; Ford, 2005; Waddell *et al.*, 2005). When children do access help, most do so from primary care or community-based facilities (Burns *et al.*, 1995; Sawyer *et al.*, 2001; Waddell *et al.*, 2002). One of the chief reasons for this gap in health services is the public's ignorance of and adverse attitude to mental disorder. Child mental health illiteracy is related to hostility to mental illness and psychiatric treatment, and the perpetuation of damaging myths about children. The mass media, potentially so influential with regard to public knowledge and attitudes, have generally not attempted to counteract myths but rather, through sensational reporting, to reinforce them.

Many prevention and promotion programmes have been implemented in primary health settings and schools. Current programmes are either universal or targeted for populations at risk (e.g., low-income families), or provided for children already suffering from mental disorder. There has been a paucity of randomized control trials addressing particular psychiatric disorders (e.g., anxiety). Most programmes have attempted to enhance general well-being or promote adaptive behavior. Though many programmes have already been implemented in community settings, there has been little examination of the efficiency and cost-effectiveness of such programmes when they are delivered to large populations (Hoagwood and Ervin, 1997).

REFERENCES

Alperstein, G. and Raman, S. (2003) Promoting mental health and emotional well-being among children and youth: A role for community child health? *Child Care Health Dev*, **29**(4), 269–74 (Review), and references therein.

American Academy of Pediatrics. (1998) The role of home-visitation programs in improving health outcomes for children and families. Council on Child and Adolescent Health. *Pediatrics*, **101**(3 Part 1):486–89.

Andrews, G. and Wilkinson, D. D. (2002) The prevention of mental disorders in young people. *Med J Aus*, **177**(Suppl.), S97–100 (Review) and references therein.

Aronen, E. T. and Kurkela, S. A. (1996) Long-term effects of an early home-based intervention. *J Am Acad Child Adolesc Psychiatr*, **35**(12), 1665–72.
Attia, M. S., Abou Nazel, M. W., Guirguis, W. W., and el Din, A. G. (1991) Impact of a mental health program on the utilization of the psychiatric clinic in sporting students' hospital. *J Egypt Public Health*, **66**(5–6), 587–08.
Baingana, F., Bannon, I., and Thomas, R. (2005) Mental health and conflicts: conceptual framework and approaches health, nutrition and population (HNP) discussion paper. Washington, DC, World Bank.
Barker, C., Pistrang, N., Shapiro, D. A. *et al.* (1993) You in mind: A preventive mental health television series. *British J Clin Psychol*, **32**(Pt 3), 281–93.
Barnet, B., Duggan, A. K., Devoe, M., and Burrell, L. (2002) The effect of volunteer home visitation for adolescent mothers on parenting and mental health outcomes: A randomized trial. *Arch Pediatr Adolesc Med*, **156**(12), 1216–22.
Barlow, J., (2005) Underdown A. Promoting the social and emotional health of children: Where to now? *J R Soc Health*, **125**(2), 64–70 (Review) and references therein.
Barlow, J., Parsons, J., and Stewart-Brown, S. (2004) Preventing emotional and behavioural problems: The effectiveness of parenting programmes with children less than 3 years of age. *Child Care Health Dev*, **31**(1), 33–42.
Bond, L., Patton, G., Glover, S. *et al.* (2004) The Gatehouse Project: Can a multilevel school intervention affect emotional wellbeing and health risk behaviours? *J Epidemiol Community Health*, **58**(12), 997–1003.
Botvin, G. J., Baker, E., Dusenbury, L. *et al.* (1995) Long-term follow-up results of a randomized drug abuse prevention trial in a white middle-class population. *JAMA*, **273**(14), 1106–12.
Bower, P., Garralda, E., Kramer, T. *et al.* (2001) The treatment of child and adolescent mental health problems in primary care: A systematic review. *Fam Pract*, **18**(4), 373–82 (see comment) (Review) and references therein.
Bull, J., McCormick, G., Swann, C., and Mulvihill, C. (2004) Ante- and post-natal home-visiting programmes: A review of reviews. Evidence briefing. London, Health Development Agency, National Institute for Health.
Burns, B. J., Costello, E. J., Angold, A. *et al.* (1995) Children's mental health service use across service sectors. *Health Aff*, **14**(3), 147–59 (see comment).
Burns, B. J., Phillips, S. D., Wagner, H. R. *et al.* (2004) Mental health need and access to mental health services by youths involved with child welfare: A national survey. *J Am Acad Child Adolesc Psychiatr*, **43**(8), 960–70.
Butler, J. R. and Hyler, S. E. (2005) Hollywood portrayals of child and adolescent mental health treatment: Implications for clinical practice. *Child Adolesc Psychiatr Clin North Am*, **14**(3), 509–22.
Carlson, M. (2001) Child rights and mental health. *Child Adolesc Psychiatr Clin North Am*, **10**(4), 825–39.
Crisp, A. H., Gelder, M. G., Rix, S. *et al.* (2000) Stigmatisation of people with mental illnesses. *Br J Psychiatry*, **177**, 4–7 (see comment).
Department for Education and Skills. (2003) *Every Child Matters*, London, Stationary Office.
Department of Health. (1998) *Our Healthier Nation: A Contract for Health*, London, Stationary Office.
Durlak, J. A. and Wells, A. M. (1997) Primary prevention mental health programs for children and adolescents: A meta-analytic review. *Am J Commun Psychol*, **25**(2), 115–52 (see comment).
Eckenrode, J., Ganzel, B., Henderson, C. R., Jr. *et al.* (2000) Preventing child abuse and neglect with a program of nurse home visitation: The limiting effects of domestic violence. *JAMA*, **284**(11), 1385–91(see comment).
Farmer, E. M. Z., Dorsey, S., and Mustillo, S. A. (2004) Intensive home and community interventions. *Child Adolesc Psychiatr Clin North Am*, **13**, 857–84.
Fayyad, J. A., Jahshan, C. S., and Karam, E. G. (2001) Systems development of child mental health services in developing countries. *Child Adolesc Psychiatr Clin North Am*, **10**(4), 745–62.
Flisher, A. J., Kramer, R. A., Grosser, R. C. *et al.* (1997) Correlates of unmet need for mental health services by children and adolescents. *Psychol Med*, **27**(5), 1145–54

Ford, T., Hamilton, H., Goodman, R., and Meltzer, H. (2005) Service contacts among the children participating in the British child and adolescent mental health surveys. *Child Adolesc Ment Health*, **10**(1), 2–9.

Glazebrook, C., Hollis, C., Heussler, H. *et al.* (2003) Detecting emotional and behavioural problems in paediatric clinics. *Child Care Health Dev*, **29**(2), 141–49.

Goodman, R., Slobodskaya, H., and Knyazev, G. (2005) Russian child mental health: A cross-sectional study of prevalence and risk factors. *Eur Child Adolesc Psychiatry*, **14**(1), 28–33.

Hacker, K., Weidner, D., and McBride, J. (2004) Integrating pediatrics and mental health: The reality is in the relationships. *Arch Pediatr Adolesc Med*, **158**(8), 833–34.

Hoagwood, K. and Erwin, H. D. (1997) Effectiveness of school-based mental health services for children: A 10-year research review. *J Child Fam Stud*, **6**(4), 435–51.

Jellinek, M. S., Murphy, J. M., Little, M. *et al.* (1999) Use of the pediatric symptom checklist to screen for psychosocial problems in pediatric primary care: A national feasibility study. *Arch Pediatr Adolesc Med*, **153**(3), 254–60.

Jorm, A. F. (2000) Mental health literacy. Public knowledge and beliefs about mental disorders. *British J Psychiatry*, **177**, 396–01 (see comment) (Review) and references therein.

Kratochwill, T.R., Albers, C. A., and Shernoff, E. S. (2004) School-based interventions. *Child Adol Psychiatr Clin North Am*, **13**(4), 885–903, vi–vii (Review) and references therein.

Lauria-Horner, B. A., Kutcher, S., and Brooks, S. J. (2004) The feasibility of a mental health curriculum in elementary school. *Can J Psychiatry*, **49**(3), 208–11.

Levav, I., Jacobsson, L., Tsiantis, J. *et al.* (2004) Psychiatric services and training for children and adolescents in Europe: Results of a country survey. *Eur Child Adolesc Psychiatry*, **13**(6), 395–01.

Lewis, O., Sargent, J., Friedrich W *et al.* (2001) The impact of social change on child mental health in Eastern Europe. *Child Adolesc Psychiatr Clin North Am*, **10**(4), 815–24.

Mabe, P. A., Turner, M. K., and Josephson, A. M. (2005) Parent managment training. *Child Adolesc Psychiatr Clin North Am*, **10**(3), 451–64.

Nation, M., Crusto, C., Wandersman, A. *et al.* (2003) What works in prevention. Principles of effective prevention programs. *Am Psychol*, **58**(6–7), 449–56 (Review) and references therein.

Navon, M., Nelson, D., Pagano, M., and Murphy, M. (2001) Use of the pediatric symptom checklist in strategies to improve preventive behavioral health care. *Psychiatr Serv*, **52**(6), 800–04.

Offord, D. R., Kraemer, H. C., Kazdin, A. E. *et al.* (1998) Lowering the burden of suffering from child psychiatric disorder: Trade-offs among clinical, targeted, and universal interventions. *J Am Acad Child Adolesc Psychiatry*, **37**(7), 686–94.

Olds, D., Henderson, C. R., Jr., Cole, R. *et al.* (1998) Long-term effects of nurse home visitation on children's criminal and antisocial behavior: 15-year follow-up of a randomized controlled trial. *JAMA*, **280**(14), 1238–44 (see comment).

Olds, D. L., Robinson, J., O'Brien, R. *et al.* (2002) Home visiting by paraprofessionals and by nurses: A randomized, controlled trial. *Pediatrics*, **110**(3) 486–96 (see comment).

Olson, C. K. and Kutner, L. A. Media outreach for child psychiatrists. *Child Adolesc Psychiatr Clin North Am*, **14**(3), 613–22.

Patterson, J., Barlow, J., Mockford, C. *et al.* (2002) Improving mental health through parenting programmes: Block randomised controlled trial. *Arch Dis Child*, **87**(6), 472–77 (see comment).

Paykel, E. S., Hart, D., and Priest, R. G. (1998) Changes in public attitudes to depression during the Defeat Depression Campaign. *British J Psychiatry*, **173**, 519–22.

Pinfold, V., Toulmin, H., Thornicroft, G. *et al.* (2003) Reducing psychiatric stigma and discrimination: Evaluation of educational interventions in UK secondary schools. *Br J Psychiatry*, **182**, 342–46.

Puura, K., Hilton, D., Mantymaa, M. *et al.* (2005) The outcome of the European early promotion project: Mother–Child interaction. *Int J Ment Health Promot*, **7**(1), 82–94.

Rahman, A., Mubbasharm, M., Gater, R., and Goldberg, D. (1998) Randomised trial of impact of school mental-health programme in rural Rawalpindi, Pakistan. *Lancet.*, **352**, 1022–25.

Reid, M. J., Webster-Stratton, C., and Baydar, N. (2004) Halting the development of conduct problems in head start children: The effects of parent training. *J Clin Child Adol Psychol*, **33**(2), 279–91.

Rones, M. and Hoagwood, K. (2000) School-based mental health services: A research review. *Clin Child Fam Psychol Rev*, **3**(4), 223–41 (Review) and references therein.

Sanders, M. R. (1999) Triple P-Positive Parenting Program: Towards an empirically validated multilevel parenting and family support strategy for the prevention of behavior and emotional problems in children. *Clin Child Fam Psychol Rev*, **2**(2), 71–90 (Review) and references therein.

Sanders, M. R. (2002) Parenting interventions and the prevention of serious mental health problems in children. *Med J Aus*, **177**(Suppl.), S87–92.

Sanders, M. R., Montgomery, D. T., and Brechman-Toussaint, M. L. (2000) The mass media and the prevention of child behavior problems: The evaluation of a television series to promote positive outcomes for parents and their children. *J Child Psychol Psychiatry*, **41**(7), 939–48.

Sanders, M. R., Tully, L. A., Turner, K. M. *et al.* (2003) Training GPs in parent consultation skills. An evaluation of training for the Triple P-Positive Parenting Program. *Aust Fam Phys*, **32**(9), 763–68.

Sawyer, M. G., Arney, F. M., Baghurst, P. A. *et al.* (2001) The mental health of young people in Australia: Key findings from the child and adolescent component of the national survey of mental health and well-being. *Aust N Z J Psychiatry.*, **35**(6), 806–14.

Serketich, W. J. and Dumas, J. E. (1996) The effectiveness of behavioral parent training to modify antisocial behavior in children: A meta-analysis. *Behav Ther*, **27**(2), 171–86.

Silk, J. S., Nath, S. R., Siegel, L. R., and Kendall, P. C. (2000) Conceptualizing mental disorders in children: Where have we been and where are we going? *Develop Psychopathol*, **12**(4), 713–35.

Spoth, R., Redmond, C., Shin, C. (1998) Direct and indirect latent-variable parenting outcomes of two universal family-focused preventive interventions: Extending a public health-oriented research base. *J Consult Clin Psychol*, **66**(2), 385–99.

Stancin, T. and Palermo, T. M. (1997) A review of behavioral screening practices in pediatric settings: Do they pass the test? *J Dev Behav Pediatr*, **18**(3), 183–94 (Review) and references therein.

Sturm, R., Ringel, J. S., and Andreyeva, T. (2003) Geographic disparities in children's mental health care. *Pediatrics*, **112**(4), e308.

Thompson, A. H., Stuart, H., Bland, R. C. *et al.* (2002) Attitudes about schizophrenia from the pilot site of the WPA worldwide campaign against the stigma of schizophrenia. *Soc Psychiatry Psychiatr Epidemiol*, **37**(10), 475–82.

US Department of Health and Human Services. (1999) Mental Health: A Report of the Surgeon General, Department of Health and Human Services, Substance Abuse and Mental Health Services Administration, Center for Mental Health Services, National Institute of Mental Health, National Institutes of Health, Rockville, MD.

Vaughan, G. and Hansen, C. (2004) 'Like minds, like mine': A New Zealand project to counter the stigma and discrimination associated with mental illness. *Aust Psychiatry*, **12**(2), 113–17.

Villani, V. S., Olson, C. K., and Jellinek, M. S. (2005) Media literacy for clinicians and parents. *Child Adolesc Psychiatr Clin North Am*, **14**(3), 523–53.

Waddell, C., McEwan, K., Shepherd, C. A. *et al.* (2005) A public health strategy to improve the mental health of Canadian children. *Canad J Psychiatry*, **50**(4), 226–33 (Review) and references therein.

Waddell, C., Offord, D. R., Shepherd, C. A. *et al.* (2002) Child psychiatric epidemiology and Canadian public policy-making: The state of the science and the art of the possible. *Can J Psychiatry*, **47**(9), 825–32.

Weist, M. D. and Albus, K. E. (2004) Expanded school mental health: Exploring program details and developing the research base. *Behav Modif*, **28**(4), 463–71.

White, D. and Pitts, M. (1998) Educating young people about drugs: A systematic review. *Addiction*, **93**(10), 1475–87.

Wilson, S. J., Lipsey, M. W., and Derzon, J. H. (2003) The effects of school-based intervention programs on aggressive behavior: a meta-analysis. *J Consult Clin Psychol*, **71**(1), 136–49.

Woolfenden, S. R., Williams, K., and Peat, J. K. (2002) Family and parenting interventions for conduct disorder and delinquency: A meta-analysis of randomised controlled trials. *Arch Dis Child*, **86**(4), 251–56 (see comment) [summary for patients in *J Pediatr.* 2002, **141**(5), 738; PMID: 12448428]. (Rcview) and references therein.

World Health Organization. (1989) United Nations Convention on the Rights of the Child. World Health Organization, Geneva.

World Health Organization. (2001) The World health report: 2001: Mental health: New understanding, new hope.World Health Organization, Geneva.

Zwaanswijk, M., Van der, E. J., Verhaak, P. F. *et al.* (2003) Factors associated with adolescent mental health service need and utilization. *J Am Acad Child Adolesc Psychiatry*, **42**(6), 692–700.

CHAPTER 3

The Epidemiology and Burden of Child and Adolescent Mental Disorder

Myron L. Belfer
Harvard Medical School, Boston MA, USA
Barry Nurcombe
The University of Queensland, Brisbane, Australia

INTRODUCTION

To fully appreciate the burden associated with child and adolescent mental disorders, it is necessary to understand the context of the child and adolescent, the developmental trajectory of normal children and those with disorder, the economic costs of psychiatric disorders, and the potential of children and adolescents with disorder to compromise society.

The ICD-10 and DSM-IV diagnostic classifications for children and adolescents are woefully inadequate and of limited applicability in epidemiological studies. There is increasing concern with their propensity to identify co-morbidity. While reflecting the complexity of disorders in real life, the tendency to identify co-morbidity is seen by some as reflecting a lack of precision in diagnostic nomenclature and processes (Maj, 2005). Rutter (2003) reviews the need to achieve a better integration of our newer biological and environmental understanding of the causation of mental disorders in children and adolescents with the diagnostic classification of disorders. The issues of the utilization of a categorical and dimensional approach to diagnosis are explored.

It is particularly important to consider the cultural dimension of disorders in children and adolescents, not only in terms of understanding the presentation of disorders, but also of understanding the potential for impairment in life functioning. The melding of an understanding of culture with epidemiology has lagged and represents an area ripe for future research.

The Mental Health of Children and Adolescents: an area of global neglect. Edited by H. Remschmidt *et al.*

In the current clinical and societal environment, the reporting of symptoms associated with disorder may be influenced by a sensitivity to pathology promoted by pharmaceutical companies and by a trend toward diagnosing disorder at earlier stages in development. The role of parents, who in the modern era may be stressed by societal, work, and economic demands, needs to be considered.

Recent reports of "epidemics" of autism have highlighted other issues (Fombonne, 2005). Sound epidemiological data now confirm that there is no evidence of an epidemic of autism anywhere in the world. However, this conclusion was reached only when evidence pointed to gaps in methodologies used in case ascertainment, the phenomenon of "diagnosis shifting" (mental retardation to autism) was clarified, and the supposed causes of the purported epidemics were not proven valid.

DISABILITY ADJUSTED LIFE YEARS

A widely utilized measure of the impact of mental disorders is the disability adjusted life year (DALY). This statistic demonstrated for adult disorders a degree of attributable disability exceeding expectations. Unfortunately, the DALY measure has been far less adequate for assessing the burden of mental disorder in children and adolescents from both a conceptual perspective and a statistical inference. First, child mental disorders were not identified as discrete disorders. Second, disability in the early years of life which might have lifelong consequences for burden was not fully considered. Had both of these factors been incorporated, child mental disorders would probably have contributed more significantly to the DALYs.

When child and adult data for neuropsychiatric disorders are aggregated, significant information is lost, especially because the effects of childhood and adolescent illness are more long-standing than illness that begins in adulthood. Thus, while the Global Burden of Disease project shows that the burden of psychiatric illness has been seriously underestimated in the past, and that five of the ten leading causes of disability worldwide in 1990 were due to psychiatric conditions (unipolar depression, alcohol use, bipolar affective disorder, schizophrenia, and obsessive-compulsive disorder) (Murray and Lopez, 1996), it can be assumed that the burden of childhood psychiatric illness is appreciably more prominent.

Even if childhood illnesses were disaggregated from those of adults, the method by which DALYs are constructed would severely underestimate the burden of disease for childhood and adolescent mental disorders. DALYs are purposely age-biased: they give the greatest weight to an individual aged 25. All other ages are calculated as a percentage of that full value. For example, one year at age 2 has only 20% of the weight of a year at age 25 (Anand and Hanson, 1997). The reason for this is to reflect social roles, as an individual at age 25 can be supporting children as well as elderly parents and is thus is of theoretically "more value" to a society. The last point to consider regarding age preference in the calculation of DALY is that it measures disease burden at one point in time only. As it is designed to do so, DALY fails to take into account the future value of child health.

Finally, the concept of DALY has the same problems that other attempts to quantify mental illness have encountered: how to incorporate societal costs. Anand and Hanson (1997) argue that Murray's definition of DALY is too narrowly defined, as the true "burden of disease" should take into consideration other people affected by mental disorder, such as, family and friends, as well as the need for public services (Anand and Hanson, 1997). As it currently stands, DALY was designed with a "strongly egalitarian flavor," and takes only sex and age into account.

THE ECONOMIC COST OF CHILD AND ADOLESCENT MENTAL DISORDERS

Child and adolescent mental disorders, more so than other illnesses, have long-standing costs to society. Children with depression (Hankin *et al.*, 1998), attention deficit hyperactivity disorder (ADHD), and conduct disorder (Scott *et al.*, 2001) have higher rates of somatic complaints (Bernstein *et al.*, 1997) and health care utilization. They also impose costs on society in terms of education, the burden on the criminal justice system and social services, associated with high-risk behavior (Mannuzza *et al.*, 1998; Knapp, 2000), and the need for informal care (Egger *et al.*, 1999). The societal impact is aggravated by lost economic productivity and potential destabilization of communities. Leibson *et al.* (2003) followed a birth cohort of children with ADHD over 9 years and found that direct medical care costs were more than double for children with ADHD ($4306 versus $1944) than those without the diagnosis, even when the analysis excluded those with hospital and emergency department admissions (Leibson *et al.*, 2001). A review of the literature on children with ADHD by Leibson (2003) shows that almost all cost analyses have estimated direct medical costs only, without reference to indirect costs.

Byford *et al.* (1999) conducted a randomized control trial of the cost-effectiveness of home-based social work intervention versus hospitalization and outpatient care for children and adolescents who deliberately poisoned themselves. They did not find a difference in direct medical costs, but recognized that there are costs associated with mental health outside of the health care system, especially as health care trends change (e.g., in the United Kingdom, where social workers have been shifted from child mental health services to district social work teams) (Byford *et al.*, 1999).

For conduct disorder, comprehensive studies have examined costs beyond the boundaries of health care. A pilot study of ten afflicted children showed that they incurred an average annual cost of over £15 000 attributable to the conduct disorder (Knapp, 2000). Knapp *et al.* (1999) examined the hidden costs of children with conduct disorder. Only 10% of the total costs to society were in the health sector; the rest fell into education (special educational needs), social welfare, family care (through effect on parental employment), and the welfare system. A follow-up into adulthood of children with antisocial behavior showed that the costs of public services were ten times higher than for those without problems as children. Long-term costs were high not only in direct medical care but also in terms of crime, foster and residential care, and expenditure of state benefits (Scott *et al.*, 2001; Knapp *et al.*, 2002).

In a recent review of economic analyses for child and adolescent mental disorder, Romeo *et al.* (2005) found 17 studies with both cost and outcome data: thirteen were cost-effectiveness analyses; four were cost-offset studies; and one was a cost-utility analysis using quality-adjusted life years gained. Besides the fact that most of these studies are technically weak, they include only health care costs and take the provider's perspective only (as opposed to the societal perspective) and thus limit the usefulness of the findings.

CONTEXTUAL CONCERNS ASSOCIATED WITH MENTAL DYSFUNCTION

Displacement

The global problem of displacement from family, home, community, and country is of enormous importance. In 1999, 21.5 million refugees were displaced by war. An additional 30 million, 80% of whom are children and women, were displaced internally. Eisenbruch *et al.* (2004) note that one out of every 275 persons is "of concern" to the United Nations High Commissioner for Refugees (2002). More than 21 million are displaced within their own country, a 25% increase on the year before. Eighty per cent of refugees are women and children (Martin, 1992). Fullilove (1996) emphasizes the importance of "place" in the healthy development of individuals. Sampson *et al.* (1997) describe the importance of the community as a mediator and contributor to the impact of violence on children and adolescents through "collective efficacy." Forced emigration and loss of parents and relatives in war often lead to abandonment. Although these stressors can demonstrate the resiliency of youth, they are known to lead to depression, suicide, and other problems.

Displacement from homes, families, communities, and countries affects children in a host of ways. In a study of the Croatian war, Zivic (1993) found significantly higher depressive and phobic symptoms in displaced children than in children in stable social conditions. In a developmental study of Israeli children exposed to Scud missile attacks, Laor *et al.* (1996) found a higher level of externalizing and stress symptoms in displaced children compared to those able to maintain family and community connections. Displaced children find themselves without the protection and support of parents. Street children depend on survival tactics including criminal activity and prostitution. Youth gangs are increasingly evident, especially in societies where there is inadequate government organization and control. More often than not, the children are the victims rather than the perpetrators of criminal activity.

Conflict

International child and adolescent mental health has become concerned with the effect of armed conflict or its aftermath. Thabet and Vostanis (1998) investigated anxiety symptoms and disorders in children living in the Gaza strip and their relation to social adversities. Children reported high rates of anxiety. Teachers reported increased rates of mental health problems that would justify clinical assessment. Anxiety, particularly pessimism, increased with age and was higher among girls. Low socioeconomic status (father unemployed or unskilled worker) was the strongest predictor of general mental health problems. Living in inner city areas or camps, both common among refugees, was strongly associated with anxiety.

Thabet *et al.* (2000) examined the mental health profile of 322 Arab children living in the Gaza strip. Western categories of mental health problems did not clearly emerge from the analysis: The main difference appeared to be in parents' perception of emotional problems of preschool children. The authors warn of the need to define meaningful diagnostic constructs for this population and culture, and revise measures for child mental health problems. Culture mediates the range of child responses (Aptekar and Stocklin, 1997). More than half of children exposed to war meet criteria for PTSD (Allwood, *et al.*, 2002). Levels of stress have been found to be related to war exposure (Smith, *et al.*, 2002). The Impact of Event Scale (IES) revealed that traumatic stress persists after the war (Dyregrov *et al.*, 2002) and is associated with a higher risk of comorbid psychiatric diagnosis (Donnelly and Amaya-Jackson, 2002).

Soldiering and prostitution

In the turmoil of some resource-poor countries, children are forced to become child soldiers and sexual slaves. Child soldiers reportedly suffer post-traumatic stress disorder (Moszynski, 2003; Derluyn, *et al.*, 2004; Kuruppuarachchi and Wijeratne, 2004; Magambo and Lett, 2004; McKay and Wessells, 2004; Singh, 2004). Horrific experiences place an as yet undefined burden on the psychological development of the victim. Understanding these experiences may shed light on the extremes to which resiliency allows healthy development. More likely, forced military service will cause permanent scarring evidenced in disturbed interpersonal relationships, distorted defenses, heightened aggression, reduced empathy, and self-destructive behavior. Data are not yet available to ascertain whether these young people have post-traumatic stress disorder in the classic sense or whether, because of the early age of induction into the culture of war, they develop in a different way as a survival response. Huge challenges face child mental health in helping to reclaim the lives of former child soldiers (Bracken *et al.*, 1996; Lamberg, 2004).

As for trafficking in children, an estimated 1 million children are forced into prostitution every year. The total number of prostituted children could be as high as 10 million (Willis and Levy 2002). Children are trafficked worldwide (International Organization for Migration, 2001; Inter-American Commission of Women, 2001). Urgent attention is paid to combating the trafficking (Asian, 2003) but the management of the psychological sequelae for the children will need further attention. Nongovernmental organizations have been taking a lead in developing programmes for children and adolescents freed from trafficking. Another issue of concern is the trafficking of children for child labor and other forms of exploitation. The International Labor Organization (1998) has taken this up as a major concern. The psychological consequences of child labor are complex and associated with the relationship of children to their families and their assumption of adult roles prematurely.

HIV/AIDS

In sub-Sahara Africa, Russia, and parts of Asia, acquired immunodeficiency syndrome (AIDS) is pandemic. Special attention needs to be given to the consequences of AIDS for children and youth. The direct impact on children and adolescents is evident in India, other parts of Asia, and Africa, where sexual exploitation has led to a high incidence of youth infection with death as a result of lack of available treatment. An estimated 1.5 million children less than 15 years old are living with human immunodeficiency virus (HIV) infection or AIDS (UNICEF, 2000). More than one-fourth of the young population in sub-Sahara Africa is infected. Among the 10 most affected countries, all in sub-Sahara Africa, approximately

6000000 children younger than the age of 15 years have lost their mother or both parents to AIDS. Those infected but struggling with the illness face the prospect of having to adjust to declining physical and mental functioning and living isolated lives. Neuropsychological dysfunction including dementia, depression, and other disorders, go largely untreated. These children and adolescents, living as orphans or in a stigmatized environment, are vulnerable because of the loss of parent figures, malnutrition, and disenfranchisement from societies that have a stigmatizing view of AIDS-affected and HIV-infected persons.

The mental health consequences are similar in the international arena and are well documented in U.S. studies (Belfer and Munir, 1997). A caution in developing countries is that recognition of the neuropsychological consequences is overshadowed by the totality of the devastation. The lack of recognition of depression, dementia, and other consequences of HIV infection contributes to the spread of the panpidemic. As documented by Carlson and Earls (1997), whether through social policy as evidenced in the Leagane children of Romania or as the consequence of the pandemic of AIDS, the rearing of children in orphanages or in other situations that deprive children of appropriate stimulation and nurturance has long-lasting consequences.

Substance abuse

Substance abuse in children and adolescents is worldwide (Belfer and Heggenhougen, 1995). In resource-poor countries, the problem is of no less importance than in Western countries. It exacts a tremendous toll in terms of morbidity and mortality. Illicit drugs, psychoactive substances not defined as drugs of abuse (e.g., khat, inhalants, and alcohol) are used by youth regardless of economic circumstance or religious prohibition. Homeless street children are particularly vulnerable to substance abuse and other high risk behavior (Raffaelli and Larson, 1999). Senayayake *et al.* (1998) studied the street children in Colombo. Family disintegration was mentioned as the cause of life on the streets by 36%; child labor was reported in 38%; 16% admitted to being sexually abused; 20% were tobacco smokers. Homeless children also are prominent among those groups using inhalants. Road accidents are common among those using drugs.

Solvent and inhalant use is associated with poor economies. In South America, inhalant use is a dominant factor in the presentation of youth affected by psychoactive substances. In Sao Paolo, Brazil, up to 25% of children age 9–18 years abuse solvents (Carlini-Cotrim and Carlini, 1988). In Sudan, gasoline is the inhalant of choice, whereas in Mexico, Brazil, and elsewhere in Latin America, paint thinner, plastic cement, shoe dye, and industrial glue are often used. Gasoline use is found on Australian aboriginal and Native Canadian reservations (Cameron and Debelle, 1984). In Mexico, three of every 1000 people between the ages of 14 and 24 years use inhalants on a regular basis (Belasso, 1978). These figures do not include two high-risk groups, the homeless population and those less than 14 years old, whose rates of inhalant abuse are much greater. Several community studies carried out in different parts of Mexico show that starting ages are as young as 5 or 6 years (Belasso, 1978). Data suggest that the percentage of young people using inhalants decreases as age increases, and other substances such as alcohol and marijuana are substituted. Inhalant use decreases as the educational level increases (Cravioto *et al.*, 1992).

Forster *et al.* (1996) studied the activities of children found wandering in the streets of Porto Alegre, Brazil, aiming to describe their drug habits and practice of thefts or mendicancy. Regular abuse of inhalants was reported much more frequently by the *street* subgroup of children, reaching a prevalence of 40%. Thievery was reported mainly by the children from the *street* group and only by the ones who used illicit drugs. Very poor children spend many hours of the day by themselves in the streets of a big city accompanied by others who are never under adult supervision. In spite of being alone for some hours a day and associating with others who use drugs, having a family and regularly attending school decreases the likelihood of delinquency and drug use.

Violence and abuse

Violence to and by children and adolescents is all too prevalent (World Health Organization, 2002). Bullying, corporal punishment and the victimization of parents by children and adolescents has now been reported worldwide. To understand child abuse one must understand the vast cultural diversity in which children and adolescents live. There is a need for greater attention to country-specific interventions (Djeddah *et al.*, 2000). What is termed "abuse" varies between cultures.

Taxonomy and classification

Munir and Beardslee (2001) are critical of the DSM and propose a developmental and psychobiologic framework for understanding the role of culture in child and adolescent psychiatry. Beauchaine (2003) notes that developmental psychopathologists have criticized categorical classification systems because they fail to account for within-group heterogeneity in cultural influences. Appendix I of DSM-IV includes an "outline for cultural formulation" to assist in evaluating the effect of cultural context on diagnosis and treatment, but the appendix does not enable cultural formulations of child and adolescent psychopathology. Novins *et al.* (1997) attempted to design cultural case formulations for American Indian children. He identified several gaps concerning cultural identity and the cultural aspects of the therapeutic relationship. Rutter (2003) discusses newer approaches to diagnosis.

Epidemiology

It is challenging to determine the epidemiology of childhood mental disorders in Western society. Internationally the problem is even more complex. Reporting systems are inadequate, the definition or recognition of disorders varies or has different interpretations, and the cultural component of what constitutes a disorder is only now being appreciated by epidemiologists and researchers. In studying the epidemiology of psychiatric disorder in children and adolescents in resource-poor countries, it is important to define not only the prevalence and incidence of disorders, but also their degree of impairment and burden of disease. No single study or set of independent studies on the epidemiology of child and adolescent disorders since 1980 is definitive or relevant to all societies. Studies carried out in the 1980s reflect the methodological deficiencies noted earlier and do not represent the current realities of the countries from which the data were reported (Odejide *et al.*, 1989; Hackett and Hackett, 1999). Weiss (2001) has defined a new epidemiological approach combining qualitative study with classic epidemiologic methods (Raguram *et al.*, 2004).

The new "cultural epidemiologic" approach has not yet been applied to child and adolescent mental disorders but it is promising.

Faced with the realities of resource-poor countries, there is a danger of becoming a diagnostic nihilist. On the contrary, responsible investigators in Western Ethiopia clearly identified disordered mental functioning that meets a set of defined criteria (Tadesse *et al.*, 1999). There is good evidence that depression, psychosis, and mania can be identified and treated. The problem arises when one considers the cultural context. Is a hallucination during a ritual a disturbance in need of treatment? If the hallucination persists, should it be treated? What diagnostic label is appropriate? Counter to prevailing belief, Giel and Van Lujik (1969) found, in the pre-HIV/AIDS era, that mental disorders were diagnosed more frequently than infectious diseases in African health centers. Recently, WHO studies of primary care showed that many patients seeking care had mental disorders, and their communities were aware of the problem (Harding *et al.*, 1980). Omigbodun (2004) documented psychosocial problems in Nigerian children and adolescents. 62.2% of new referrals to the clinic had experienced significant psychosocial stressors in the year preceding presentation. Problems with primary support (e.g., separation from parents to live with relatives), disruption of the family, abandonment by mother, psychiatric illness in a parent, and sexual/physical abuse occurred in 39.4%. Significantly more children and adolescents with disruptive behavior and disorders like enuresis, separation anxiety, and suicidal behavior had psychosocial stressors when compared to children with psychotic conditions, autistic disorder and epilepsy.

Prevalence

Epidemiological reports of the more esoteric disorders are a distraction from the significant burden of disease that needs to be addressed in the mainstream of care. In most studies, methodological inadequacies and other constraints do not permit these studies to be applied to programme planning or needs assessment. However, most countries today have access to appropriate epidemiologic study guidelines; it is a matter of setting a national priority and allocating resources to ascertain the data. For example, Malhotra (1998) used a sophisticated three-stage assessment of the epidemiology of disorders in Indian school children aged 4–12 years. In this study, assessments by teachers, parents, and clinicians were compared. Teacher assessment on the Rutter B scale had a low concordance rate with clinical assessment. When children tested positive on both the teacher and parent assessment, there was a diagnostic concordance rate of 92.3% on the clinical assessment. The evidence pointed to a prevalence rate of psychiatric disorder between 7 and 20%. Diagnoses included enuresis, mental retardation, and epilepsy. Overall, a conservative estimate of severe psychiatric disorder in India is 10% of the population younger than age 14 years, representing 35 million children (1998).

Giel *et al.* (1981) demonstrated in four countries (Sudan, Philippines, Colombia, and India) that between 12 and 29% of children aged 5–15 years had mental health problems. The types of disorder identified in these resource-poor countries were no different from those encountered in industrialized countries. Mothers readily reported the symptoms that made diagnoses possible. Thabet and Vostanis (1998) reported anxiety symptoms and disorders among children living in the Gaza Strip comparable to previous epidemiologic research in Western societies. There were high rates of anxiety disorders and school-related mental health problems. Thabet and Vostanis found the same prevalence rate (21%) of anxiety-related disorders as Kashani and Orvaschel did (1990). Thabet and Vostanis (1998) state that their findings do not support the commonly held belief that, in non-Western societies, anxiety and other mental health symptoms are predominantly expressed through somatic symptoms. Citing Nikapota (1991) they state that child mental health symptoms do not differ significantly across cultures; culture-specific mental health disorders are rare.

Tadesse *et al.* (1999) reported a prevalence of 17.7% of childhood behavioral disorder in Western Ethiopia. Behavioral disorders were more frequent in boys than in girls. Their data were gathered with a version of the Reporting Questionnaire for Children developed by WHO. Hackett *et al.* (1999) and Bird *et al.* (1989) found an excess of male patients with externalizing disorders, reflecting the Western view of a male predisposition to externalizing disorders. The findings of comparability with Western epidemiologic data are at odds with some older studies and may reflect new social and economic realities.

What of attention deficit hyperactivity disorder, autism, and anorexia nervosa? The diagnosis and treatment of these disorders highlight both the weakness and strength of having an international perspective. The recognition and labeling of disorders come as a result of improved international communication. However, the process of assessment must take into account a host of cultural and formal diagnostic criteria. This is too often ignored. Cultural concepts of what is normal or abnormal and how parents perceive the presence or absence of disorder (Hackett and Hackett, 1999) must be considered. In the case of eating disorders, there is clear evidence that incidence is affected by Western influences (Becker, 1995). In the diagnosis of ADHD, pharmaceutical companies are a major source of both public and professional understanding and contribute to the awareness of the problem for which formal diagnostic procedures are required. The influence of public awareness and concerns about diagnosis requires further study.

In a study of adolescents in Bahrain with Adjustment Disorder, al-Ansari and Matar (1993) examined the life stressors that precipitated referral to a child psychiatry unit. Disappointment in relationships with a family member or friend of the opposite sex was a main stressor. Eating disorders are rare in resource-poor countries such as India (Khandelwal *et al.*, 1995), but anecdotal evidence suggests that with globalization and migration rates are increasing (Littlewood, 1995). Autism is reported in affluent and resource-poor countries (Lotter, 1978; Gupta, 2001; Yeargin-Allsopp and Boyle, 2002),with a cross-national consistency (Lotter, 1978; Chung *et al.*, 1990; Takei, 1996). However, high rates of autism, almost 200 times higher than in the general population of children, have been reported among boys born in Sweden to Ugandan mothers (Gillberg *et al.*, 1995). This finding in light of the analysis by Fombonne (2005) requires further investigation.

SPECIFIC MENTAL DISORDERS

Post-traumatic stress disorder

For children and adolescents, there are conflicting views on the impact of trauma on mental functioning (Mollica *et al.*, 1997; Weine, *et al.*, 1998; Sack *et al.*, 1999). The resiliency of children over the long term is apparent, but individual investigators identify specific consequences of trauma, particularly depression, externalizing behavior, and PTSD (Laor *et al.*, 1996). Diagnosis does not coincide with functional status according to Sack *et al.* (1995). Sack *et al.* (1999) show the persistence of PTSD and also demonstrate its sometimes delayed onset. However, over time children affected by PTSD appeared to function well. Terr (1983) demonstrated the persistent effect on children of traumas with lasting functional deficits. Studies from Kuwait (Abdel-Mawgoud, 1997) and Iran (Almqvist and Brandell-Forsberg, 1997) also showed the persistence of PTSD. Thabet and Vostanis (1998), in the Gaza Strip, found that the prevalence of at least mild PTSD among children aged 6–11 years of at least mild PTSD was 73%; 39% presented with moderate to severe PTSD symptoms. Ahmad (1992) reported that 25% of displaced Kurdish children had PTSD. Weine *et al.* (1998) found similar rates in Bosnian adolescents who moved to the United States during the Balkan war of the 1990s.

Conduct disorder and delinquency

A Sri Lankan study of the adjustment in children using the Strengths and Difficulties Questionnaire (Goodman), with parent, teacher, and child informants, found problems consistent with other international studies of child mental health. Compared with Muslim and Singhalese children, Tamil children were rated as more hyperactive and emotional with more severe conduct problems and total behavioral difficulties. The relationship between behavioral adjustment and Tamil ethnicity was associated with the longstanding ethnic conflict in Sri Lanka. It supports the need for child and adolescent health services in civil war-torn countries (Prior, M., *et al*, 2005).

A descriptive survey of Flemish delinquent adolescents found a significant difference between ethnic groups on self-report scores (Vermeiren *et al.*, 2000). Tramontina *et al.* (2001) evaluated the association between DSM-IV conduct disorder (CD) and school dropout in a sample of students from the state schools in Porto Alegre, Brazil. The prevalence of DSM-IV CD was higher in the school-dropout group than in controls. The odds ratio for school dropout was higher in the presence of DSM-IV CD, even after controlling for potential confounding factors such as family structure and income.

Depression

Childhood depression is gaining prominence (World Health Organization, 2004). A cross-cultural evaluation of depression in children in Egypt, Kuwait, and the United States (Becker, 1995) showed similar clinical patterns. As noted elsewhere, depression and its variants are seen in children and adolescents worldwide. Depressive and anxiety disorders should not be overshadowed by the attention currently given to PTSD and ADHD in developing countries in the aftermath of natural disaster and conflict.

Suicide

Youth suicide is pervasive. In Western countries, suicide is overwhelmingly associated with defined mental illness. It is the second leading cause of death for American Indian and Alaska Native youth (Borowsky, 1999). Elsewhere in the world, it can be very difficult to identify the mental illness associated with the suicidal act. In the face of overwhelming helplessness, suicide may appear to be the only escape, with no clearly labeled mental illness. Studies of suicide in the West have focused on risk factors associated with cognitive distortions, substance use, and familial factors (Shaffer, 1988). In some resource-poor countries, the balance in determining suicidal risk may rest with environmental stressors and the perception of "no way out." Unrealistic expectations for success or happiness may often be more determinant of suicidal angst than reality (Bertolote, 2003). According to Murthy (2000), the traditional protective effect of religion in certain cultures does not operate in the younger generation.

Chan *et al.* (2001) and Chan (2003) regard suicide in contemporary China as a response to globalization, in which "Chinese" values are closely identified with the global culture. The high suicide rate is a reflection not of psychiatric disorder but of socio-cultural factors. Suicide is viewed by those without demonstrable mental illness as a solution to personal dilemmas that thwart expectations. From this perspective, in India and in other resource-poor countries, the motive of the suicidal individual is not to achieve an exalted goal, but rather to have enough dowry to marry, not to be isolated because of rape, or to be successful in passing an examination. The alteration in emphasis is important in the consideration of intervention strategies and training. A survey of adolescent health in nine Caribbean countries has identified risk and protective factors predisposing to suicide attempts (Blum, *et al.*, 2003).

Disabilities, mental retardation, and epilepsy

Disability – physical or mental – is all too common in resource-poor countries, especially after conflict. In Cambodia, for example, about 1 out of every 40 have physical disabilities, 20–35 children per thousand children below age 18 years might be mentally retarded (102 000–178 500) and 2–4 individuals per thousand have severe mental disorders (20 400–40 800), and 14–60 per thousand have epilepsy (154 000–408 000) (UNESCO, 2003).

In resource-poor countries mental retardation and epilepsy dominate child mental health services. In the 1980s, prevalence rates of mental retardation in resource-poor countries were estimated to be 8–12 per 1000 for children aged 3–10 years (Narayanan, 1981; Belmont, 1984; Tao K, 1988). Mental retardation and epilepsy are the most common mental disorders in India (Malhotra and Chaturvedi, 1984). The rate of serious mental retardation in some resource-poor countries ranges from 5 to 16.2 per 1000 population (Stein *et al.*, 1986), significantly higher than the rate in the West. Cerebral palsy and postnatal causes of mental retardation are much more common in transitional societies than in developed countries. Untreated epilepsy impedes participation in society. Unfortunately, although the cost of medication is relatively low, access to care is limited. The care of the mentally retarded varies widely in resource-poor countries. In some a special effort is made to provide meaningful vocational education, especially in agrarian economies. All too often, the moderately and severely retarded are relegated to substandard institutions where disease and premature death are rife.

CONCLUSION

Child and adolescent mental disorders are unquestionably ubiquitous and burdensome. The burden of child and adolescent mental disorders can be documented from many perspectives. We are yet to understand the toll on society. It is a challenge to disseminate the tools needed for epidemiologic research and assessment of the "burden of disease." Refined diagnosis and assessment of burden will hopefully lead to the implementation of policies to support mental health promotion, prevention, and treatment.

REFERENCES

Abdel-Mawgoud, M., al-Haddad, MK (1997) Heroin addiction in Bahrain: 15 years experience. *Addiction*, **91**(12):1859–64.

Ahmad, A. (1992) Symptoms of post-traumatic stress disorder among displaced Kurdish children in Iraq: victims of man-made disaster after the Gulf War. *Nordic J Psychiatry*, **46**:314–19.

Almqvist, K. and Brandell-Forsberg, M. (1997) Refugee children in Sweden: Post-traumatic stress disorder in Iranian preschool children exposed to organized violence. *Child Abuse Negl*, **21**(4), 351–66.

Anand, S., Hanson, K. (1997) Disability-adjusted life years: a critical review. *J Health Econ*, **16**(6):685–02.

al-Ansari, A. and Matar, A. M. (1993) Recent stressful life events among Bahraini adolescents with adjustment disorder. *Adolescence*, **28**(110), 339–46.

Aptekar, L. and Stocklin, D. (1997) Children in particularly difficult circumstances, in *Handbook of Cross-Cultural Psychology* (J. C. Triandis and W. W. Lambert), Vol. I, Allyn & Bacon, Boston, USA, pp. 377–12.

Allwood, M. A., Bell-Dolan, D., and Husain, S. A. (2002) Children's trauma and adjustment reactions to violent and nonviolent war experiences. *J Amer Acad Child Adolesc Psychiatry*, **41**(4), 450–57.

Asian, D. B. (2003) Combating trafficking of women and children in South Asia – Regional synthesis paper for Bangladesh, India, and Nepal. Manila, Asian Development Bank.

Beauchaine, T. P. (2003) Taxometrics and developmental psychopathology. *Dev Psychopathol*, **15**(3), 501–27.

Becker, A. E. (1995) *Body, Self and Society – The View from Fiji*, University of Pennsylvania Press, Philadelphia.

Belasso, G. (1978) The international challenge of drug abuse: The Mexican experience, in The International Challenge of Drug Abuse (ed R. C. Petersen) (National Institute on Drug Abuse), 19th Edition, Department of Health, Education, and Welfare, Public Health Service, Alcohol, Drug Abuse, and Mental Health Administration, National Institute on Drug Abuse, Division of Research, Rockville, MD.

Belfer, M. and Heggenhougen, K. (1995) Substance abuse, in *World Mental Health: Problems and Priorities in Low-Income Countries* (eds R. Desjarlais, L. Eisenberg, B. Good, and A. Kleinman), Oxford University Press, New York, pp. 87–115.

Belfer, M. L. and Munir, K. (1997) Acquired immunodeficiency syndrome, in *Textbook of Child and Aadolescent Psychiatry*, 2nd Edition (ed J. M. Wiener), American Academy of Child and Adolescent Psychiatry, Washington, D.C.

Belmont, L. (1984) The international pilot study of severe childhood disability – Final report – *Screening for Severe Mental Retardation in Developing Countries*, Bishop Bekkers Institute, Utrecht.

Bertolote, J. (2003) Department of Mental Health and Substance Abuse, World Health Organization, Geneva, Switzerland. Personal Communication.

Bird, H. R., Gould, M. S., Yager, T. *et al.* (1989) Risk factors for maladjustment in Puerto Rican children. *J Amer Acad Child Adolesc Psychiatry*, **28**(6), 847–850.

Blum, R. W., Halcon L., Beuhring T. *et al.* (2003) Adolescent health in the Caribbean: Risk and protective factors. *Am J Public Health*, **93**(3), 456–60.

Borowsky, I.W., Resnick, M.D., Ireland, M., Blum, R.W. (1999) Suicide attempts among American Indian and Alaska Native youth: risk and protective factors. *Arch Pediatrics Adolesc Med*, **153**(6), 573–80.

Bracken, P. J., Giller, J. E., and Ssekiwanuka, J. K. (1996) The rehabilitation of child soldiers: Defining needs and appropriate responses. *Med Confl Surviv*, **12**(2), 114–25.

Byford, S., Harrington, R., Torgerson, D., Kerfoot, M, Dyer, E, Harrington, V., Woodham, A, Gill, J., McNiven, F. (1999) Cost-effectiveness analysis of a home-based social work intervention for children and adolescents who have deliberately poisoned themselves. Results of a randomized control trial *Brit J Psychiatry*, **174**:56–62.

Cameron, F. J. and Debelle, G. D. (1984) No more Pacific island paradises. *Lancet*, **1**(8388), 1238.

Carlini-Cotrim, B. and Carlini, E. A. (1988) The use of solvents and other drugs among children and adolescents from a low socioeconomic background: A study in Sao Paulo, Brazil. *Int J Addict*, **23**(11), 1145–56.

Carlson, M. and Earls, F. (1997) Psychological and neuroendocrinological sequelae of early social deprivation in institutionalized children in Romania, in *The Integrative Neurobiology of Affiliation* (eds C. S. Carter, I. I. Lederhendler, and B. Kirkpatrick), Academy of Sciences, New York, pp. 419–28.

Chan, K. P., Hung, S. F., and Yip, P. S. (2001) Suicide in response to changing societies. *Child Adolesc Psychiatr Clin North Am*, **10**(4), 777–95.

Chan, K. (2003) Hong Kong, China. Personal Communication.

Chung, S. Y., Luk, S. L., and Lee, P. W. (1990) A follow-up study of infantile autism in Hong Kong. *J Autism Dev Disord*, **20**(2), 221–32.

Cravioto, P., Anchondo, R. L., and de la Rosa, B. (1992) Risk factors associated with inhalant use among Mexican juvenile delinquents, in *Epidemiologic Trends in Drug Abuse* (ed B. S. Johnson) (National Institute on Drug Abuse, Community Epidemiology Work Group), U.S. Department of Health and Human Services, Public Health Service, Alcohol, Drug Abuse, and Mental Health Administration, Division of Epidemiology and Prevention Research, National Institute on Drug Abuse, pp. 472–77.

Derluyn, I., Broekaert, E., Schuyten, G., and De, T. E. (2004) Post-traumatic stress in former Ugandan child soldiers. *Lancet*, **363** (9412), 861–63 (see comment).

Djeddah, C., Facchin, P., Ranzato, C., and Romer, C. (2000) Child abuse: Current problems and key public health challenges. *Soc Sci Med*, **51**(6), 905–15.

Donnelly, C. L. and Amaya-Jackson, L. (2002) Post-traumatic stress disorder in children and adolescents: Epidemiology, diagnosis and treatment options. *Paediatr Drugs*, **4**(3), 159–70.

Dyregrov, A., Gjestad, R., and Raundalen, M. (2002) Children exposed to warfare: A longitudinal study. *J Trauma Stress*, **15**(1), 59–68.

Eisenbruch, M, de Jong, J, and van de Put, W. (2004) Bringing order out of chaos: Identification, management and prevention of psychosocial and mental health problems of refugees and victims of organized violence within primary care. *J Trauma Stress*, **17**(2), 123–31.

Egger, H.L., Costello, E.J., Erkanli, A., Angold, A. (1999) Somatic complaints and psychopathology in children and adolescents: stomachaches, musculoskeletal pains, and headaches. *J Am Acad Child Adolesc Psychiatry*, **38**(7):852–60.

Fombonne, E. (2005) Epidemiology of autistic disorder and other pervasive developmental disorders. *J Clin Psychiatry*, **66**(Suppl. 10), 3–8.

Forster, L. M., Tannhauser, M., and Barros, H. M. (1996) Drug use among street children in southern Brazil. *Drug Alcohol Depend*, **43**(1–2), 57–62.

Fullilove, M. T. (1996) Psychiatric implications of displacement: Contributions from the psychology of place. *Am J Psychiatry*, **153**, 1516–23.

Giel, R. and van Lujik, N. (1969) Psychiatric morbidity in a small Ethiopian town. *Rev Med Psychosom Psychol Med*, **11**(4), 435–56.

Giel, R., de Arango, M. V., Climent, C. E. *et al.* (1981) Childhood mental disorders n primary health care: Results of observationa in four developing countries. *Pediatrics*, **68**(5), 677–83.

Gillberg, C., Schaumann, H., and Gillberg, I. C. (1995). Autism in immigrants: Children born in Sweden to mothers born in Uganda. *J Intellect Disabil Res*, **39**(Part 2), 141–44.

Gupta, N. (2001) Austism: Some conceptual issues. *Indian Pediatr*, **38**(9), 1065–67 (comment).

Hackett, R. and Hackett, L. (1999) Child psychiatry across cultures. *Int Rev Psychiatry*, **11**(2), 225–35.

Hackett, R. J., Hackett, L., Bhakta, P., and Gowers, S. (1999) The prevalence and associations of psychiatric disorder in children in Kerala, South India. *J Child Psychol Psychiatry*, **40**(5), 801–07.

Hankin, B.L., Abramson, L.Y., Moffitt, T.E., Silva, P.A., McGee, R., Angell, K.E. (1998) Development of depression from preadolescence to young adulthood: emerging gender differences in a 10-year longitudinal study. *J Abnorm Psychol*, **107**(1):128–40.
Harding, T. W., De Arango, M. V., Baltazar, J. *et al.* (1980) Mental disorders in primary health care: A study of their frequency and diagnosis in four developing countries. *Psychol Med*, **10**(2), 231–41.
Inter-American Commission of Women. (2001) Trafficking of women and children for sexual exploitation in the Americas – An introduction to Trafficking in the Americas.
Khandelwal, S. K., Sharan, P., and Saxena, S. (1995) Eating disorders: An Indian perspective. *Int J Soc Psychiatry*, **41**(2), 132–46.
International Labor Organization, International Program on the Elimination of Child Labor. (1998) Combating trafficking in children for labour exploitation in the Mekong sub-region: A proposed framework for ILO-IPEC action and proceedings of a Mekong sub-regional consultation. ILO/IPEC.
International Organization for Migration. (2001) Trafficking in women and children from the Republic of Armenia: A study. International Organization for Migration, Yerevan.
Kashani, J. H. and Orvaschel, H. (1990) A community study of anxiety in children and adolescents. *Am J Psychiatry*, **147**(3), 313–18.
Knapp, M., Scott, S., Davis, J. (1999) The cost of antisocial behavior in younger children. *Clinical Child Psychology Psychiatry*, **4**(4):457–73.
Knapp, M. (2000) Schizophrenia costs and treatment cost-effectiveness *Acta Psychiatr Scand Suppl*, (407):15–18.
Knapp, M., McCrone, P, Fombonne, E, Beecham, J, Wostear, G. (2002) The Maudsley long-term follow-up of child and adolescent depression: 3. Impact of comorbid conduct disorder on service use and costs in adulthood *Br J Psychiatry*, **180**:19–23.
Kuruppuarachchi, K. and Wijeratne, L. T. (2004) Post-traumatic stress in former Ugandan child soldiers. *Lancet*, **363**(9421), 1648 (comment).
Lamberg, L. (2004) Reclaiming child soldiers' lost lives. *JAMA*, **292**(5), 553–54.
Laor, N., Wolmer, L., Mayes, L. C. *et al.* (1996) Israeli preschoolers under Scud missile attacks. A developmental perspective on risk-modifying factors. *Arch Gen Psychiatry*, **53**(5), 416–23.
Leibson, C.L., Katusic, S.K., Barabaresi, Wm.J. *et al.* (2001) Use and costs of medical care for children and adolescents with and without attention deficit/hyperactivity disorder. *JAMA*, **285**(1), 60–66.
Leibson, C.L., Long, K.H. (2003) Economic implications of attention-deficit hyperactivity disorder for healthcare systems. *Pharmacoeconomics*, **21**(17):1239–62.
Littlewood, R. (1995) Psychopathology and personal agency: Modernity, culture change and eating disorders in South Asian societies. *Br J Med Psychol*, **68**(1), 45–63.
Lotter, V. (1978) Childhood autism in Africa. *J Child Psychol Psychiatry*, **19**(3), 231–44.
Magambo, C. and Lett, R. (2004) Post-traumatic stress in former Ugandan child soldiers. *Lancet*, **363**(9421), 1647–48 (comment).
Maj, M. (2005) The aftermath of the concept of "Psychiatric Comorbidity." *Psychother Psychosom*, **74**:67–68.
Malhotra, S., Chaturved, S. (1984) Patterns of childhood psychiatric disorders in India. *Indian Pediatric J*, **51**, 235–40.
Malhotra, S. (1998) Challenges in providing mental health services for children and adolescents in India in *Designing Mental Health Services and Systems for Children and Adolescents – A Shrewd Investment* (eds J. G. Young and P. Ferrari), Brunner/Mazel, Philadelphia, pp. 321–34.
Mannuzza, S., Klein, R.G., Bessler, A., Malloy, P. LaPadulla, M. (1998) Adult psychiatric status of hyperactive boys grown up. *Am J Psychiatry*, **155**(4):493–98.
Martin, F. (1992) *Refugee Women*, Zed Press, London.
Mawgoud, M. (1997) A survey of fears associated with Iraqi aggression among Kuwaiti children and adolescents: A factorial study 5.7 years after the Gulf War. *Psychol Rep*, **81**(1), 247–55.
McKay, S. and Wessells, M. G. (2004) Post-traumatic stress in former Ugandan child soldiers. *Lancet*, **363**(9421), 1646–47 (comment).
Mollica, R. F., Poole, C., Son, L. *et al.* (1997). Effects of war trauma on Cambodian refugee adolescents' functional health and mental health status. *J Am Acad Child Adol Psychiatry*, **36**(8), 1098–106.
Moszynski, P. (2003) Child soldiers forgotten in Angola. *Br Med J*, **326**(7397), 1003.

Munir, K. M. and Beardslee, W. R. (2001) A developmental and psychobiologic framework for understanding the role of culture in child and adolescent psychiatry. *Child Adol Psychiatr Clin North Am*, **10**(4), 667–77.

Murray, C.J., Lopez, A.D. (1996) The incremental effect of age-weighting on YLLs, YLDs, and DALYs: a response. *Bull World Health Organ*, **74**(4):445–46.

Murthy, R. S. (2000) Approaches to suicide prevention in Asia and the Far East, in *International Handbook of Suicide and Attempted Suicide* (eds K. Hawton and K. Van Heeringen), John Wiley & Sons, Ltd, London, pp. 625–37.

Narayanan, H. (1981) A study of the prevalence of mental retardation in Southern India. *Int J Mental Health*, **10**, 128–36.

Nikapota, A. D. (1991) Child psychiatry in developing countries. *Br J Psychiatry*, **158**, 743–51.

Novins, D. K., Bechtold, D. W., Sack, W. H. *et al.* (1997) The DSM-IV outline for cultural formulation: A critical demonstration with American Indian children. *J Am Acad Child Adol Psychiatry*, **36**(9), 1244–51.

Odejide, A. O., Oyewunmi, L. K., and Ohaeri, J. U. (1989) Psychiatry in Africa: An overview. *Am J Psychiatry*, **146**(6), 708–16.

Omigbodun, O. O. (2004) Psychosocial issues in a child and adolescent psychiatric clinic population in Nigeria. *Soc Psychiatry Psychiatr Epidemiol*, **39**(8), 667–72.

Prior, M., Virasinghe, S., and Smart, D. (2005) Behavioural problems in Sri Lankan school children: associations with socio-economic status, age, gender, academic progress, ethnicity and religion. *Social Psychiatry Psychiatric Epidemiol*, **40**(8), 654–62.

Raffaelli, M. and Larson, R. W. (1999). *Homeless and Working Youth Around the World – Exploring Developmental Issues*, Jossey-Bass, San Francisco.

Raguram, R., Raghu, T. M., Vounatsou, P., and Weiss, M. G. (2004) Schizophrenia and the cultural epidemiology of stigma in Bangalore, India. *J Nerv Ment Dis*, **192**(11), 734–44.

Romeo, R., Byford, S. Knapp, M. (2005) Annotation: Economic evaluations of child and adolescent mental health interventions: a systematic review. *J Child Psychol Psychiatry*, **46**(9):919–30.

Rutter, M. (2003) Categories, dimensions, and the mental health of children and adolescents. *Ann N Y Acad Sci*, **1008**, 11–21.

Sack, W. H., Clarke, G. N., Kinney, R. *et al.* (1995) The Khmer Adolescent Project. II: Functional capacities in two generations of Cambodian refugees. *J Nerv Ment* Dis, **183**(3), 177–81.

Sack, W. H., Him, C., and Dickason, D. (1999) Twelve-year follow-up study of Khmer youths who suffered massive war trauma as children. *J Am Acad Child Adolesc Psychiatryr*, **38**(9), 1173–79.

Sampson, R. J., Raudenbush, S. W., and Earls, F. (1997) Neighborhoods and violent crime: A multilevel study of collective efficacy. *Science*, **277**(5328), 918–24.

Scott, S., Knapp, M., Henderson, J. et al. (2001) Financial cost of social exclusion: follow-up study of anti-social children into adulthood. *Brit Med J*, **322**, 191–95.

Senanayake, M. P., Ranasinghe, A., and Balasuriya, C. (1998) Street children – a preliminary study. *Ceylon Med J*, **43**(4), 191–93.

Shaffer, D. (1988) The epidemiology of teen suicide: an examination of risk factors. *J Clin Psychiatry*, **49**(Suppl):36–41.

Singh, S. (2004) Post-traumatic stress in former Ugandan child soldiers. *Lancet*, **363**(9421), 1648 (comment).

Smith, P., Perrin, S., Yule, Wm. *et al.* (2002) War exposure among children from Bosnia-Hercegovina: Psychological adjustment in a community sample. *J Trauma Stress*, **15**(2), 147–56.

Stein, Z., Durkin, M., and Belmont, L. (1986) "Serious" mental retardation in developing countries: An epidemiologic approach. *Ann N Y. Acad Sci*, **477**, 8–21.

Tadesse, B., Kebede, D., Tegegne, T., and Alem, A. (1999) Childhood behavioural disorders in Ambo district, western Ethiopia. I. Prevalence estimates. *Acta Psychiatr Scand Suppl*, **397**, 92–97.

Tadesse, B., Kebede, D., Tegegne, T., and Alem, A. (1999) Childhood behavioural disorders in Ambo district, western Ethiopia. II. Validation of the RQC. *Acta Psychiatr Scand Suppl*, **397**, 98–101.

Takei, N. (1996) Childhood autism in Japan. *Br J Psychiatr*, **169**(5), 671–72 (comment).

Tao, K. (1988) Mentally retarded person's in the People's Republic of China: A review of epidemiological studies and services. *Am J Ment Retard*, **93**, 193–99.

Terr, L. C. (1983) Chowchilla revisited: The effects of psychic trauma four years after a school-bus kidnapping. *Am J Psychiatry*, **140**(12) 1543–50.
Thabet, A. A. and Vostanis, P. (1998) Social adversities and anxiety disorders in the Gaza Strip. *Arch Dis Child*, **78**(5), 439–42.
Thabet, A. A., Stretch, D., and Vostanis, P. (2000) Child mental health problems in Arab children: Application of the strengths and difficulties questionnaire. *Int J Soc Psychiatry*, **46**(4), 266–80.
Tramontina, S., Martins, S., Michalowski, M. B. *et al.* (2001) School dropout and conduct disorder in Brazilian elementary school students. *Can J Psychiatry*, **46**(10), 941–47.
UNESCO (2003) Focus on ability and celebrate diversity – Highlights of the Asian and Pacific decade of disabled persons 1993–2003. New York, United Nations.
UNICEF. (2000) The State of the World's Children. UNICEF, New York.
UNHCR. Refugees by Numbers 2001 Edition. http://www unhcr.com
UNHCR, Refugees by Numbers, United Nations High Commissioner for Refugees, Geneva, 2002
UNICEF. (2003) Innocenti Research Centre. Trafficking in human beings, especially women and children, in Africa. UNICEF Innocenti Research Center, Florence, Italy.
Vermeiren, R, De, C. A., and Deboutte, D. (2000) A descriptive survey of Flemish delinquent adolescents. *J Adol*, **23**(3), 277–85.
United Nations, Economic and Social Commission for Asia and the Pacific. (2003). Focus on ability, celebrate diversity – Highlights of the Asian and Pacific decade of disabled persons, 1993–2003. United Nations, New York.
Weine, S. M., Vojvoda, D., Becker, D. F. *et al.* (1998) PTSD symptoms in Bosnian refugees 1 year after resettlement in the United States. *Am J Psychiatry*, **155**(4), 562–64.
Weiss, M. G. (2001) Cultural epidemiology: An introduction and overview. *Anthropology Med*, **8**(1), 5–29.
Willis, B. M. and Levy, B. S. (2002) Child prostitution: Global health burden, research needs, and interventions. *Lancet*, **359**(9315), 1417–22.
World Heallth Organization. (2002) World Report on Violence and Health, World Health Organization, Geneva, Switzerland.
World Health Organization. (2004) *WHO Guide to Mental and Neurological Health in Primary Care – A Guide to Mental and Neurological Ill Health in Adults, Adolescents and Children*, 2nd Edition, Royal Society of Medicine Press, London.
Yeargin-Allsopp, M. and Boyle, C. (2002) Overview: the epidemiology of neurodevelopmental disorders. *Ment Retard Dev Dis Res Rev*, **8**(3), 113–16.
Zivciç, I. (1993) Emotional reactions of children to war stress in Croatia. *J Am Acad Child Adolesc Psychiatry*, **32**(4), 709–13.

CHAPTER 4

Disseminating Child and Adolescent Mental Health Treatment Methods: An International Feasibility Study

The Integrated Services Programme (ISP) Task Force

The ISP Task Force is a Working Committee of the World Psychiatric Association (WPA) Presidential Global Programme on Child Mental Health. The Task Force included the following members (alphabetically) José J. Bauermeister, John Fayyad, Richard Harrington, Kimberly Hoagwood, Jack (S.F.) Hung, Peter S. Jensen, Kelly Kelleher, Laura Murray, Cheryl So, and site directors Alan Apter and Orit Krispin (Tel Aviv, Israel) John Fayyad (Lebanon), Luis Augusto Rohde and Paulo Knapp (Porto Alegre, Brazil), and Amira Seif El Din (Alexandria, Egypt).

BACKGROUND

Across the world, one in five children have emotional and behavioral conditions severe enough to interfere with their ability to grow and to learn. Over the last decade, scientists have generated a host of discoveries concerning the causes, consequences, and treatment of childhood mental disorders; yet there has been relatively little attempt to assist countries worldwide to apply newly developed techniques to the prevention and intervention with children's mental health problems.

The WPA Presidential Programme on Child Mental Health, launched in 2002, decided to develop a comprehensive set of tools to address different countries' needs for systematic, evidence-guided treatment of child and adolescent mental health problems. Designed for broad application and future scalability, the WPA Presidential Programme includes three components: community awareness, prevention, and integrated services. Each of these components was developed by a task force of international experts, under the guidance of a steering committee, and implemented in multiple sites in different countries. This report describes the ISP and its implementation across four countries.

The Mental Health of Children and Adolescents: an area of global neglect. Edited by H. Remschmidt *et al.*

THE VISION AND PURPOSE OF THE ISP

The purpose of the ISP was to enable willing sites across different countries, along with their clinical leadership and staff, to implement an integrated, evidence-based system of care. The system of care would be tailored to the mental health needs of the population at that site within a given country, based on its local resources. Clinicians and clinical leaders would be provided detailed consultation and support in implementing the ISP. As the ISP was developed for use by those sites participating in the WPA Presidential Programme, the materials, manuals, and accompanying process were designed to be applicable in other sites, in the future. It was hoped that the interventions would be adaptable to the mental health needs of different countries, and appropriate to the parents, teachers, health care workers, and other community leaders within those countries.

As many clinical needs might have been addressed, ISP developers chose to focus on the diagnostic tools and implementation methods for treating two broad categories of common psychological problems in school-age children, namely, the "internalizing" and "externalizing" disorders. *Internalizing disorders* are thus named, because they are experienced by the child, but may not always be apparent to others. These conditions encompass the DSM-defined mood and anxiety disorders, as well as sub-threshold symptom constellation involving principally sadness, depression, thoughts about death, anxiety, worries, fears, the physiological symptoms of anxiety (e.g., shortness of breath or increased heart rate), fear-based avoidance of normative experiences (e.g., attending school), and fears of specific objects or situations. In contrast, the other major type of problem (*externalizing disorders*) is characterized by a persistent pattern age-inappropriate inattentive, hyperactive and impulsive behavior that interferes significantly with daily functioning. "Externalizing" problems can also refer to impatience, difficulty delaying responses, the tendency to interrupt or intrude on others, or to display a pattern of negativistic, defiant, disobedient, hostile, aggressive, deceitful, and antisocial behavior. When severe, externalizing behavior can be directed toward authority figures and violate the basic rights of others or important societal rules.

The internalizing and externalizing behavior problems in children are found in all cultures, although their manifestations vary in accordance with sociocultural factors. The two types of behavior problems tend to co-occur (for example, an anxious-depressed child may also show inattention–hyperactivity–impulsivity and defiance-aggression). Thus, given the frequency of overlap, it was thought to be necessary to develop an intervention for both major problem types, to allow clinicians the flexibility to deal with the most commonly occurring problems. However, the ISP was not designed to address the types of difficulty presented by very young children, or the very severe psychiatric disorder, such as psychosis, autism, schizophrenia, or extreme conduct disorder.

The ISP thus was planned to provide health care workers a flexible, practicable method of treating the two major problem types. The intervention should be adaptable to different countries, cities, and localities, depending on the amount of health care funding and school resources available, the nature and intensity of the problems that these children present, and the social preferences and other cultural factors important within the particular community.

Should a given locality have few resources, the ISP provides a modest but feasible intervention, in school, health care, or community settings. If the locality has greater health care resources, the ISP is compatible with more comprehensive evaluation and treatment, including medical-psychiatric diagnostic assessment and additional treatment, as required.

THE ISP APPROACH

The ISP Task Force prepared three manuals, two on the specific treatment of internalizing and externalizing problems of childhood, and one on overall programme implementation. Both intervention manuals were designed to be brief (8–12 sessions) and to involve both child and parents. Both were drawn from the current literature concerning evidence-based intervention, (viz., cognitive behavior therapy for anxiety/depression and behavior therapy/parent training for child disruptive behavior). Please see Bauermeister *et al.* (2006) for a more extensive report on how these manuals were developed and translated.

Key child mental health leaders, most often child psychiatrists known to be the members of the Task Force through relationships with the World Health Organization or the World Psychiatric Association, were contacted and invited to participate in the programme. Of six potential sites and child mental health leaders contacted, four actually participated (see acknowledgments for ISP Task Force Site Directors). A modest amount of support (generally less than $5000) was available for each site to offset local expenses.

The overall ISP approach involved the steps as follows:

- Manual development and translation (Bauermeister *et al.*, 2006)
- Training of clinics, clinicians, clinical supervisors, and other clinical staff in implementing evidence-based assessment and intervention (EBAIs) (Murray *et al.*, 2006)
- Implementation of the EBAIs, including
  - systematic evaluation and assessment of children presenting with mental health problems, with the assessments to include standardized rating scales; (Hoagwood *et al.*, 2006; So *et al.*, 2006)
  - standardized assessments together with other appropriate clinical information to determine level and type of care, based upon algorithms and principles of care, as clinically appropriate to the local culture and situation;
  - provision of mental health care for children with internalizing and externalizing problems and their families, based on the principles and procedures described in the two accompanying manuals, as ethically and culturally appropriate in the particular setting (Bauermeister *et al.*, 2006).
- Continuing technical assistance provided by the ISP Task Force (Murray *et al.*, 2006)
- Evaluation of the nature and extent of implementation of EBAIs (Hoagwood *et al.*, 2006) participating clinics and staff
- Data collection, analysis, and report write-up (Hoagwood *et al.*, 2006).

LESSONS LEARNED

Below, we present some of the "lessons learned" from this enterprise, a "first" for all those involved, beginning first with some of the issues pertaining to manual development, followed by lessons learned from the challenges faced during the training of participants in widely dispersed locales and with many languages.

Developing adaptable, flexible, and culturally appropriate treatment manuals

The manuals are organized in two levels. Level I, usually consisting of 2–3 sessions, was designed for those children and families who could benefit from psychoeducation and support alone, delivered by people who are not mental health clinicians. Level II, consisting of another 4–6 sessions, involves direct treatment designed for sites, settings, and countries that have existing mental health resources.

Each of the manuals is accompanied by guidelines and materials required to train professional groups, not only mental health therapists but also teachers, school administrators, and clinic directors. Each of the manuals was derived from evidence-based treatments with substantial data on efficacy. With this evidence base, the ISP Task Force adapted materials from So's detailed and comprehensive manuals developed for Hong Kong parents (So, 1997) and children (So *et al.*, 2004) together with materials adapted from other manuals (Arnold *et al.*, 1997). The internalizing disorders treatment manual was adapted from treatment manuals developed and implemented for children experiencing anxiety, depression, and post-traumatic symptoms following the New York City 9/11/2001 disaster. These 9/11 manuals in turn were derived from a synthesis of evidence-based treatment manuals first designed by Stark *et al.* (1991), Wood *et al.* (1996), and Layne *et al.* (2005).

The manuals were designed for youths with mild to moderate problems. The externalizing manual is primarily for children aged 6–12 years, whereas the internalizing manual is for children aged 8–14 years. The treatment manuals emphasize that clinician require training and continuing supervision by experienced clinicians. They also indicate when and for which children they should or should not be applied. A particular therapeutic technique should not be applied without careful planning and adaptation to the values of each locality (Bauermeister *et al.*, 2006).

In addition to providing programme components matching different countries' resources and needs, manuals were adapted for the values, beliefs, and practices of the family culture (Bauermeister *et al.*, 2006; Forehand and Kotchick, 1996). Parenting practices and psychosocial processes occur within the larger context of a local or national culture. Consequently, each site was encouraged to accomplish the necessary adaptation by being sensitive to the cultural values of parents and children and collaborating working with them. The latter, among other things, required the parents and therapists to develop a supportive, reciprocal relationship based on the therapist's knowledge and the parent's strengths and perspectives (Jensen, 2006).

The treatment manuals were implemented in the four sites by mental health professionals who volunteered to participate. Although in some localities such as Porto Alegre, few adaptations were needed, in others, several modifications were made or recommended. These adaptations (see below) are not necessarily associated with true cultural values, as it is difficult to disentangle individual differences, socioeconomic variables, and contextual factors from cultural influences. They do point out, however, the importance of the beliefs and practices of participating families, and the likelihood of site-to-site variations, both within and across different cultures (Bauermeister *et al.*, 2006; Murray *et al.*, 2006; So *et al.*, 2006).

Our experiences illustrated the importance of using culturally relevant language. For example, although manuals were translated into Arabic by the Alexandria site, the two other Arabic sites needed to modify the Egyptian translation to convey the intended meaning. On the contrary, in some instances, other seemingly "American" words, such as the English acronym "ACTION," did not need to be translated, as the word was understood in several other cultures and carried additional value because young people understood it and liked it. Similarly, other factors such as stigma and barriers treatment seemed to exist in all sites, though some aspects of treatment, such as the acceptability of medication treatment, varied considerably.

Although no site experienced a need for *extensive* modifications of the content of the therapy, minor to moderate changes were required in every site. Nonetheless, observations by staff at participating sites consistently indicated that the treatment programmes and accompanying manuals could be successfully implemented. Therapists shared the same cultural background of the participants and could promptly identify cultural issues requiring adjustments to the manuals.

Training for evidence-based interventions in cross-cultural contexts: challenges and solutions

The task of providing training and supervisory services to therapists in the participating sites was complicated by several environmental and economic constraints (Murray *et al.*, 2006). The following challenges were encountered: providing supervision across widely spaced time zones, geographies, and languages; the inability to provide the kind of relationship usually required in psychotherapy supervisions; the need for a credible evidence-based programme that could address training needs beyond those of clinicians alone (e.g., the needs of clinic staff and administrators); the simultaneous implementation of two new evidence-based programmes; considerable site-to-site variation in terms of previous training, resources, and staff capacity; the need for an adaptation of manuals developed principally in the United States for populations of limited ethnic diversity; the logistic difficulty and related quality assurance of supervisory conference calls; and the need for the ISP to provide a sustainable system for the continuation of evidence-based treatment after the ISP Task Force has withdrawn.

To address these problems, the ISP Task Force concluded that the training/supervision model, if it were to be ultimately disseminable, must combine some face-to-face contact with other exchanges (e.g., e-mail, web conference, and telecommunication). A one-and-one-half day, face-to-face training ("Helping Challenging Children" programme) was provided for supervisors and therapists from each participating site at a central location (Berlin). In addition to teaching the principles of behavioral therapy (BT), training promoted role-playing of the major therapeutic techniques involved in the "Helping Challenging Children" manual (Bauermeister *et al.*, 2006; Murray *et al.*, 2006).

After the face-to-face training, the ISP Task Force conducted monthly international supervision teleconferences with participating supervisors and therapists. More frequent teleconferences (i.e., twice a month) were arranged before therapy sessions were started, gradually tapered to once monthly, after implementation at each site had become smoother. Local-site supervisors continued to provide weekly face-to-face supervision for the therapists in their home countries (Murray *et al.*, 2006).

At the initial stage face-to-face training provided a good opportunity for members from each site to get to know the members of the ISP Task Force and maintain a personal relationship with them. The way each clinician provided mental health services within the larger context of his or her culture was extensively discussed during training later. Personal relationships and resultant group cohesion facilitated a better understanding of the cultural issues involved.

Training was designed to prepare qualified mental health professionals to deliver the interventions. All therapists had to be credentialed according to the standards of local government, regulatory authorities, or professional organizations. The training modules were not designed to substitute for formal training in the clinical disciplines of child psychiatry or child psychology. Once they had been trained, therapists were encouraged to use designated sections of the ISP manuals and materials to provide psychoeducation for schools, parents, and community leaders.

Considering the different complexity of therapeutic skills required for the two treatment programmes, the ISP Task Force decided that training for externalizing problems should be provided before that for internalizing problems, and that sites should have 3–4 months' experience with the first manual before learning the second. The precise timing of the transition was tailored to each site, depending upon the availability of mental health personnel and their previous experience with EBAIs. In addition, to ensure treatment adherence and competence of therapists, ISP manuals contained checklists to allow supervisors to provide systematic supervision in their home countries (Bauermeister *et al.*, 2006).

Because of the poor quality of conference calls (e.g., when the operator failed to set up the call, when calls were disconnected during conferences, poor sound quality, etc.) and because participants had different mother tongues, they were encouraged to e-mail questions or case vignettes to the ISP Task Force prior to each teleconference. This strategy gave participants more time to peruse materials and allowed them to participate actively in the teleconference. Tracking difficult or illustrative cases regularly during each teleconference also helped therapists to develop a better understanding of the ISP manuals.

Although different challenges arose throughout training and supervision, most problems were solved with the concerted effort of all participating sites. The ISP distance training/supervision model could act as a blueprint for future international training programmes. Nonetheless, future studies will need to determine whether EBAIs are sufficient to ensure treatment fidelity and to find out whether such methods are effective in different cultural and geographic settings (Bauermeister *et al.*, 2006; Murray *et al.*, 2006).

Challenges and successes

The four international sites had diverse organizational structures and developed different methods of implementing the ISP (So *et al.*, 2006). Each had different starting points, organizational structures, and financing mechanisms, and each experienced its own problems and successes. However, a common theme for success was a prior favorable relation with stakeholders, staff, and administrators at the site, which seemed to ensure the degree of support and commitment that all sites saw as critical. The availability of consistent fiscal support for the project (through government sponsored programmes, for example) was related to the ease of recruitment of staff and their acceptance of the project.

Common themes within some school-based sites were difficulties with parental involvement and teacher acceptance. Both school-based sites (Tel Aviv and Alexandria) suggested that future implementation studies should provide more training for teachers to facilitate their involvement, perhaps augmented by giving them a tangible benefit in return. Several sites suggested that poor parental involvement was due to the setting (e.g., services offered in schools), whereas others suggested that the traditional cultural roles could be obstructive. The most obvious contrast was between Brazil and the other three sites: Brazil had a massive infrastructure staffed with professionals and a mechanism for funding participants. The other sites were less well endowed.

An overview of the four international sites participating in this feasibility study sheds light on the multiple factors that must be considered in cross-cultural implementation. Organizational structures are diverse. Organizations embrace sociopolitical issues, security situations, and differences in the availability of trained professionals. Materials must be translated and adapted for the local dialect. Cultural factors (e.g., mistrust of psychological services and the different roles of family members) must also be taken into account (So *et al.*, 2006).

Our study emphasizes the uniqueness of implementation at each location, suggesting that a general guideline of how to think through implementation will be especially important for international work and dissemination. Although the step-by-step therapy manuals were useful in all sites, it was evident that the adaptation and implementation of manualized psychosocial therapy requires concerted attention to the unique organizational, cultural, and social factors operating in particular sites.

CONCLUSION

We have been heartened by what we learned from each other during programme implementation (Bauermeister *et al.*, 2006; Hoagwood *et al.*, 2006; Jensen, 2006; Murray *et al.*, 2006; So *et al.*, 2006). Although most EBAIs were developed for English-speaking, "Western" societies, we were impressed by the degree to which many therapeutic principles and procedures were appropriate in settings very different from those for which they were first developed. Nevertheless, important adaptations were necessary, even critical in a number of instances, highlighting to each of us the extent to which an "evidence-base" depends on a partnership between clinicians, researchers, and families, all of whom have something to teach each other, particularly when EBAIs are taken out to the "real world" and into different societies. This was an important step in our learning process. On behalf of the children affected worldwide by mental health problems, we trust that the step will be one of many more.

ACKNOWLEDGMENTS

The authors thank the clinicians and therapists who contributed their time, dedication, and expertise to this project and provided additional input and comments for this paper:

Lisiane Lyzkowski and Maria G. Machado, Porto Alegre (Brazil); Wafaa Mohamed Saad and Mohamed Osman Ebrahim, Alexandria (Egypt); Muhammed El Heib and Sami Hamdan, Tel Aviv (Israel); and Lynn Farah and Youmna Cassir, Beirut (Lebanon).

For more information about this report, contact Peter S. Jensen, M.D.; Center for the Advancement of Children's Mental Health, Unit #78; Department of Child Psychiatry, NYSPI/Columbia University, 1051 Riverside Drive, New Cork, NY, 10032, USA; Phone: 212 543-5334; Fax: 212 543-5260; E-mail: pj131@columbia.edu

REFERENCES

Arnold, L. E., Abikoff, H. B., Cantwell, D. P. *et al.* (1997) NIMH collaborative multimodal treatment study of children with ADHD (MTA): Design, methodology, and protocol evolution. *J Atten Disord*, **2**(3), 141–58.

Bauermeister, J. J., So, C. Y. C., and Jensen, P. S. (2006) Integrated Services Program (ISP) Task Force. Development of adaptable and flexible treatment manuals for externalizing and internalizing disorders in children and adolescents. *Braz J Psychiatry*, **28**(1), 67–71.

Forehand, R. and Kotchick, B. A. (1996) Cultural diversity: A wake-up call for parent training. *Behav Ther*, **27**, 187–206.

Hoagwood, K. E., Kelleher, K., Murray, L. K., and Jensen, P. S. (2006) Integrated Services Program Task Force. Implementation of evidence-based practices for children in four countries: A project of the World Psychiatric Association. *Braz J Psychiatry*, **28**(1), 59–66.

Jensen, P. S. (2006) Integrated Services Program (ISP) Task Force. Disseminating child & adolescent mental health treatment methods: An international feasibility study. *Braz J Psychiatry*, **28**(1), 1–2.

Layne, C., Saltzman, W., Goldman, E., and Stark, K., (2005) Macquarie University, and the Integrated Psychotherapy Consortium. Post-traumatic stress symptoms intervention manual. New York State Office of Mental Health, Project Liberty Enhanced Services Program.

Murray, L. K., Fayyad, J., Jensen, P. J. *et al.* (2006) Integrated Services Program (ISP) Task Force. An examination of cross-cultural systems implementing evidence-based assessment and intervention approaches. *Braz J Psychiatry*, **28**(1), 76–79.

So, C. Y. C. (1997) *Parent Training for Attention-Deficit/Hyperactivity Disorder*. Unpublished manuscript. Kwai Chung Hospital, Hong Kong.

So, C. Y. C., Hung, J. S. F., Bauermeister, J. J., and Jensen, P. S. (2006) Integrated Services Program (ISP) Task Force. Training of evidence-based assessment and intervention approaches in cross-cultural contexts: Challenges and solutions. *Braz J Psychiatry*, **28**(1), 72–75.

So, C. Y. C., Leung, P. W. L., and Hung, S. F. (2004) *Enhancement of Learning Behavior Project: Cooperation Between Schools, Families, and Community*, 2nd Edition, Kwai Chung Hospital and Department of Psychology, The Chinese University of Hong Kong, Hong Kong.

Stark, K. D., Rouse, L. W., and Livingston, R. (1991) Treatment of depression during childhood and adolescence: Cognitive behavioural procedures for the individual and family, in *Child and Adolescent Therapy: Cognitive-Behavioural Procedures* (ed P. C. Kendall), Guilford, New York, pp. 165–206.

Wood, A. J., Harrington, R. C., and Moore, A. (1996) Controlled trial of a brief cognitive-behavioural intervention in adolescent patients with depressive disorders. *J Child Psychol Psychiatry*, **37**, 737–46.

CHAPTER 5

Prevention of Mental Health Disorders in Children and Adolescents

CHAPTER 5.1

The Principles of Prevention in Child and Adolescent Mental Health

Barry Nurcombe
The University of Queensland, Brisbane, Australia

THE PREVALENCE OF PSYCHIATRIC DISORDER IN CHILDREN AND ADOLESCENTS

In a survey of 52 studies, Roberts *et al.* (1998) found that the average prevalence of psychiatric disorder in children and adolescents was 15.8%, with a range of 11–22%.

Sawyer *et al.* (2000) surveyed a representative sample of 4500 Australian school children aged 4–17 years, using the Child Behavior Checklist (CBCL) (Achenbach, 1991), The Diagnostic Interview Schedule for Children (DISC-IV) (Shaffer *et al.*, 2000), and The Child Health Questionnaire (CHQ) (Landgraf *et al.*, 1996). Adolescents aged 13–17 years also completed the Center for Epidemiologic Studies Depression Scale (CES-D) (Radloff, 1977) and the Youth Risk Behavior System Questionnaire (YRBS) (Brener *et al.*, 1995). Sawyer *et al.* (2000) found that 14.7% of children and 13.1% of adolescents were in the clinical range. Children and adolescents with mental health problems had a poorer quality of life, lower self-esteem, worse school performance than those who did not, and were a greater burden to their families. Adolescents with mental health problems reported high rates of suicidal behavior, smoking, drinking, and drug use. Few psychiatrically disturbed children were receiving any professional treatment, and those who did receive help usually obtained it from general practitioners, school counselors, or pediatricians. Very few had attended a specialized mental health service or clinician.

Remschmidt *et al.* (1998) found that between 1.9 and 3.9% of children and adolescents under 18 years of age, living in three German counties, had attended mental health services within a one-year period. Of a sample of 1969 representative subjects aged between 6 and 18 years, the prevalence of mental disorder was 12.7% (according to the CBCL; Achenbach and Edelbrock, 1983). Only 3.3% had received specialized treatment. Assuming a 5% rate of treatment necessity, 34% of those who needed some kind of treatment were untreated.

The Mental Health of Children and Adolescents: an area of global neglect. Edited by H. Remschmidt *et al.*

These sobering statistics indicate that, even if primary diagnostic and therapeutic services were effective, and even if the links between primary and specialized professional services were efficient, there are far too many seriously disturbed families for existing facilities to serve. Furthermore, empirical support for different kinds of mental health treatments outside of laboratory studies is lacking (Weisz *et al.*, 1995), and the dropout rate from community services alarmingly high (Nurcombe *et al.*, 2005). For these reasons, the idea of prevention has been promoted. Prevention aims to avert or divert unfavorable developmental trajectories in such a way as to reduce the incidence or severity of psychopathology and promote mental health.

RISK AND RESILIENCE

A number of *risk factors* are known to be associated with later psychiatric disorders. They vary from *biological* (e.g., genetic or chromosomal abnormality, exposure to intrauterine toxins such as alcohol or nicotine, premature birth, exposure to toxins such as lead during early development, and chronic physical disability such as epilepsy or brain injury) and *temperamental* (e.g., behavioral inhibition or difficult temperament) to *familial* (e.g., parental depression, alcoholism and antisocial personality; disorganized infant–parent attachment; coercive child rearing; single-parent or blended families; marital discord and domestic violence; physical abuse, sexual abuse, and neglect), *socioeconomic* (e.g., poverty, membership of a disadvantaged minority group), and *catastrophic* (e.g., civilian disaster or war).

Protective factors counterbalance risk. It is known, for example, that an easy, likeable temperament, above-average intelligence, good support from at least one parent, a cohesive family environment, and social capital in the form of good schools, adequate community resources for sport and skill-building, and good employment prospects protect otherwise vulnerable individuals from psychiatric disorder. Protective factors act by moderating the effect of risk factors or by promoting alternative, compensatory processes that enhance self-esteem and a sense of personal effectiveness.

Prevention, thus, might work by eliminating risk factors (e.g., the cessation of smoking or drinking during pregnancy), by decreasing their impact (e.g., reducing the incidence of premature birth by providing good antenatal care and nutrition for socially disadvantaged women), or by enhancing protective factors (e.g., providing good schools and social opportunities).

In reality, most outcomes have multiple determinants. Psychopathology following child sexual abuse, for example, is associated with the following three groups of *moderating factors*: (a) antecedent factors such as the quality of child–parent attachment prior to the abuse; (b) the nature of the abuse experience (repeated, coercive, intrafamilial genital penetration being the most adverse); and (c) the quality of parental support after the child discloses the abuse. Moderating factors operate through the following *mediating factors*: (a) whether the child has sustained post-traumatic stress disorder; (b) the child's attitude toward self and others; and (c) the child's coping methods (denial, dissociation, distraction, and repetition – compulsion being the most pathogenic).

Preventive intervention that aims to reduce the incidence of psychopathology after child sexual abuse might therefore focus on improving the quality of family support to the child, counteracting the child's adverse attitudes toward herself and others, helping the child to assimilate and cognitively reconstruct memories of abuse, treating post-traumatic stress disorder, and promoting healthy self-assertiveness and self-protection. Prevention that aims to stop sexual abuse from occurring in the first place relies upon promoting community awareness, teaching children to avoid or report perpetrators, and treating as soon as possible sexually abused boys, a proportion of whom will otherwise grow up to be sexual perpetrators as adults.

THE GOALS AND TYPES OF PREVENTION

Prevention in child and adolescent mental health refers to intervention that aims to eliminate, or reduce the incidence of, or ameliorate the severity of, general or specified psychopathology in the population as a whole or in particular groups that are at risk of developing psychiatric disorder or impairment.

Preventive intervention can be classified according to when in the course of the development of a psychiatric disorder the intervention is applied. *Primary prevention* refers to intervention in normal populations to avert future mental ill-health (e.g., school-based alcohol and drug education). *Secondary prevention* focuses on special at-risk groups in order to stave off the development of psychopathology (e.g., the treatment of sexually abused children). The term *tertiary prevention* (the early treatment of patients with established psychiatric disorders) has fallen into disuse.

An alternative classification system has been proposed by the Institute of Medicine (1994), in accordance with the population served. *Universal prevention* is offered to the entire population of a particular area (e.g., good antenatal care). *Targeted prevention* is offered to particular groups. *Targeted indicated prevention* is directed at groups who are identified as being at risk by virtue of biological markers or symptom patterns (e.g., epilepsy or highly aggressive preschool children). *Targeted selective prevention* is aimed at children at increased risk by virtue of their membership of a vulnerable subgroup (e.g., the children of highly stressed, economically disadvantaged, single mothers), or because they are about to experience a life transition or stressful event (e.g., change of schools or divorce).

Prevention can also be classified in accordance with the *level* and *timing* of intervention. The level of intervention refers to whether intervention is delivered to the individual, the family, the peer group, the school, or the community as a whole. Timing refers to the developmental period when the intervention occurs: antenatal, infancy, preschool, middle childhood, adolescence, or adulthood.

Take, for example, the following programme. Olds *et al.* (1986) successfully reduced the incidence of child maltreatment by delivering a nurse-home-visiting programme to mothers who were at risk of abusing their children by virtue of adolescent pregnancy, poverty, or single parenthood. The programme began antenatally and continued until the child was two-years old. This was a primary, targeted, selective prevention of family-level type, delivered in the antenatal-infancy period.

DEVELOPMENTAL DISCONTINUITY, DIVERGENT DEVELOPMENT, AND EQUIFINALITY

Discontinuity refers to breaks or changes in development that lead to a different outcome. For example, a number of studies have shown that a proportion of children who have been seriously sexually abused have no discernible psychopathology at the time of ascertainment.

However, Gomez-Schwartz *et al.* (1990) found that, when assessed 18 months later, many previously asymptomatic children had developed serious psychopathology.

Divergent development refers to the way that a single stressor can lead to a variety of later outcomes (e.g., child sexual abuse is linked to disturbed self-concept, chronic emotional distress, self-harm, substance abuse, dissociative disorder, somatoform disorder, sexual problems, and revictimization or sexual perpetration in adulthood).

Equifinality or *convergent development* refers to the way that a variety of risk factors affecting the child at different periods of development can lead to the same outcome. For example, antisocial behavior in male adolescents is predicted by genetic background, disorganized attachment, coercive child rearing, aggressive behavior in early childhood, depression of verbal intelligence, learning problems, gravitation toward delinquent companions in late childhood, and early initiation into alcohol and drug use. Some of these risk factors may be causative whereas others represent points on the longitudinal development toward the undesirable end point.

It is important to determine whether a risk factor is *causal* (e.g., genetic factors in attention deficit hyperactivity disorder) or a *noncausal correlate* (e.g., abnormal saccadic eye movements in schizophrenia). Prevention should be aimed at those causal factors that are accessible for intervention. Furthermore, a single risk factor can play different parts in the causation of psychiatric disorder. Family dysfunction, for example, can precede sexual abuse, increase the likelihood that it will occur, be precipitated by the disclosure of abuse, and aggravate its effect (Spaccarelli, 1994).

The possibility of adverse and favorable *reciprocal interactions* should be considered. For example, premature children raised by disadvantaged parents are more likely to develop impaired intelligence and learning problems than are those raised in families that provide good social and language stimulation to the child during infancy and the preschool period. Preventive intervention might, for example, intervene to generate progressively more and more favorable interactions between premature child and mother.

SCHOOL DROPOUT: A POTENTIAL FOCUS FOR INTERVENTION

To exemplify the reasoning behind prevention programmes, the problem of school dropout will be discussed.

Prevatt and Kelly (2003) state that 11% of American high school students leave school without a diploma or credential. The adverse outcomes of failure to finish high school include low income as an adult, life-dissatisfaction, alienation, depression, gang-membership, alcohol and drug abuse, and violent or criminal behavior. Half of all welfare families are headed by parents who dropped out of high school and half the prison population dropped out of school. The problem is serious and prevalent. What is its cause and what can be done about it?

A wealth of previous studies have documented the following factors as associated with dropping out from high school: poverty, minority status, single parenthood, child maltreatment, poor health care, family disruption, parental mental illness, learning problems, chaotic school atmosphere, alcohol and substance use, adolescent pregnancy, etc. Poverty (low SES) is probably a noncausal marker for causative problems such as adverse parenting and failure of the family to value education. Chaotic school atmosphere probably aggravates the problem (i.e., is a moderating factor) whereas learning problems mediate it.

How can these risk factors be combined to generate a valid theoretical model that could guide preventive intervention?

Battin-Pearson *et al.* (2000) tested five theoretical models of early high school dropout, as follows:

- *Academic Mediation.* In this theory, poor academic achievement is described as the mediator of dropout. Other variables such as deviant affiliation, individual psychopathology, and poor family socialization are regarded as moderating factors which predict dropout via poor academic achievement. Low allegiance to the school is hypothesized as the result of poor achievement.
- *General Deviation.* Delinquent attitudes and behavior, drug use, early sexual behavior, and adolescent pregnancy, all regarded as indicators of personal deviance, predict dropout.
- *Deviant Affiliation.* Before leaving school, dropouts typically gravitate toward deviant peers. Other dropouts have been rejected by their peers. Does deviant affiliation have its effect on dropout directly or is its effect mediated through poor academic performance?
- *Poor Family Socialization.* Family disruption, poor parenting, parental psychopathology, negative parental attitudes to education, and low parental expectation that the child will succeed are likely to affect academic performance, but may also predict dropout directly.
- *Structural Strains.* This theory relates school dropout to demographic factors such as low SES and membership of a minority ethnic group.

Battin-Pearson *et al.* (2000) used latent-variable structural equation modeling to examine whether poor academic achievement at 14 years of age mediates the effects of general deviance, low school bonding, low parental expectations, deviant affiliation, and demographic factors in predicting dropout at 16 years of age. If so, the implication is that preventive efforts should concentrate on academic achievement. If not, then some or all of the other five factors must also be addressed.

As expected, poor academic achievement was a strong predictor of dropout and mediated the effects of all five factors on dropout. However, general deviance, poor bonding to school, and SES also had direct effects on dropping out. Partial support was found for all five models, but none was fully adequate to explain the data. A causal chain model that combines poor family socialization, poor academic performance, general deviance, and deviant affiliation is most likely to generate an effective preventive intervention.

EMPIRICALLY BASED PROGRAMMES FOR THE PREVENTION OF HIGH SCHOOL DROPOUT

Prevatt and Kelly (2003) conducted a literature search and found 217 articles on dropout prevention. They located 16 preventive studies in peer-reviewed journals which involved an empirical analysis of effectiveness and included measurement of dropping out as one of the dependant variables. Five of these studies employed a control or comparison group and yielded a strong or promising outcome. These five studies will now be summarized.

Meyer (1984) implemented *Direct Instruction Follow Through* with minority group third-grade children. The 3–4-year programme combined a direct-instruction mathematics, reading and language programme with vigilant monitoring of school progress, heavy emphasis on basic skills instruction, and focused teacher training. The average dropout rate in the experimental group was 28%, compared with 46% for the control group.

Curiel *et al.* (1986) evaluated the outcome of a bilingual education programme for Mexican–American English-speaking students followed from Grades 7 through 11, after they had received bilingual education during the first six grades of school. The dropout rate in programme participants was 23.5% compared with 43% in the comparison group.

Pearson and Banerji (1993) implemented *The Ninth Grade Programme* in six high schools. This programme was a rather loose amalgam of ability grouping, tutoring, a buddy system, class orientation, study skills, and teacher-as-advisor meetings. The proportion of treatment students who dropped out decreased over the 3 years of the programme from 10.3 to 4.4%.

Sinclair et al (1998) evaluated the effectiveness of *The Check and Connect Programme.* In this programme, adult monitors worked for several years with the 25 families assigned to each of them, tracking academic progress and checking for behavior indicating potential dropout (e.g., tardiness, truancy, disciplinary problems). Students were provided with feedback about their progress and assisted with problem solving. If the student had serious academic or behavior problems, written contracts were drawn up, tutoring was arranged, and a cognitively oriented problem-solving programme implemented. The treatment group had a 9% dropout rate in the ninth grade, compared with 30% in the control group.

Temple *et al.* (2000) investigated the effect of *The Chicago Child–Parent Center and Expansion Programme* on dropout rates at 17 years of age. This programme operated from prekindergarten to the third grade and provided language stimulation, parent involvement, parent training, social support for families, and volunteer assistance in classroom activities and field trips. The design of the evaluation was quasi-experimental (i.e., students were not assigned randomly to the treatment and comparison groups). The dropout rate in the treatment group was 22.8%, and in the comparison group 32.6%.

All these interventions were of targeted, indicated, primary prevention type. Four of the programmes (Meyer, 1984; Curiel *et al.*, 1986; Pearson and Banerji, 1993; Sinclair *et al.*, 1998) were delivered at the individual level, in middle or late childhood, whereas one programme (Temple *et al.*, 2000) involved children and families in early childhood. Two of the programmes (Meyer, 1984; Sinclair *et al.*, 1998) placed a heavy emphasis on classroom instruction and were clearly based on the academic mediation model. One programme (Curiel *et al.*, 1986) that was heavily influenced by the structural strains model focused on bilingual education. One programme (Pearson and Banerji, 1993) was based on an amalgam of the general deviance and academic mediation models. Temple *et al.* (2000) based their intervention on a combination of the academic mediation and deviant socialization models.

Prevatt and Kelly (2003) noted that most of the programmes in their general review were based on prior research but that few were grounded in an explicit theoretical model. The widespread use of school-wide or classroom-wide intervention made random assignment difficult or impossible, and shifted the focus from targeted individuals to targeted systems. The measurement of outcome was problematic as it usually relied upon school records the reliability of which was uncertain. Other criticisms were leveled at the lack of sophistication in statistical analyses (e.g., failure to report effect sizes or power analyses) and inadequate descriptions of the interventions applied.

THE CHARACTERISTICS OF SUCCESSFUL INTERVENTION PROGRAMMES

Nation *et al.* (2003) reviewed prevention programmes across four areas: substance abuse, risky sexual behavior, school failure, and delinquency and violence. Nine qualities characterized programmes that were effective are as follows:

- *Comprehensiveness.* Successful programmes employ combinations of interventions to increase awareness and promote skills and are directed at individual, family and school-system levels. Risk factors are addressed and protective factors enhanced or promoted.
- *Variation in teaching methods.* Most effective programmes emphasize skill-building through interactive instruction and practical experience.
- *Adequate dosage.* Good interventions last long enough and are sufficiently intense to have an effect: The greater the needs of the participants, the longer the duration of the programme and the more intensive it must be. Booster programmes are provided to enhance prior skills learned or to introduce new, developmentally appropriate skills.
- *Theoretical model.* Effective interventions are grounded in explicit theoretical models of the interaction between risk and protective factors, and how these factors might be eliminated, ameliorated, or enhanced.
- *The promotion of positive relationships.* Parent–child, child–teacher, and peer relationships are addressed, and positive adult models (e.g., mentors) provided.
- *Appropriate timing.* Effective interventions are delivered before the participants have developed the targeted problem to a full extent, thus giving the intervention the opportunity to alter pathogenic developmental trajectories. Furthermore, the intervention is developmentally appropriate; in other words, it is tailored to the cognitive and social development of the participants.
- *Sociocultural relevance.* Intervention programmes that reflect local community norms, cultural beliefs, and practices increase the receptiveness of participants and families. Successful programmes take into account the individual needs of participants. One-size-fits-all programmes work best for those who least need them and may actually be harmful for those most in need of intervention.
- *Outcome evaluation.* Effectiveness is based on evaluation, not anecdote or fashion. Good programmes incorporate continuous quality improvement through the feedback of outcome data.
- *Staff training and support.* Effective programmes pay close attention to the selection, training, supervision, and continuing support of staff. The opinions of staff should be sought concerning the implementation and evaluation of the programme. High staff turnover, conflict, and demoralization sabotage effective intervention. Supervision and the provision of treatment manuals counteract the tendency of some staff to drift off the treatment model. In other words, an attempt is made to ensure that the programme is delivered with fidelity.

THE NEED FOR RESEARCH

Excellent reviews of the effectiveness of preventive intervention have been provided by Durlak and Wells (1997), Carr (2002), and Reppucci *et al.* (1999).

In many prevention studies, the follow-up period was too brief to assess the long-term impact of the intervention. Few researchers have attempted to replicate findings or to examine the validity of their programmes in other populations or settings. More information is needed concerning the effect of the quality of implementation (e.g., treatment fidelity) on outcome, and whether matching the programme to the individual, developmental and sociocultural characteristics of participants enhance effectiveness, and which of the components of the programme are effective.

Future programmes should be based on explicit theoretical models derived from empirical research into how risk and protective factors interact in causal chains to produce undesirable outcomes. Intervention programmes should have clear goals and objectives, operationalized methods of intervention, treatment manuals to assure standardization, and multi-modal outcome evaluation. Future studies should determine which participants benefit from a programme and which do not.

PLANNING AN EFFECTIVE PROGRAMME

The first requirement is to choose a problem that is serious and prevalent in your community. Consider whether the community would be receptive to the idea of prevention or, if not, whether prevailing attitudes could be changed. Consider whether your interest in the problem and your current position allow you the authority and time to get the job done.

Next, choose your planning team. Best of all are those people who you know have the skills (e.g., in particular intervention techniques, programme design, or statistical analysis) required to form a balanced design team. Mavericks and egocentrists should be avoided; a high degree of collaboration is required.

Find out what is known about the risk and protective factors associated with the problem. Have any theoretical models been proposed? If so, which one, in your opinion, best encompasses the interactive chain of factors that produces the undesirable outcome. If none of the available models is adequate, construct your own model and base the design of the intervention upon it.

Choose the timing and level of the intervention. Generally speaking, the earlier an adverse developmental trajectory is diverted, the better it is. Generally, targeted interventions are better than universal interventions. Universal interventions often fail to reach those most in need and expend their energy on those who do not need them. However, universal educational programmes can create a social environment favorable for targeted intervention. Decide whether your programme will be directed toward the individual child, the family, or a social system such as a classroom or school. Generally, multiple levels are preferable.

Parent education and involvement is likely to enhance the effect of a child-directed programme. How will you decide which children should be targeted? What screening instruments are required?

Make sure that your programme is suitable for the sociocultural group for which it has been designed. Consult with others who have implemented programmes for the group. You may need to add a cultural consultant to your team. Recruit team members and clinicians from the ethnic group involved.

Seek the advice of a statistician consultant (or, better still, ask one to join the team). You need to find out how many subjects are required, and what is the power of your design to find a clinically significant effect. What evaluation instruments will you use, and for how long will you follow up your results?

What resources will you need in terms of staff, equipment, travel, etc.? What support will you need from senior administrators (e.g., politicians, government department heads), local administrators (e.g., school principals), and local staff (e.g., teachers, physicians, hospital staff) to recruit subjects and pursue the programme? Work out how you will advertise the programme to those who need to know, including the parents of the children to whom the programme is to be offered. Attract as many allies as possible. Journalists can be very helpful. Never refuse an opportunity to speak about your programme on radio, television, or in the press. Design a programme web site to publicize the programme and disseminate information about the problem it addresses.

Estimate the costs and seek funding for your project. Your programme will need to be piloted, if possible, to eliminate mistakes and refine the intervention. If possible, try to recruit clinician-implementers from existing staff. Thus, it will be a community-based rather than a laboratory study that you will implement, and the results will have more ecological validity. If you seek support from a research-funding agency, the design of your programme should include a well-chosen control group, random assignment if feasible, comprehensive outcome measures, a power analysis, and pilot data.

If you are to recruit subjects from schools or mental health agencies, for example, you will need top-level and local authority and support to do so. However, referral sources often forget about intervention projects, particularly if their staff changes. They will need to be reminded through regular visits, written information, and scientific presentations.

All long-term projects are affected by attrition due to change of residence, parental, or child resistance to the programme or premature self-termination. If possible, it is desirable to include self-terminators in the outcome evaluation. Even an abbreviated evaluation can be helpful.

At the outset, as the project proceeds, and when it has been evaluated, disseminate knowledge about the problem in general, the nature of your project, and the results of intervention. Your target audiences are the administrators from whom you seek authority and funding, the local managers from whom you seek collaboration, your referral sources, the subject families, and the general public.

COST-EFFECTIVENESS AND COST-BENEFIT ANALYSES

The aim of prevention is to intervene early in order to avert later more serious problems. School dropout, adolescent pregnancy, juvenile delinquency, drug abuse, suicide in adolescence or young adulthood, and post-traumatic adjustment problems, for example, are serious social problems. Not only do they limit personal productivity, but also they are arduous (if not impossible) to reverse or control. Antisocial behavior, for example, requires expensive (and largely ineffective) control and management by the police, probation, and correctional systems. It is reasonable, therefore, to ask whether the cost of prevention and its likelihood of success outweigh the cost of the undesirable outcome.

Durlak (1997) points out that there is no standard procedure for cost analysis: no agreement about what is a cost, or what is a benefit, or how to compare them. Furthermore, costs vary with the setting of implementation.

Yates (1998) has described the mathematical principles of *cost-effectiveness analysis* (CEA) and *cost-benefit analysis* (CBA). CEA compares costs to outcomes as they are measured in human services and social sciences. CBA compares costs to programme outcomes that are measured in the same units as costs (e.g., dollars). *Cost-offsets* are funds that other agencies or individuals do not have to spend because of what an intervention accomplished. For example, for each child diverted from antisocial behavior as an adult, there are cost-offsets for the public and for the police and correctional systems. *Benefits* are the resources generated by the programme (e.g., the income earned by individuals who might otherwise have been incarcerated).

CEA and CBA compare costs and outcomes separately, or combine them in the form of a single index such as a ratio. Ratios of benefits divided by costs are easy to present and comprehend. If benefits exceed costs, a programme is potentially supportable. Lipsey (1984) surveyed delinquency prevention programmes and found benefit-cost ratios varying from 0.17 to 8.79. Many analyses, however, fail to include personal benefits accruing from successful intervention such as improved quality of life. It is difficult to attach a dollar value to such an outcome. The quality of life index (Miller and Galbraith, 1995) was designed to do so.

In CEA a detailed list is provided of all costs and benefits, some expressed in monetary terms (e.g., wages), and others in descriptive form (e.g., the hours required to complete an intervention programme or greater vocational attainment). External benefits (e.g., reduction of insurance premiums, fewer motor vehicle accidents) should also be considered.

Durlak (1997) points out a danger: Politicians and administrators may be so transfixed by the cost of an intervention that they ask for it to be curtailed in intensity, duration, or quality. It is often a mistake to do so. It could be argued that token programmes do little good and can ultimately do harm if it is found that time and money have been ineffectually expended.

THE ETHICS OF INTERVENTION

It is important not to claim more benefit from a proposed prevention programme than it can deliver. Unfulfilled promises lead to the disillusionment of referring agents, clinicians, and funding agencies. Similarly, intervention programmes that have no empirical basis (e.g., those that rely upon education alone) should not be supported. Researchers and administrators have the responsibility to ensure that the scarce amount of money available for prevention (said to be no more than 3% of the U. S. health budget) is well spent.

THE FUTURE

To date, no preventive programmes have tackled the major DSM-IV categories of schizophrenia, bipolar disorder, manic depressive disorder, or obsessive compulsive disorder. The prevention of these conditions will depend on greater knowledge of their genetics and the gene-environment interactions that predict them. Most preventive programmes today target risky behavior (e.g., smoking, drinking, drug use, unprotected sexual activity, school dropout, suicidal behavior), parenting problems (e.g., coercive parenting, parents at risk of physically abusing their children, maternal depression), problems associated with chronic physical illnesses (e.g., asthma and diabetes), the prevention of cognitive delay in premature infants or socially disadvantaged preschool children, and the prevention of psychopathology following psychological trauma.

Recent meta-analyses or reviews of the literature (e.g., Durlak and Wells, 1997; Reppucci *et al.*, 1999; Carr, 2002) make it clear that a number of primary and secondary prevention programmes are both clinically beneficial and cost-effective. The programmes that work have definable characteristics (e.g., an empirically based theoretical model; clear goals and objectives; standardized interventions; good staff training, supervision, and support; outcome measurement). Universal programmes are generally of insufficient intensity and duration to reach those most in need.

In the future, the emphasis will pass to targeted programmes that operate on multiple levels (child, family, school, and community), with sensitivity to the sociocultural group or groups involved. Funding bodies will increasingly demand that proposed prevention programmes be empirically based, and that operating programmes be accountable for their results.

The dissemination and adoption of effective programmes is a serious problem. Rotheram-Borus and Duan (2003) recommend that private enterprise models of marketing and dissemination be adopted by prevention experts, and that experts collaborate with marketing organizations in disseminating their programmes. Dissemination requires programmes to be presented in such a way as to be understandable and acceptable to clinicians, the public, policy makers, and funding bodies.

REFERENCES

Achenbach, T. M. (1991) Manual for the Child Behaviour Checklist/4-18 and 1991 Profile, University of Vermont, Burlington VT.

Achenback, T. M., and Edelbrock, C. (1983). *Manual for the Child Behaviour Checklist and Revised Child Behaviour Profile.* Burlington VT: University of Vermont. Department of Psychiatry.

Battin-Pearson, S., Newcomb, M. D. Abbott, R. D. *et al.* (2000) Predictors of early high school dropout: A test of five theories. *J Educ Psychol*, **92**, 568–82.

Brener, N. D., Collins, J. L., Kann, L. *et al.* (1995) Reliability of the youth risk behaviour survey questionnaire. *Am J Epidemiol*, **141**, 575–80.

Carr, A. (2002) *Prevention: What works with children and adolescents?* Brunner-Routledge, Hove, UK.

Curiel, H., Rosenthal, J. A., and Richek, H. G. (1986) Impacts of bilingual education on secondary school grades, attendance, retentions and dropouts. *Hisp J Behav Sci*, **8**, 357–67.

Durlak, J. A. and Wells, A. M. (1997) Primary prevention mental health programs for children and adolescents: A meta-analytic review. *Am J Commun Psychology*, **25**, 115–43.

Durlak, J. A. (1997) *Successful Prevention Programs for Children and Adolescents*, Plenum, New York.

Gomez-Schwartz, B., Horowitz, J. M., Cardarelli, A. P.and Souzier, M. (1990) The aftermath of child sexual abuse: 18 months later, in *Child Sexual Abuse, The Initial Effects* (eds B. Gomez-Schwartz, J. M. Horowitz and A. P. Cardarelli), Sage, Newbury Park CA.

Institute of Medicine (1994) *Reducing Risks for Mental Disorders: Frontiers for Preventive Intervention Research*, National Academy Press, Washington DC.

Landgraf, J. M., Koetz, L. and Ware, J. E. (1996) *The CHQ User's Manual*, 1st Edition, The Health Institute, New England Medical Center, Boston MA.

Lipsey, M. W. (1984) Is delinquency prevention a cost-effective strategy? A California perspective. *J Res Crime Delinquency*, **21**, 279–302.

Meyer, L. A. (1984). Long-term academic effects of Indirect Instruction Project Follow-Through. *Elem School J*, **84**, 380–94.

Miller, T. R. and Galbraith, M. (1995) Injury prevention counselling by pediatricians: A benefit-cost comparison. *Pediatrics*, **96**, 1–4.
Nation, M., Crusto, C., Wandersman, A. *et al.* (2003) What works in prevention: Principles of effective prevention programs. *Am Psychol*, **58**, 449–56.
Nurcombe, B., Bickman, L., de Andrade, A. *et al.* (2007) Attrition from a community-based treatment program for sexually abused children and adolescents. *J Am Acad Child Adolesc Psychiatry*, submitted for publication.
Olds, D. L., Henderson, C. R., Chamberlin, R., and Tatelbaum, R. (1986) Preventing child abuse and neglect: A randomised trial of nurse-home visitation. *Paediatrics*, **78**, 65–78.
Pearson, L. C. and Banerji, M. (1993) Effects of a ninth-grade dropout prevention program on student academic achievement, school attendance, and dropout rates. *J Exp Educ*, **61**, 247–56.
Prevatt, F. and Kelly, F. D. (2003) Dropping out of school: A review of intervention programs. *J School Psychology*, **41**, 377–95.
Radloff, L. S. (1977) The CES-D scale: A self-report depression scale for research in The general population. *Applied Psychological Measurement*, **1**, 385–401.
Remschmidt, H., Schmidt, M. H., and Walther, R. (1998) Survey of the utilization of psychiatric services for children and adolescents in Germany in *Designing Mental Health Services for Children and Adolescents: A Shrewd Investment* (eds J. G. Young and P. Ferrari), Brunner/Mazel, Philadelphia PA.
Reppucci, M. D., Woolard, J. L., and Fried, C. S. (1999) Social, community and preventive interventions. *Ann Rev Psychol*, Annual, 38–58.
Roberts, R. E., Attkisson, C. C., and Rosenblatt, A. (1998) Prevalence of psychopathology among children and adolescents. *Am J Psychiatry*, **155**, 715–25.
Rotheram-Borus, M. J., and Duan, N. (2003) Next generation of preventive interventions. *J Am Acad Child Adolesc Psychiatry*, **42**, 518–26.
Sawyer, M. G., Kosky, R. J., Graetz, B. W. *et al.* (2000) The national survey of mental health and wellbeing: The child and adolescent component. *Aust NZJ Psychiatry*, **34**, 214–20.
Shaffer, D., Fisher, P., Lucas, C. *et al.* (2000) NIMH Diagnostic interview schedule for children, Version IV (NIMH DISC-IV): Description, differences from previous versions, and reliability of some common diagnoses. *J Am Acad Child Adolesc Psychiatry*, **39**, 28–38.
Sinclair, M. F., Christenson, S. L., Evelo, D. L. and Hurley, C. M. (1998) Dropout prevention for youth with disabilities: Efficacy of a sustained school engagement procedure. *Exceptional Children*, **65**, 7–22.
Spaccarelli, S. (1994) Stress, appraisal, and coping in child sexual abuse: A theoretical and empirical review. *Psychol Bull*, **116**, 340–62.
Temple, J. A., Reynolds, A. J. and Miedel, W. T. (2000) Can early intervention prevent high school dropout? Evidence from the Chicago Child-Parent Centres. *Urban Education*, **35**, 31–56.
Weisz, J. R., Weiss, B., Ham, S. S. *et al.* (1995) Effects of psychotherapy with children and adolescents revisited: A meta-analysis of treatment outcome studies, *Psychol Bull*, **117**, 450–68.
Yates, B.T. (1998) Formative evaluation of costs, cost-effectiveness and cost benefit: Cost procedure, process, outcome analysis in *Handbook of Applied Social Research Methods* (eds L. Bickman and D. J. Rog), Sage, Thousand Oaks, CA.

CHAPTER 5.2

Evidence-Based Primary Prevention Programmes for the Promotion of Mental Health in Children and Adolescents: A Systematic Worldwide Review

Martine F. Flament, Hien Nguyen and Claudia Furino
The University of Ottawa Institute of Mental Health Research, Canada
Howard Schachter
The University of Ottawa Evidence-Based Practice Centre, Canada
Cathy MacLean
The Royal Ottawa Mental Health Center, Canada
Danuta Wasserman, Norman Sartorius, and Helmut Remschmidt
The WPA Presidential Programme on Child Mental Health

INTRODUCTION

In both industrialized and developing countries, it has been estimated that one in four people will be affected by a mental or behavioral disorder at some stage in life; presently, around 450 million people worldwide suffer from mental disorders, causing mental disorders to be one of the leading causes of disability (WHO, 2001b). Many mental disorders of adulthood begin during childhood or adolescence. For example, depressive disorders, the fourth most prevalent disease in the world, often has its onset in the school-age years (WHO, 2001b). Community-based studies have estimated the overall prevalence of child and adolescent mental disorders to be around 20% (Verhulst, 1995; Bird, 1996; WHO, 2005). Among children visiting

The Mental Health of Children and Adolescents: an area of global neglect. Edited by H. Remschmidt *et al.*

primary care facilities in various countries, 12–29% suffer from a psychiatric disorder; of those, only 10–22% are identified by primary health workers, suggesting that the majority of children in need do not receive proper diagnosis and care (Giel *et al.*, 1981).

In many countries, mental health services for youth represent a subset of adult mental health services or child health services, rather than a distinct category requiring unique and specified policies and funding (WHO, 2005). Furthermore, treatment seeking among this population is a limiting factor for appropriate care, as children and adolescents are less capable than adults of advocating for themselves, and seldom decide alone to seek health services. Their readiness to report mental and emotional problems to parents or teachers may be stifled by the stigma and discrimination linked to mental illness, ever present though varying across countries and cultures. Of note, the stages of emotional, cognitive, and social development are defined and perceived diversely around the world. For example, the concept of adolescence is not universally adopted; in many countries, the end of childhood is followed immediately by adulthood (WHO, 2005).

Currently, no country in the world has a clearly defined mental health policy for children and adolescents (Shatkin and Belfer, 2004), and only 34 countries (7% of countries worldwide) have identifiable mental health policies (WHO, 2005). The paucity of recognizable policies directed at mental health among youth results in significant costs to the families of these children, and to society at large. For example, it has been shown that children, with depression and conduct disorders generate high costs during childhood and adulthood (Knapp *et al.*, 2002). Moreover, the costs of antisocial behavior among adults are ten times greater for those who were seriously antisocial in childhood than for those who were not (Scott *et al.*, 2001). Although these findings suggest that interventions in childhood or adolescence will lead to cost savings in adulthood, their cost-effectiveness has yet to be supported by documented research.

OBJECTIVE

Our objective was to conduct a systematic qualitative review concerning evidence-based prevention programmes that foster mental health or aim to prevent the occurrence of mental disorders in infants, children, and adolescents.

An initial search of the literature found several reviews relating to primary prevention programmes in children and youth (Barlow and Coren, 2000; Barlow and Coren, 2001; Beardslee and Gladstone, 2001; Miller *et al.*, 2002; Pratt and Woolfenden, 2002; McBride, 2003; Skara and Sussman, 2003; Barlow and Coren, 2004). Although some were conducted systematically (Barlow and Coren, 2000; Barlow and Coren, 2001; Pratt and Woolfenden, 2002; McBride, 2003; Barlow and Coren, 2004), these reviews considered programmes dealing with only specific disorders, such as depression (Beardslee and Gladstone, 2001), eating disorders (Pratt and Woolfenden, 2002), or substance abuse (Skara and Sussman, 2003). The current review uses a systematic method to identify and qualitatively describe both general and disorder-focused primary prevention programmes available for infants, children, and adolescents. To our knowledge, this task had not yet been undertaken.

METHOD

Defining the search area

The terms of the search were defined as follows:

Prevention: The term can be categorized threefold into *primary prevention*, which is meant to intercept the onset of an illness; *secondary prevention*, intended to decrease the duration of or minimize the symptoms or effects of an illness that is already underway; and *tertiary prevention*, which seeks to rehabilitate or restore previous adaptability in people seriously affected by an illness (Institute of Medicine, 1994; Kolvin, 1994; El-Hazmi, 1997; WHO, 2002; WHO, 2003; WHO, 2004a; WHO, 2004b). For the purpose of our project, only *primary prevention* will be considered.

Intervention: Often used in the literature interchangeably with treatment, the term *intervention* is interpreted in this study as having a preventive aim.

Programme: In order to take into consideration the variability in health care resources, diagnostic procedures, and treatment practices across cultures and around the world, this term is interpreted in its most fundamental sense: any organized intervention approach that could be implemented effectively in industrialized as well as developing countries.

Mental disease: This term is understood as all mental disorders identified and defined by the two widely accepted current diagnostic classifications: *International Classification of Diseases*, 10th edition (ICD-10; WHO, 1992) and *Diagnostic and Statistical Manual for Mental Disorders*, 4th edition (DSM-IV; APA, 1994).

Mental health: The simplest interpretation of this term, the absence of mental disease, is employed but is elaborated to be more consistent with the view that health is a state comprised of positive qualities and not merely the lack of infirmity (WHO, 2001a). Mental health is additionally defined by subjective quality of life and adaptation to the environment. Our analysis includes not only programmes that focus on clinically significant mental disorders, but also those that address preclinical factors that could jeopardize mental health, such as substance use, school dropout, conduct problems, and programmes that aim to foster mental health in general.

Infants, children, and adolescents: All preventive programmes, primarily targeting infants, children up to the age of 12 years, and adolescents up to the age of 19 years inclusively, are included in this analysis. Programmes that have been applied to both children/adolescent and adult populations are also included.

Evidence: Due to the general paucity of sound empirical work in the area, we accepted for the current review both structured and unstructured evaluations of programme efficacy. Both community and laboratory assessments are included, but they are differentiated from each other. Community-based evaluations are regarded as superior to those conducted solely in laboratory settings, as the latter may not be ecologically valid. Subjective reports of the use and perceived effects of a programme were considered sufficient for analysis, but regarded as at the lowest level of evidence.

Search strategies

Several complementary strategies were employed to search for relevant programmes.

We searched the computerized scientific literature databases (up to June 17, 2004) most relevant to psychiatry, psychology, and community research: Medline (1966–June Week 2, 2004); PsycInfo (1872–May Week 3, 2004); ERIC (1966–May, 2004); and SocioFile (1974–May, 2004). The search strategy was developed in accordance with the definitions given above for the terms of the search, with selected keywords to cover all the mental disorders of infancy, childhood, or adolescence (the full list of keywords may be obtained from the corresponding author). For practical reasons, only material for which at least some documents were accessible in the English or French language were included in our review.

We also contacted directly persons or groups known to us as having developed prevention programmes within specific organizations or communities (e.g., the YouthNet Programme and Better Beginnings, Better Futures, in Ontario, Canada).

Due to the relevance of interventions to a variety of domains, we broadened the search to additional resources, such as the United Nations Children's Fund (UNICEF), World Psychiatric Association (WPA), United States Substance Abuse and Mental Health Services Administration (SAMHSA), and World Health Organization (WHO) web sites, where we conducted searches using the aforementioned keywords.

In order to access a wider range of intervention programmes as well as international resources, we also conducted general Internet searches with the same keywords, using SCIRUS and Google as search engines. The names of specific programmes derived from the Internet search were subsequently used as key words for additional searches in the scientific literature databases. This strategy was used to address the inconstant reliability of Internet sources. Conversely, programmes identified through the scientific literature were used as key words for Internet searches, using SCIRUS and Google as search engines.

Because multiple databases were searched, it was likely that a record would be indexed by more than one database and, consequently, would appear more than once in our search results. To identify and remove duplicate records, all records were downloaded into a citation management programme (Reference Manager®).

Selection of programmes for analysis: Inclusion/exclusion criteria

Level 1 assessment: Selecting relevant abstracts

Each record generated from the search was judged for inclusion at the first level by two independent reviewers (HN and CF). Records included an abstract and key words, in addition to a citation. Material generated from the Internet searches was entered into this level of assessment as records, the URL address serving as its citation, and the full document serving as the abstract. At this level, criteria for inclusion were as follows: records describing programmes which aimed to promote mental health or prevent mental disorder(s), or to identify, or prevent, or treat risk factors; and those describing programmes applied to infant, child, and/or adolescent populations. The abstract was excluded if it described a narrative review, letter, editorial, commentary, systematic review, or an opinion piece that did not also include original data. At level 1, a record would not be retained for further analysis if there was consensus between the reviewers that it either failed to meet one or more inclusion criteria, or met the exclusion criterion.

Level 2 assessment: Selecting relevant articles
Records that passed Level 1 assessment were then reviewed in accordance with the full articles, by the two independent reviewers (HN and CF). Level 2 assessment used the same inclusion and exclusion criteria as Level 1, with the addition of a further inclusion criterion: that the report evaluated the effectiveness of the programme. In all articles for which consensus could not be achieved between the reviewers from the Level 2 assessment forms, the reviewers discussed the pros and cons, in the presence of a third party (MFF), until agreement was reached.

Level 3 assessment: Grouping articles by programme
Articles that survived the first two levels of assessment underwent a third assessment by a committee of three reviewers, in which individual reports were grouped by programme. If a programme described in one article was also described in a second article with any modification, the two articles were regarded as representing two distinct programmes and were analyzed as such. From this point onward, articles were no longer analyzed as individual articles, but as sets of articles that described programmes.

Liaising with programme developers
The lead developers for each programme were contacted by electronic mail, when possible, and by regular mail otherwise, to ask them to provide additional information for review. Of the 47 authors approached, 8 could no longer be reached at the contact information given on the report, and 12 did not respond. Of the 27 authors contacted who responded to our request, 9 could not offer any additional information, and 18 forwarded supplementary material. Additional information regarding the programme forwarded by programme developers was entered into the review at Level 1 assessment and proceeded through each level, as with reports generated from the literature search.

Level 4 assessment: Data abstraction
Each programme was first summarized by one of the two independent primary reviewers (HN or CF), using a data abstraction form designed by the authors to ensure thoroughness and provide an easily readable outline (form available on request). For each prevention programme, descriptive information was derived solely from the text of the articles retained. The initial summary and original programme information were then reviewed by a second person (MFF).

RESULTS

General principles

From our search and by referral, we were able to identify several key reviews of primary prevention principles and concepts (WHO, 2002). A common and recurring theme was the dimorphism inherent to preventive research. Programmes can seek to *prevent mental disorders* or to *promote mental health* (WHO, 2002; WHO, 2004a; WHO, 2004b). Although these goals can seem to be opposing, it is important for programme developers to understand that prevention and promotion are overlapping and complementary (WHO, 2002). Prevention programmes can be classified in three dimensions, the first being the level of intervention, the second the way in which the population is selected for intervention, and the third the overall goal with respect to harm minimization.

In terms of level of intervention, a prevention programme can be delivered at the *individual level* by offering services directly to the target population without seeking to alter the environment, or at the *ecological level*, attempting to change individuals indirectly by modifying the environment (Durlak and Wells, 1997).

To classify target populations, we followed the selection taxonomy proposed by the Institute of Medicine (IOM, Institute of Medicine, 1994), which is based on Gordon's (1987) operational classification of disease prevention. The IOM model divides preventive care into three strategies: *universal*, *selective*, and *indicated*. *Universal strategies* address entire populations with the aim of preventing or delaying the onset of disease, and are delivered to large groups without prior screening. Universal programmes assume that all members of a population share the same general risk and are equally capable of benefiting from the information and skills provided by prevention, even though the likelihood of occurrence of the actual disorder may vary greatly among individuals. *Selective strategies* target subsets of the total population deemed to be at risk for a disease by virtue of their membership to a particular subgroup in the population. Risk groups may be identified on the basis of biological, psychological, social, or environmental risk factors. Selective prevention targets an entire subgroup regardless of the degree of risk of any individual within the group, because the subgroup as a whole is considered to be at high risk. As such, an individual's personal risk is not specifically assessed or identified. *Indicated strategies* are designed to prevent the onset of disease in individuals who do not meet clinical criteria for a disorder, but who are showing early signs or symptoms at a subclinical level. Indicated programmes address risk factors associated with the individual and place less emphasis on assessing or addressing environmental influences.

As defined earlier, prevention strategies can be distinguished as *primary*, *secondary*, or *tertiary*, depending on the overall goal they seek to achieve regarding a specific mental disorder. Only *primary prevention*, which seeks to prevent the disorder, is considered in the present review.

Over the past decade, research in the field has indicated an increase in both the number of programmes, and the efforts for rigorous standardized process-outcome evaluation (Kolvin, 1994; Reppucci, Woolard, and Fried, 1999; Carr, 2002; WHO, 2004a). Experts in prevention research agree that, though *randomized controlled trials* (RCT) are difficult to implement in the context of prevention programmes, because many curricula are delivered by class, school, or even by community (WHO, 2004a), RCTs remain the empirical "gold standard" (Kolvin, 1994; Reppucci, Woolard, and Fried, 1999; Carr, 2002; WHO, 2004a). However, for the reasons mentioned in the definition of the search area, both structured and unstructured evaluations of programme efficacy were retained for our review, including *quasi-experimental designs* (intervention group versus control group without random allocation of subjects to one or the other), *within-subject pre- post-intervention comparisons*, *informal surveys*, and, at the lower level of evidence, *anecdotal clinical reports*.

Our analysis of the objectives and contents of programmes' evaluation studies used the categorization system implemented by Breton *et al.* (2002) in a review of Canadian suicide programmes, and based on the framework proposed earlier by Champagne *et al.* (1986). Evaluation can be classified under two broad categories: *normative evaluation* and *evaluative research*. *Normative evaluation* refers to administrative programme monitoring, and focuses on applying norms and criteria to a programme's structure, processes, and results. *Evaluative research* is based on a scientific approach and includes six types of analysis: *strategic analysis*, which examines the appropriateness of addressing a specific health problem, and the pertinence of the chosen method of intervention; *programme analysis*, which addresses programme theory, or the chain of causal assumptions linking programme elements to desired outcomes, and the capacity of the programme elements to achieve these outcomes; *productivity analysis*, which determines whether the resources available are sufficient to produce a required outcome; *programme effects analysis*, which addresses a particular health problem; *efficiency analysis*, which examines the relationship between the financial resources used and the effects obtained; and *implementation analysis*, which explores how variations in the level of implementation and the environmental context affect the impact of the programme.

Evidence-based primary prevention programmes

Results from the search strategy

The search strategy generated 1131 records. The progress of these records through the various phases of the review is illustrated in Figure 5.2.1. Of the 1131 records entered into the initial assessment, 960 were excluded because they did not describe a programme that promotes mental health/prevents mental disorders/targets a risk factor for a mental disorder; or did not describe a programme that has been applied to infant/child/adolescent populations; or because they were narrative reviews, systematic reviews, letters, opinion pieces, editorials, or commentaries which did not also include original data. Of the 171 records deemed relevant, 5 were excluded because the corresponding full report could not be accessed in either French or English (Sorensen, 1989; Struzzo, 1999; Buddeberg-Fischer *et al.*, 2000; Nyden *et al.*, 2000; Kraus *et al.*, 2003). The full contents of the remaining 166 records were retrieved and entered into the second level of assessment. The second relevance assessment screening excluded 96 reports, based on the criteria described above. The 70 reports retained were grouped according to the programme they described. In the end, 47 unique primary prevention programmes were identified and reviewed.

Disorders targeted

The programmes retrieved targeted a variety of specific disorders. Most were aimed at preventing substance abuse (n = 18) and depression or anxiety (n = 11). The remaining programmes sought to prevent eating disorders (n = 6), behavioral or conduct disorders (n = 3), post-traumatic stress disorder (n = 3), and suicide (n = 3). The three programmes that did not indicate a specific disorder or targeted several unrelated disorders were classified as promoting mental health in general.

For each programme, a number of key features were identified and reviewed using our data abstraction form. These features are summarized in Tables 5.2.1–5.2.13, in which

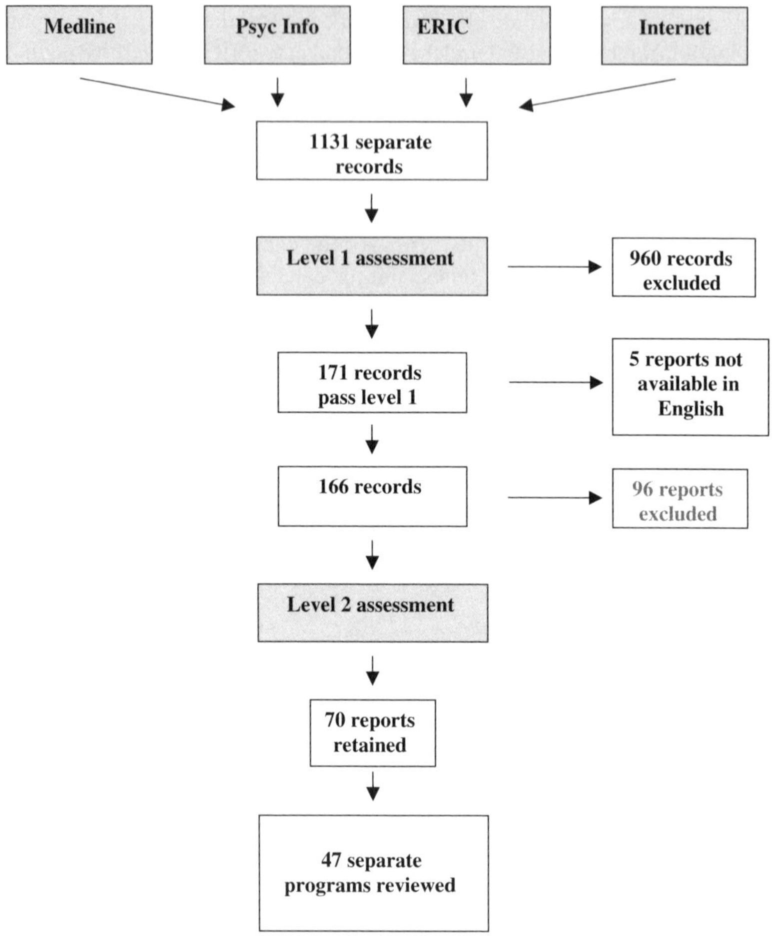

Figure 5.2.1 The results of the literature search

programmes are grouped according to the disorders targeted. The full data abstraction record for any programme can be obtained by request to the corresponding author.

Countries where the programmes were implemented

Fourteen countries in all were associated with the 47 separate programmes. The United States generated the most programmes ($n = 33$), followed by Canada ($n = 7$), Australia ($n = 7$), the Netherlands ($n = 3$), the United Kingdom ($n = 3$), Norway ($n = 3$), Germany ($n = 2$), Belgium ($n = 1$), Italy ($n = 1$), and China ($n = 1$). Four programmes (*PATHS*, *FRIENDS*, *Penn Prevention Programme*, and *Go Girls*) have been implemented in more than one country. The *PATHS* programme (Greenberg *et al.*, 1995; Kam *et al.*, 2003) has been implemented in eight different countries: the United States, Belgium, United Kingdom, Norway, Canada, Australia, and Israel. The *FRIENDS* programme

Table 5.2.1 Programmes targeting substance abuse – programme outline

Name, Institute, Country[a], Reference	Target population, Age, Sex	Theoretical orientation →Objectives	Description	Setting, Manual, Providers (Training)
Safe Haven City of Detroit Department of Health, Bureau of Substance Abuse *USA* (Aktan *et al.*, 1996)	Selective (African–American children who have a substance using parent) 6–12 years old with their parent Males and females	– Parental alcoholism and use of illicit drugs increase risk of alcoholism, drug use initiation, drug use/misuse in children via both biological and environmental risk factors – Family skills training has been reported to reduce risk factors and substance use in children of substance users →To reduce risk factors for substance use in families where one parent is a known substance user, by increasing parenting efficacy, parent-child bonding, child-school bonding, family cohesion, positive family communication, family expressiveness and organization	– 12 weekly sessions *Programme elements* • parents' training: teach more appropriate methods to cope with children's behaviors and increase number of positive interactions • children's skills training: teach prosocial skills such as coping with loneliness, making choices, controlling anger, recognizing feelings, coping with peer pressure • family skills training: teach parents to set limits appropriately and reward good behavior	Community English manual (Aktan *et al.*, 1994) African–American substance use counselors (3-day training in programme philosophy and curriculum)
Coalition for Youth Quality of Life (CYQL) Project University of Montreal *Canada* (Dedobbeleer and Desjardins, 2001)	Universal 9–25 years old Males and females	– Alcohol and drug use are result of interaction between predisposing personal and social factors – Ecological and participatory approach →To prevent alcohol and other drug abuse among youth through coalition built with 15 partners, including public health organizations, community organizations, schools, police, parents, youth representatives	– 3-year intervention programme *Programme elements* • youth educational programme • parent educational programme • alternatives to drugs and alcohol use programme • youth mobilization, support systems for youth in trouble • skills development programme • competence enhancement programme	School, community No manual Task force members (training in programme development, youth needs, substance abuse, and possible strategies of intervention)

(*continued*)

Table 5.2.1 *(Continued)*

Name, Institute, Country[a], Reference	Target population, Age, Sex	Theoretical orientation →Objectives	Description	Setting, Manual, Providers (Training)
Effective Classroom Management (ECM) Training Pacific Institute for Research and Evaluation, Lafayette, CA *USA* (Moskowitz *et al.*, 1983; Malvin *et al.*, 1984)	Universal 11–15 years old Males and females	– Affective education and humanistic psychology – Previous research has found association between self-attitudes, social competency, attitudes toward institutions, and adolescent drug abuse – Teachers should become more sensitive to emotional needs of students →To prevent adolescent substance abuse by exposition to teachers trained in ECM	– Teacher training: 12 two-hour training sessions – No programme implemented directly with students *Programme elements* • teaching techniques in communication, problem-solving, classroom discipline, self-esteem enhancement • trainer observing teacher in classroom and providing feedback	School No manual Teachers and specialists in health education
Healthy School and Drugs Netherlands Institute of Mental Health and Addiction *The Netherlands* (Cuijpers *et al.*, 2002)	Universal 12–18 years old Males and females	– Bandura (1996) social cognition theory and McGuire (1985) model of behavioral change, adapted (De Vries, Weijts, and Kok, 1992) – Intention and behavior depend on three determinants: attitude, social influence, self-efficacy →To prevent substance abuse via a multicomponent programme	– 3-year programme consisting of five components *Programme elements* • Committee to plan activities • educational lessons about tobacco, alcohol, marijuana, ecstacy, gambling • formulation of school drug regulations • development of system for early detection of students with drug problems • parental involvement in drug prevention at school	School Manual available (no language or reference specified) Teachers

"Here's Looking At You, Two" (HLAYT) Villanova University *USA* (Green and Kelley, 1989)	Universal 5–19 years old Males and females	– Incidence of alcohol and drug abuse problems among young people can be reduced if they achieve one or more of the following: (1) higher levels of self-esteem; (2) improved coping skills; (3) effective interpersonal decision-making; (4) more facts and substantive knowledge about drugs and chemical dependence →To increase drug and alcohol knowledge and to decrease adolescent drug and alcohol use through one or more pathways	– Comprehensive school curriculum for grades K through 12 which can be taught as a unit *Programme elements* • programme to educate parents and assist them in dealing with family substance abuse problems • student assistance programme that identifies and refers at-risk students • absenteeism prevention programme to identify students who are chronically absent and work with them and their families • student leadership programme	School No manual Teachers (30-h training)
"I'm Special" (ISP) The Drug Education Center, Inc., University of North Carolina *USA* (Kim, McLeod, and Shantzis, 1990)	Universal 7–10 years old Males and females	– Personal growth theories (Briggs, 1970; Maslow, 1970; Satir, 1972; Kaplan, 1980); social control theory (Briar and Piliavin, 1965; Kornhouser, 1978); and social learning theory (Bandura, 1977) →To develop child's sense of uniqueness and self-worth, healthy social skills, and effective group cooperation	– 9 weekly 45–50 min in-class sessions *Programme elements* • each session begins with goal statement written in understandable language • teacher designs session appropriate to needs of class • each session concludes with processing questions that help review lesson	School English manual (Lesesne, 1986) Teachers, school health personnel (20-h training)
Keep A Clear Mind (KACM) University of North Florida *USA* (Werch, 1991)	Universal 8–12 years old Males and females	– Social skills training model – Four major factors influence children's substance use: (1) parental drug using; (2) parental attitudes, normative standards, and beliefs about drugs; (3) family management techniques; (4) parent–child communication	– 4 weekly in-class sessions *Programme elements* • each lesson provides brief introduction to weekly topic, followed by five activities to be completed at home with a parent	School, community No manual Teachers

(*continued*)

Table 5.2.1 *(Continued)*

Name, Institute, Country[a], Reference	Target population, Age, Sex	Theoretical orientation →Objectives	Description	Setting, Manual, Providers (Training)
		→To help children develop specific skills to refuse and avoid "gateway" drug use	• activities include answering simple questions about drugs; listing reasons not to use drugs; writing "no" statements to resist social pressure; selecting best way to refuse and avoid drugs; completing contracts to refuse/avoid drugs	
Peer-managed Self-control Programme for Prevention of Alcohol Abuse in American Indian High School Students Florida Mental Health Institute *USA* (Carpenter, Lyons, and Miller, 1985)	Indicated (American Indians nominated as at-risk by teachers) 14–20 years old Males and females	– Social learning paradigm – Peer group plays important role in development of abusive drinking – Excessive alcohol ingestion is socially acquired, overlearned; habitual pattern of behavior maintained by reinforcing contingencies →To prevent alcohol abuse in American Indian adolescent population by providing peer-mediated self-control training	– Ten 2-h sessions divided in two 50-min components with 20-min break *Programme elements* • first and last session are informal get-togethers to complete knowledge test and drinking profile • first 50-min component: lecture by alcohol educator (preferably American Indian) • second 50-min component: group discussion led by peer counselor or alcohol educator	School English manual (Lyons, Carpenter, and Strelich, 1981) Peer counselors, adult alcohol educator
Personal Growth Class (PGC) University of Washington *USA* (Eggert *et al.*, 1994)	Selective (at-risk or current school-dropouts, low GPA) 14–18 years old Males and females	– Social-network-support perspective, utilizing concepts and processes derived from integrated model of strain, social learning, and control theories – Behavior is a function of the individual within a network of social relationships	– 90 daily 55-min in-class sessions (one school semester) – Offered as structured elective class within regular school curriculum *Programme elements* • self-esteem enhancement unit • decision-making unit • personal control unit • interpersonel communication unit	School English manual (no reference)

		– Peer network structure, teacher-student relationships, and school context are associated with initiation and progression of drug involvement, truancy, school failure →To diminish risk factors associated with school strain and deviant peer bonding while enhancing protective factors by developing life skills and pro-social school bonding →To increase drug use control, school performance, and mood management	• classroom observer (school counselor and programme director) monitoring and reinforcing programme implementation	Teachers, school nurses (3-day training workshop on programme philosophy, design, and rationale for central goals)
Project ALERT The RAND Corporation *USA* (Ellickson and Bell, 1990; Bell, Ellickson, and Harrison, 1993)	Universal 11–14 years old Males and females	– Social influence model of prevention: initial substance use is a social phenomenon – Bandura (1977) self-efficacy theory – Health belief model to build resistance and motivation by education regarding negative impact of drugs on health →To curb adolescent drug use by motivating young people to resist drugs and helping them acquire the skills to do so	– Seventh grade curriculum (eight bi-weekly in-class lessons) and eighth grade booster lessons (three lessons) *Programme elements* • lessons on current effects of drugs, how to identify pro-drug pressures and acquire a repertoire of strategies for resisting those pressures • role-playing, psychodrama, written responses to practice how to say "no" • small group discussions • question–answer exercises	School No manual Teachers

(*continued*)

Table 5.2.1 *(Continued)*

Name, Institute, Country[a], Reference	Target population, Age, Sex	Theoretical orientation →Objectives	Description	Setting, Manual, Providers (Training)
Project Northland University of Minnesota *USA* (Komro *et al.*, 1994; Komro *et al.*, 1996; Perry *et al.*, 1996; Komro *et al.*, 2001; Perry *et al.*, 200); Perry *et al.*, 1993)	Universal 10–19 years old Males and females	– Social-influence model defining alcohol use by adolescents as socially learned, and functional behavior – Alcohol use is a social behavior embedded in larger framework of community norms and social support systems that regulate occurrence of these behaviors →To prevent or delay onset of alcohol use among young adolescents, as well as reduce use among those who are already drinkers	– Seven year, school-wide programme *Programme elements* • parent involvement • education programmes • behavioral curricula • peer participation • community task force activities	School, community No manual Peer leaders, teachers (trained to plan, organize and promote alcohol-free activities)
Start Taking Alcohol Risks Seriously (STARS) University of North Florida *USA* (Werch, 1996)	Selective (inner-city youth) 11–14 years old Males and females	– Multicomponent Motivational Stages (McMOS) prevention model which posits continuum of stages in alcohol-use habits acquisition and change – Model founded on health belief model, social learning theory, and self-control theory →To prevent alcohol use among inner-city youth, using primary health care practitioners to offer brief consultation sessions	– Brief initial health consultation followed by six weekly individual follow-up consultations *Programme elements* • messages to heighten youths' awareness of prevention issues • youth asked to perform prevention behavior and skills, with feedback from healthcare provider	School No manual Nurses (provided with consultation protocols)
Self Management and Resistance Training (SMART)	Universal 11–13 years old Males and females	– Social influences approach to prevention – Many young people begin using drugs due to poor self-perception – Drug use provides escape from stress	– Consists of two programmes: SOCIAL and AFFECT (each with 12 weekly in-class sessions)	School No manual Providers not specified

University of Southern California *USA* (Hansen *et al.*, 1988; Graham *et al.*, 1990)		– Students committed to a set of values will not use drugs as long as their values are kept salient – Decision to use drugs often based on emotional reasons →To prevent the use of gateway drugs (tobacco, alcohol, marijuana) in adolescents	*Programme elements* • SOCIAL component: offering social skills to resist drug offers, teach students about various sources of social pressure to use drugs, with role-playing opportunities to practice these skills • AFFECT component: training in basic resistance skills, decision-making skills, values clarification, stress management	
Drug Abuse Resistance Education (DARE) University of Minnesota *USA* (Perry *et al.*, 2003; Lynam *et al.*, 1999)	Universal 11–13 years old Males and females	– Multicomponent approach to prevention →To equip elementary, middle and high school children with knowledge about drug abuse, consequences of abuse, and skills for resisting peer pressure to experiment with drugs, alcohol, and tobacco	– Ten weekly in-class sessions *Programme elements* • skills to resist influences to use drugs and handle violent situations • character building and citizenship skills • accurate information about drugs, alcohol, and tobacco • good decision-making skills • how to recognize and resist peer pressure. • ideas for positive alternatives to drug use	School No manual Police officers (trained in elementary school DARE curriculum, and having taught at least two semesters of middle and junior high school curriculum)
Highly role-specified (HRS) alcohol prevention programme University of Bergen *Norway* (Wilhelmsen, Laberg, and Klepp, 1994)	Universal 12–13 years old Males and females	– Social-cognitive theory – Changes in behavior follow from changes in cognitive structures such as self-efficacy and outcome expectations – Theory of reasoned action advocating that attitudes and norms influence intention to act	– Ten weekly in-class sessions over 2 month period *Programme elements* • student elected peer leaders • classroom teacher and peer leaders implement preplanned activities	School Manual (no language or reference specified) Teachers and peer leaders (trained to cooperate for programme implementation)

(*continued*)

Table 5.2.1 *(Continued)*

Name, Institute, Country[a], Reference	Target population, Age, Sex	Theoretical orientation →Objectives	Description	Setting, Manual, Providers(Training)
		→To create consciousness of existing social norms for alcohol use and to resist drinking	• four main topics: (1) alcohol use and local traditions; (2) norms for alcohol use; (3) managing drinking pressure; (4) attitudes toward alcohol use • role-playing to practice resisting pressure to drink	
Hope House Hope House Inc., Albany, NY *USA* (Krupka and Knox, 1985)	Universal 12–14 years old Males and females	– Brief exposure to natural field sites, such as prisons, have profound impact on "next generation down" adolescents →To correct knowledge, idealizing attitudes and nonchalance about substance use by exposing students to substance user therapeutic communities, and didactic presentations about substance abuse	– Educational sessions about substance abuse in health class – 90-min visit to residential treatment centre (Hope House) *Programme elements* • human relationships unit: substance abuse curriculum • field visit: tour and lunch with clients in treatment, where clients' experiences with substance abuse are discussed	School No manual Providers not specified
Tuning Into Health (TITH) Alcoholism Foundation of Manitoba *Canada* (Ambtman *et al.*, 1990)	Universal 6–15 years old Males and females	– Inadequate knowledge of consequences of drug abuse results in inappropriate attitudes and behavior – Drug abuse occurs as result of inappropriate values and inadequate decision-making skills – Substance abuse caused by deficient psychosocial skills	– Three components: early years (grades 2,3), middle years (grades 4,5,6), junior high (grades 7,8) *Programme elements* • early years: hazardous products and medicines • middle years: drugs and decisions, drugs and influence, smoking • junior high: alcohol, tobacco, prescription drugs, other drugs	School English manual (Strople and Koss, 1986; Sarachuk and Koss, 1986) Teachers

		→To reduce future incidence of problems associated with drugs by helping students to understand what drugs are, their effects on body, factors that influence people to use drugs, decision-making as way to deflect influences that promote drug use, and alternatives to drug use		
Stress Management and Alchohol Awareness Programme (SMAAP) George Mason University *USA* (Roosa, 1989; Short *et al.*, 1995)	Selective (children with alcoholic parent) 9–12 years old Males and females	– Stress process model stating that high levels of stress in environment contribute to risk of mental health problems – Other environmental factors or personality factors can either increase or decrease person's vulnerability to stress →To improve putative mediators of mental health problems in children of alcoholics.	– Eight weekly 1-h group (N = 8–10) sessions *Programme elements* • brief lectures, group discussions, role playing, home work assignments • teaching child effective ways of dealing with stress, self-esteem enhancement strategies, alcohol knowledge, emotion- and problem-focused coping, social support seeking strategies	School English manual (Ayers *et al.*, 1989) Teachers, social workers, graduate students (40-h training)

[a]The country in italic indicates where the programme was developed.

Table 5.2.2 Programmes targeting substance abuse – programme evaluation

Name, Institute, Country[a], Reference	Design →Objectives [type of evaluation] Methods, (*outcome measures*)	Significant results programme versus control	
		Positive results	Negative/unexpected results
Safe Haven City of Detroit Department of Health, Bureau of Substance Abuse *USA* (Aktan *et al.*, 1996)	Within-subject comparison: N = 88 parents and N = 88 "targeted" children Within-subject matched comparison: N = 56 (n = 27 "high" drug users, n = 29 "low" drug users, based on parent self-report of drug use frequency) →to evaluate effectiveness of programme for all participants →to compare degree of effectiveness for low and high drug using parents →to evaluate how well programme can be delivered [Analysis of programme effects, normative evaluation of process] Comparisons pre-, post-programme, 6- and 12-month follow-up (*FES; CBCL; authors' self report measure for parent functioning and programme satisfaction; attendance based on observation by trainers*)	• in children, reduction in prevalence of conduct disorders, delinquent behavior, social withdrawal, and externalizing problems • in parents, decrease in depression and improvement in perceived efficacy as parents • family cohesion improved • drop in illegal drug use for total sample and parents in high using group • staff successful in recruiting families and implementing programme • high-drug using parents reported increase in amount of time spent with children	• participant involvement did not predict outcome • no effect on family conflict, family relationship, family organization
Coalition for Youth Quality of Life (CYQL) Project University of Montreal *Canada* (Dedobbeleer and Desjardins, 2001)	Quasi-experimental: N = 791 (number per group not reported) Group assignment by school →To evaluate effectiveness of programme after two years of implementation [Analysis of programme effects] Comparisons pre-programme, 18-, and 30-month follow-up (*RSES; CI; PBI; authors' self-report measures for frequency of alcohol use and misuse; attitudes toward alcohol*)	• improvement in self-esteem and relationship with father in sixth graders at 18-month follow-up	• no significant effects on awareness of alcohol and drug problems, involvement in substance use prevention activities, relationship with mother, decision making skills, leisure activities • no significant impact on alcohol use

Effective Classroom Management (ECM) Training Pacific Institute for Research and Evaluation, Lafayette, CA *USA* (Moskowitz *et al.*, 1983; Malvin *et al.*, 1984)	Quasi-experimental: *N* = 273 (*n* = 190 to Programme, *n* = 83 to Control) Group assignment by school →To evaluate effect of teachers with ECM training on students' drug abuse [Analysis of programme effects] Comparisons pre-programme and 3-year follow-up (*SQ; DAS*)		• no evidence that greater exposure to ECM-trained teachers was associated with more favorable student outcomes • boys in experimental group held more pro-drug attitudes and were more involved in alcohol and cocaine use
Healthy School and Drugs Netherlands Institute of Mental Health and Addiction *The Netherlands* (Cuijpers *et al.*, 2002)	Quasi-experimental design: *N* = 1930 in 12 schools (*n* = 1156 – nine schools – to Programme, *n* = 774 – three schools – to Control) Group assignment by school →To examine effects of programme after 3 years [Analysis of programme effects] Comparisons pre-programme, 1-, 2- and 3-year follow-up (*authors' self-report measures of tobacco and alcohol use*)	• in both groups, proportion of students using tobacco, alcohol, and cannabis increased during study • after 3 years, significant effect of intervention on frequency of smoking and alcohol use, and number of drinks per week • proportion of students using marijuana lower in first 2 years (no longer significant at 3 years) • positive effects on knowledge about substance use	
"Here's Looking At You, Two" (HLAYT) Villanova University *USA* (Green and Kelley, 1989)	Quasi-experimental: *N* = 2703 (*n* = 1698 to Programme, *n* = 1005 to Control) Group assignment by class →To evaluate effectiveness of programme after 1 year [Analysis of programme effect] Comparisons pre-programme and 1-year follow-up (*EQA -self-esteem, coping, decision-making-; authors' self-report measure about understanding dangers of drug abuse*)	• students in programme showed increase in knowledge about drugs and alcohol • at primary education level, increase in knowledge, self-esteem, and improved decision-making	• no significant effect on decision-making, self-esteem, or coping skills of middle schoolers • coping skills increased in control group

(*continued*)

Table 5.2.2 (*Continued*)

Name, Institute, Country[a], Reference	Design →Objectives [type of evaluation] Methods, (*outcome measures*)	Significant results programme versus control Positive results	 Negative/unexpected results
		• in middle-school, increased knowledge level	• beyond increasing knowledge about substance abuse, programme produced very little effect on underlying attitudes critical to changing substance abuse behaviors
"I'm Special" (ISP) The Drug Education Center, Inc., University of North Carolina *USA* (Kim McLeod, and Shantzis, 1990)	Within-subject design: $N = 270$ →To evaluate short-term effects of programme [Analysis of programme effects] Comparisons pre-programme and 4-month follow-up (*SCAT Inventory*)	• positive attitudinal change experienced by students (student–teacher relationship, self-esteem, attitude toward school, basic social values, perception of family cohesiveness) • decrease in alcohol and drug use and related problem behaviors	
Keep A Clear Mind (KACM) University of North Florida *USA* (Werch, 1991)	Quasi-experimental: $N = 511$ students and $N = 1022$ parents (number per group not reported) Group assignment by class →To investigate effects of programme on students and parents [Analysis of programme effects] Comparisons pre- and post-programme (*authors' self-report measures for student substance use; parental communication regarding drug resistance; intentions, beliefs, and knowledge about drugs*)	• mothers reported more recent communication with their children about how to refuse or avoid drugs, greater frequency of these types of discussion, as well as greater discussion with children about how to resist peer pressure to drink, smoke, and use drugs	• no effect on parental drug-related knowledge • no effect on paternal communication with child about avoiding/refusing drugs or resisting peer pressure to use drugs • no effect on students' self-efficacy, family expectations, alcohol- and drug-related knowledge

		• fathers reported greater communication with children about how to resist peer pressure to drink alcohol and smoke, and were more motivated to help their children avoid drug use • students perceived less peer use of alcohol, tobacco, and marijuana, and reported less susceptibility to peer pressure to experiment with cigarettes • KACM was favorably assessed by parents, teachers and children	• no effect on intentions to use alcohol, cigarettes, marijuana in future
Peer-managed Self-control Programme for Prevention of Alcohol Abuse in American Indian High School Students Florida Mental Health Institute *USA* (Carpenter, Lyons, and Miller, 1985, 1985)	RCT: N = 30 (n=12 Programme, n = 8 Peer counseling only, n = 10 No treatment control) →To evaluate effectiveness of peer-mediated self-control training programme with adolescent American Indian high-risk population [Analysis of programme effects] Comparisons pre-, post-programme, 4-, 9-, and 12-month follow-up (*SEI, blood alcohol content; authors' self-report measures for alcohol consumption, frequency of use, attitudes, and knowledge about alcohol*)	• in programme, decrease in quantity and frequency of drinking, and peak blood alcohol levels • improvement maintained at 4- and 12-month follow-up	• no group differences observed in knowledge and attitudes about alcohol
Personal Growth Class (PGC) University of Washington *USA* (Eggert *et al.*, 1994)	Quasi-experimental: N = 259 (n = 101 Programme, n = 138 Control) Group assignment by class →To determine effect of programme on school performance and drug involvement [Analysis of programme effects] Comparisons pre-, post-programme and 5-month follow-up (*DISA; RSES; DPBS; school records*)	• decrease in drug control problems and consequences • improvement in actual and perceived school performance • improvement in self-esteem	• no effect on progression of drug use • no effect on male bonds to deviant peers • effects declined at follow-up

(*continued*)

Table 5.2.2 *(Continued)*

Name, Institute, Country[a], Reference	Design →Objectives [type of evaluation] Methods/outcome measures	Significant results programme versus control: Positive results	Significant results programme versus control: Negative/unexpected results
		• increased bonding relationships with teachers • females exhibited attenuated bonds to deviant peers	
Project ALERT The RAND Corporation *USA* (Ellickson and Bell, 1990; Bell, Ellickson, and Harrison, 1993)	Quasi-experimental: *N* = 6527 from 30 schools (*n* = 10 schools received ALERT led by adult educator, *n* = 10 schools received ALERT led by adult educator and teen leader, *n* = 10 schools received no programme) Group assignment by school →To evaluate short- and long-term effectiveness of school-based drug-prevention programme [Analysis of programme effects, implementation analysis] Comparisons pre-programme, 3-, 12-, 15- and 24-month follow-up (*authors' self-report measures for knowledge of substance use, and resistance self-efficacy*)	• modest reduction in drinking • reduced levels of cigarette use • initial use of marijuana reduced by one third and current use reduced by 50–60% • teen leader condition reduced frequency of pro-drug beliefs compared with control group in the ninth graders • programme equally successful for schools with high and low levels of minority student enrolment • effects on cognitive risk factors (perceived consequences of drug use, normative beliefs, resistance, self-efficacy) persisted at 24-month follow-up	• programme did not help smokers • effects on drinking disappeared at 12-month • effects on drug use disappeared at 24-month • in adult educator only condition, all beneficial effects disappeared at 24-month
Project Northland University of Minnesota	Quasi-experimental: *N* = 2419 from 20 school districts (*n* = 1270 from 10 school districts to Programme, *n* = 1149 from 10 school districts to Control)	• lower tendency to use alcohol at 2- and 3-year	• no effect on cigarette use, smokeless tobacco use (e.g., chewing tobacco), or marijuana use

USA (Komro *et al.*, 1994; Komro *et al.*, 1996; Perry *et al.*, 1996; Komro *et al.*, 2001; Perry *et al.*, 2002); (Perry *et al.*, 1993)	Group assignment by school district →To assess long-term impact of programme on alcohol and substance use [Analysis of programme effects] Comparisons pre-programme, 1-, 2- and 3-year follow-up (*authors' self-report measures for alcohol and other drug use, attitudes and knowledge about drug use*)	• percentage students reporting using alcohol in past month and past week lower at 2-year • 27% reduction in use of "gateway" drugs • more likely to report that could resist alcohol at party or dance at 2-years • lower score on peer influence at 2-year • fewer students saw peer drinking as normal at 2- and 3-year • association between student involvement with planning activities, and lower rate of alcohol use	• no effect on self-efficacy or perceived access
Start Taking Alcohol Risks Seriously (STARS) University of North Florida *USA* (Werch, 1996)	RCT: $N = 138$ ($n = 68$ to Programme, $n = 70$ to Control) →To examine effectiveness of STARS programme in preventing alcohol use among inner-city youth [analysis of programme effects] Comparisons pre-programme and 3-month follow-up (*authors' self-report measures for alcohol and drug use*)	• greater reduction in heavy alcohol use	• no difference between groups in percentage of alcohol users • no effect on measures of alcohol frequency, quantity, drinking consequences, and intentions to drink • no effect on 30-day, 7-day use, or 30-day heavy use
Self Management and Resistance Training (SMART)	Quasi-experimental: $N = 5070$ from 16 schools ($n = 6$ schools to SMART, $n = 6$ schools to Affect management only, $n = 12$ schools to No treatment control) Group assignment by school	• prevention programmes are efficacious in reducing the onset of drug use 1 year following implementation	• minimal programme effect for previous drug and alcohol users

(*continued*)

Table 5.2.2 *(Continued)*

Name, Institute, Country[a], Reference	Design →Objectives [type of evaluation] Methods/outcome measures	Significant results programme versus control: Positive results	Significant results programme versus control: Negative/unexpected results
University of Southern California *USA* (Hansen *et al.*, 1988; Graham *et al.*, 1990)	→To assess effects of programme and determine if sex and ethnicity predict outcome [Analysis of programme effects] Comparisons pre-programme, 12- and 24-month follow-up (*author's self-report measures for lifetime and recent cigarette, alcohol, and marijuana use; breath analysis for cigarette use*)	• effect was strongest for cigarettes, intermediate for alcohol, and weakest for marijuana • Program effective for females only • onset of smoking and alcohol use in use in nonusers lower for SMART cohort • lower alcohol use in SMART cohort compared to control	• AFFECT management only had negative impact which became more pronounced at 24-month follow-up
Drug Abuse Resistance Education (DARE) University of Minnesota *USA* (Perry *et al.*, 2003; Lynam *et al.*, 1999)	Quasi-experimental design: $N = 6237$ from 24 schools ($n = 8$ schools to DARE, $n = 8$ schools to DARE Plus - additional peer-led component, $n = 8$ schools to Control) →To evaluate effects of DARE and DARE Plus programmes on drug use and violence [Analysis of programme effects] Comparisons pre-programme, 10- and 22-month follow-up (*authors' self report measures for alcohol, tobacco, marijuana, and other drug use, expectancies about drug use*)	• DARE Plus enhanced effect of curriculum for boys (reduced increase in tobacco, alcohol, multidrug use and victimization) • DARE Plus reduced increase in tobacco use and violence when compared to DARE only curriculum	• DARE alone curriculum did not demonstrate any significant behavioral effect
Highly role-specified (HRS) alcohol prevention programme	Quasi-experimental design: $N = 12$ schools ($n = 4$ to HRS, $n = 4$ to LRS -low role-specified-programme, $n = 4$ to Control)	• students in HRS condition had more positive results than had those in LRS and comparison condition	

University of Bergen *Norway* (Wilhelmsen, Laberg, and Klepp, 1994)	Group assignment by school →To determine if increased student involvement in school-based prevention programme reduce student' alcohol use, and influence cognitive structures related to alcohol use [Analysis of programme effects] Comparisons pre-programme and 3-month follow-up (*authors' self-report measures for alcohol use, behavioral intentions, knowledge, attitudes, and perceptions about alcohol*)	• significantly less alcohol use and stronger norms to abstain from drinking among students in HRS condition • students in HRS condition had less alcohol use and stronger attitudes, norms, and intention to abstain than in LRS condition • in pre-post analysis, HRS yielded changes in positive direction, but not LRS • LRS not effective when tested against control condition	
Hope House Hope House Inc., Albany, NY *USA* (Krupka and Knox, 1985)	Within-subject design: $N = 313$ students →To determine if brief encounter with substance disorder patients, combined with didactic presentations about substance abuse, produce changes in students' knowledge and attitudes about substance abuse [Analysis of programme effects] Comparisons pre-programme and 3-week follow-up (*authors' self-report measures for student alcohol use, family alcohol use, attitudes toward and knowledge about alcohol*)	• After visiting treatment center, students regard substance abusers in less idealized terms; substance abuse is viewed more like any other sickness and it is correctly seen as affecting all social strata	
Tuning Into Health (TITH) Alcoholism Foundation of Manitoba *Canada* (Ambtman *et al.*, 1990)	Quasi-experimental design (outcome evaluation): $N = 2{,}092$ students from 31 schools ($n = 1101$ to Programme, $n = 991$ to Control); Group assignment by school Survey (process evaluation): $N = 500$ teachers →To evaluate effect of programme on students' knowledge about drugs →To determine teacher satisfaction with design and implementation of programme [Analysis of programme effects, normative evaluation of process]	• in urban schools, greater increase in knowledge about drugs and less drug use in all grades • greater improvement in knowledge about drugs and drug use in grades 3, 4, and 5 • 84% of teacher respondents rated goals as "very clear"; 93% judged programme as complete with no need to add content	• 1/4 teachers reported need for further training • inconsistent effects in rural schools

(*continued*)

Table 5.2.2 (*Continued*)

Name, Institute, Country[a], Reference	Design →Objectives [type of evaluation] Methods/outcome measures	Significant results programme versus control	
		Positive results	Negative/unexpected results
	Comparisons pre-programme and 3-month follow-up (*authors' self-report measures for knowledge of programme elements, and teachers' experience with teaching the programme*)		
Stress Management and Alchohol Awareness Programme (SMAAP) George Mason University *USA* (Roosa, 1989; Short *et al.*, 1995)	Quasi-experimental: $N = 271$ students from 13 schools Eight schools received SMAAP alone ($n = 181$ students), five schools received SMAAP plus personal trainer ($n = 60$) Schools assigned to receive either programme immediately →To evaluate effect of programme on coping and emotional problems in children who perceive parents as problem drinkers [Analysis of programme effects] Comparisons pre-programme, 2-, 5-, and 8-month follow-up (*CAB; AEQ-A; SPPC; CDI; YSRCHS; BRS; authors' self-report measures for concern about parental drinking, and knowledge of programme content; programme attendance*)	• increase in use of positive coping strategies • teachers' reports of children's moodiness improved for those receiving SMAAP • greater improvement on social and emotion-focused coping strategies • no difference between groups with and without personal trainer • long-term effect	• no effect on self-esteem • no effect on depression or antisocial behaviors, as reported by students or teachers

AEQ-A: Alcohol; **BRS:** Behavior Rating Scale; **CAB:** Coping Assessment Battery; **CBCL**: Achenbach and Eldelbrock Child Behavior Checklist; **CDI:** Children's Depression Inventory; **CI:** Coping Inventory; **DAS:** Drug and Alcohol Survey; **DISA:** Drug Involvment Scale for Adolescents; **DPBS:** Deviant Peer Bonding Scale; Expectancies Questionnaire-Adolescent Form; **EQA:** Educational Quality Assessment; **FES**: Moos Family Environment Scale; **PBI:** Parental Bonding Inventory; **RCT:** Randomized controlled trial; **RSES:** Rosenberg Self-esteem Scale; **SCAT Inventory:** Self-Concept Attitudinal Inventory; **SEI:** Self Esteem Inventory; **SPPC:** Self-perception Profile for Children; **SQ:** Student Questionnaire; **YSRCHS:** Youth Self-Report Child Hostility Scale

[a]The country in italic indicates where the programme was developed.

Table 5.2.3 Programmes targeting depression/anxiety – programme outline

Name, Institute, Country[a], Reference	Target population, Age, Sex	Theoretical orientation →Objectives	Description	Setting, Manual, Providers (Training)
YouthNet Children's Hospital of Eastern Ontario (CHEO) *Canada* (Manion *et al.*, 1997a; Manion *et al.*, 1997b)	Universal 13–20 years old Males and females	– young people may be prone to mental illness due to sense of isolation from their community – based on suicide-specific classification of Emile Durkheim, specifically "egoistic" and "anomic" definitions of suicide →To promote awareness and increase communication among youth regarding mental health and mental illness →To empower youth to develop connections with "youth-friendly" professionals →At macroscopic level, to decrease sense of isolation by enabling youth to interact with other youth →At microscopic level, to link at-risk youth with mental health services in community	– Bilingual programme run by youth for youth *Programme elements* • youth focus groups: run by youth facilitators (18–25 years) to address stress experienced by youth • newsletter (YouthFax): written in youth-friendly language by youth; art, poetry, stories, opinions, questions sent in by youth • pens and paints project: encouraging youth to develop alternative means of self-expression and coping • project free ride: giving underprivileged youth opportunity to enjoy snowboarding	Community No manual Youth facilitators
Penn Prevention Programme **(Penn Resiliency Programme)** University of Pennsylvania *USA*, Canada, China, Australia (Jaycox *et al.*, 1994; Gillham *et al.*, 1995; Gillham *et al.*, 1999)	Indicated (high scores on CDI and CPQ, combined with high degree of parental conflict at home) 10–13 years old Males and females	– consistent with theories of social cognition – children with depressive symptoms tend to have more pessimistic explanatory style (tend to attribute internal, global, and stable causes to negative events) – these negative cognitions lead to self-fulfilling prophecies which reinforce and maintain depression →To use cognitive-behavioral techniques proactively to teach coping strategies and enhance sense of mastery and competency in children at-risk for depression	12 weekly $1\frac{1}{2}$ -hour sessions *Programme elements* • cognitive component • social problem-solving component • in-session instruction with weekly homework assignments	School English manual (Gillham *et al.*, 1995) Doctoral psychology students

(continued)

Table 5.2.3 (*Continued*)

Name, Institute, Country[a], Reference	Target population, Age, Sex	Theoretical orientation →Objectives	Programme description	Setting, Manual, Providers (Training)
Preventive Interventions for Families with Depression Judge Baker Chidren's Center and Children's Hospital, Boston *USA* (Beardslee *et al.*, 1997)	Selective (parent with affective disorder) 8–15 years old Males and females	– developmental psychology – development of psychopathology in at-risk children is a dynamic interplay between familial, biological, social, cognitive factors →To encourage resilient behavior and attitudes via enhanced family functioning	6–10 sessions led by trained clinicians *Programme elements* • direct link is made between knowledge about causes and symptoms of depression, treatment options, and individual life and family experiences	Clinical English manual (Beardslee *et al.*, 1992) Social workers, psychologists
School-based Primary Prevention of Depressive Symptomatology in Adolescents (Behavioral Skill-Training Intervention) Oregon Health Sciences University *USA* (Clarke *et al.*, 1993)	Universal 13–16 years old Males and females	– based on behavioral theory of depression, encouraging adolescents to increase their daily rates of pleasant activities to help prevent onset or exacerbation of depressive mood →To prevent depressive symptomatology and depressive disorders in adolescents through training to increase pleasant activities	– Five 50-min sessions *Programme elements* • curriculum on symptoms, causes and treatments of depression, as well as behavioral methods of increasing pleasant activities • introductory lesson: lecture and 20-min videotape about depression • subsequent lessons: training to increase rate of pleasant activities	School English manual (Clarke, 1991) Health class teachers(2-h training in administration of curriculum, and scripted manual)

School-based Primary Prevention of Depressive Symptomatology in Adolescents (Educational Intervention) Oregon Health Sciences University *USA* (Clarke *et al.*, 1993)	Universal 13–16 years old Males and females	– lectures and discussions emphasizing treatable nature of depression, and encouraging adolescents to seek intervention →To prevent depressive symptomatology and depressive disorders through nonintrusive educational intervention	– Three 50-min sessions *Programme elements* • three structured lectures and two 20-min videotapes about depression • curriculum on symptoms, causes and treatments of depression • no specific behavioral skill-training	School English manual (Clarke, 1991) Health class teachers (2-h training in administration of curriculum, and scripted manual)
Queensland Early Intervention and Prevention of Anxiety Project (QEIPAP) Queensland Health Promotion Council *Australia* (Dadds *et al.*, 1997)	Indicated (features of anxiety disorder or nonspecific anxiety sensitivity) 7–14 years old Males and females	– cognitive behavioral model – centered on Kendall's FEAR plan, in which each child implements their own plan for coping using FEAR framework: F-feeling good by learning to relax; E-expecting good things to happen through positive self-talk; A-actions to take in facing fear; R-rewarding oneself →To intervene for children who are disorder-free but show mild anxious features, using CBT strategies	– Ten weekly 1–2-h group ($N = 5–12$) sessions *Programme elements* • CBT groups during class time • parent sessions at weeks 3, 6, and 9, to teach parents what children are learning and how they can encourage them to use strategies learned	School English manual (Barrett *et al.*, 1994) Clinical psychologists (1-day training workshop)

(*continued*)

Table 5.2.3 *(Continued)*

Name, Institute, Country[a], Reference	Target population, Age, Sex	Theoretical orientation →Objectives	Programme description	Setting, Manual, Providers (Training)
Ease of Handling Social Aspects in Everyday Life-training (LISA) University of Tubingen *Germany* (Possel *et al.*, 2004a; Possel *et al.*, 2004b)	Universal 13 years old Males and females	– social information-processing model of social competence – behavior is consequence of information-processing sequence in reaction to situational stimuli – during encoding, selective perception filters relevant aspects of stimuli – depressed children process information with a bias toward those aspects that are consistent with their negative self-schema →To illustrate relationship between cognition, emotion, and behavior; explore and change dysfunctional cognitions; train self-assured behavior; train social competence skills → Cognitive modules to enable students to challenge automatic thoughts →Social modules to facilitate adaptive social behavior	– Ten weekly 1.5-hour group (N = 8–24) sessions *Programme elements* • cognitive part: based on cognitive therapy approach; designed to decrease dysfunctional and increase functional cognition • social part: training of new functional behaviors in role plays • girls and boys segregated by sex	School German manual (Possel *et al.*, 2004b) Psychologists, graduate students (having gone through programme as participants and studied manual and materials for procedures)
Family Styles Project University of Michigan *USA* (Garvin Leber, and Kalter, 1991)	Selective (children of divorce) 5–12 years old Males and females	– parental divorce constitutes immediate and major disequilibrium in life of children, affecting social, cognitive, and emotional development →To prevent low self-esteem and acting-out →To normalize common experiences of children of divorce	– 8–10 weekly sessions (depending on child age of child) *Programme elements* • addressing immediate disruption and trauma of parental separation, and longer term challenges of divorce process (e.g., interparental conflict, reduced parental contact, parental dating, and remarriage)	Clinical English manual (Kalter *et al.*, 1988) Adult co-leaders

		→To provide supportive forum in which children can experience and rework stressful aspects of postdivorce life →To assist in development of coping strategies →To share with parents concerns of children	• group discussion and role-playing on divorce-related issues	
Stress Inoculation Training for Adolescents University of Wisconsin-Milwaukee *USA* Hains *et al.*, 1992	Selective (students in competitive preparatory schools) 15–17 years old Males and females	• for those who have difficulty managing stress, training in various cognitive and behavioral coping strategies as part of intervention package may alleviate negative stress reactions →To help adolescents cope with both major life stress events and daily stressors	15 sessions *Programme elements* • Three overlapping phases: (1) education phase, to teach techniques to reconceptualize negative emotional arousal; (2) skill acquisition phase, to learn how to deal with newly developed conceptualizations; (3) rehearsal phase, to practice applying new skills in stressful situations	School English manual (Hains and Szyjakowski, 1990) Clinicians
Prevention Programme for Anxious-Withdrawn Preschoolers University of Maine, University of Sherbrooke *Canada* (LaFreniere and Capuano, 1997)	Indicated (children exhibiting emotional/behavioral problems, based on SCBE) 2–6 years old Males and females	– mothers of anxious-withdrawn children tend to be overcontrolling and intrusive, particularly in situations that call for mutuality and negotiation, rather than exercise of parental authority →To prevent anxiety and emotional disturbance in children by improving maternal skills	– 20 sessions, in four phases, over 6 months *Programme elements* • targeting group of mothers on basis of child's emotional/behavioral problems • multifaceted intervention for mothers without direct intervention with children • caregiver-focused education on child's developmental needs • determination of specific objectives	School French manual (Capuano, 1995) Graduate students

(*continued*)

Table 5.2.3 (*Continued*)

Name, Institute, Country[a], Reference	Target population, Age, Sex	Theoretical orientation →Objectives	Programme description	Setting, Manual, Providers (Training)
FRIENDS for Children Pathways Health and Research Centre/ (Griffith University, Brisbane) *Australia*, USA, Germany, Canada, Netherlands, UK, Ireland, Portugal, New Zealand (Barkley *et al.*, 2000; Lowry-Webster, Barrett, and Dadds, 2001; Shortt *et al.*, 2001; Barrett and Turner, 2001; Barrett *et al.*, 2003; Lowry-Webster, Barrett, and Lock, 2003)	Universal 7–16 years old Males and females	– based on theoretical model which addresses cognitive, physiological, and behavioral processes that interact in development, maintenance and experience of anxiety – core components of CBT (exposure, relaxation, cognitive strategies, contingency management) →To reduce incidence of serious mental disorders, emotional distress and impairment in social functioning, by teaching children and youth how to cope with and manage anxiety	– Ten weekly 75-min group sessions Two booster sessions, 1- and 3-month after programme completion *Programme elements* • FRIENDS is acronym for strategies taught: F-feeling worried; R-relax and feel good; I-inner thoughts; E-explore plans; N-nice work so reward yourself; D-don't forget to practice; S-stay calm, you know how to cope now • CBT strategies for coping with anxiety • Family skills component: 6-h sessions with parents matched to content of children's sessions	School English, German and Dutch manual (www.friendsinfo.net) Teachers (1 day group-training session provided by accredited FRIENDS trainer) cost=£34/child for term 1; £24/child for term 2

CBT: Cognitive behavior therapy; **CDI:** Children's Depression Inventory; **CPQ:** Child's Perception Questionnaire; **SCBE:** Social Competence and Behavior Evaluation
[a]The country in italic indicates where the programme was developed.

Table 5.2.4 Programmes targeting depression/anxiety – programme evaluation

Name, Institute, Country[a], Reference	Design →Objectives [type of evaluation] Methods(*outcome measures*)	Significant results programme versus control	
		Positive results	Negative/unexpected results
YouthNet Children's Hospital of Eastern Ontario (CHEO) *Canada* (Manion *et al.*, 1997a; Manion *et al.*, 1997b)	Informal survey with focus groups: $N = 1091$ →To informally obtain feedback on programme's philosophy [Normative evaluation of programme structure] (*self-report measures of self-esteem, depression, suicidal ideation, stress*)	Positive feedback on programme's philosophy	More formalized evaluation of impact of programme impact under development
Penn Prevention Programme (Penn Resiliency Programme) University of Pennsylvania *USA*, Canada, China, Australia (Jaycox *et al.*, 1994; Gillham *et al.*, 1999; Gillham *et al.*, 1995)	Quasi-experimental: $N = 143$ ($n = 69$ to Programme, $n = 49$ to Control) in original study (Jaycox *et al.*, 1994) reduced to $N = 118$ ($n = 69$ to Programme, $n = 49$ to Control) in subsequent reports Groups selected by school district →To determine immediate and long-term effects of programme on depressive symptoms and attributional style [Analysis of programme effects; programme analysis] Comparisons pre-, post-programme, 6-, 12-, 24-, 30-, and 36-month follow-up (*CDI; RCDS; CASQ; teacher report of classroom behavior, self-discipline, peer relations*)	• fewer depressive symptoms at post-test and follow-up • less likely to attribute negative events to stable and enduring causes at post-test • more optimistic explanatory style at follow-up • ability to explain negative events with less stable explanations associated with decrease in depressive symptoms at post-test and follow-up • better classroom behavior reported by teachers • greater increase in depressive symptoms in control group	• programme's benefits on depressive symptoms faded after 2 years, but effect on explanatory style maintained • depressive symptoms increased in both groups as children got older

(*continued*)

Table 5.2.4 (*Continued*)

Name, Institute, Country[a], Reference	Design →Objectives [type of evaluation] Methods (*outcome measures*)	Significant results programme versus control	
		Positive results	Negative/unexpected results
Preventive Interventions for Families with Depression Judge Baker Chidren's Center and Children's Hospital, Boston *USA* (Beardslee *et al.*, 1997)	RCT: $N = 37$ families (19 to Programme, 18 to Control) →To assess effectiveness of programme in improving parental awareness, family communication and child's knowledge [Programme analysis; normative evaluation of process] Comparisons pre- and post-programme (*SADS-L; RDC; BDI; DAS; FRI; SII; ratings of overall satisfaction with programme*)	• larger number of overall changes, higher levels of change regarding communication about illness with children • more children reported better understanding of parental affective illness • parents in both groups reported satisfaction with the intervention	
School-based Primary Prevention of Depressive Symptomatology in Adolescents (Behavioral Skill-Training Intervention) Oregon Health Sciences University *USA* (Clarke *et al.*, 1993)	RCT: $N = 380$ ($n = 190$ to Programme, $n = 190$ to Control) →To determine if programme is associated with reduction in depressive symptoms and high scoring depressive "cases" [Analysis of programme effects] Comparisons pre-, post-programme, and 12-week follow-up (*CES-D*)		• no significant main effects found for depression knowledge, treatment seeking, or attitudes about depression

School-based Primary Prevention of Depressive Symptomatology in Adolescents (Educational Intervention) Oregon Health Sciences University *USA* (Clarke *et al.*, 1993)	RCT: $N = 622$ ($n = 361$ to Programme, $n = 261$ to Control) →To determine if the programme is associated with a reduction in depressive symptoms and high scoring depressive "cases" [Analysis of programme effects] Comparisons pre-, post-programme, and 12-week follow-up (*CES-D*)		• no significant main effects found for depression knowledge, treatment seeking, or attitudes about depression
Queensland Early Intervention and Prevention of Anxiety Project (QEIPAP) Queensland Health Promotion Council *Australia* (Dadds *et al.*, 1997)	Quasi-experimental: $N = 128$ ($n = 61$ to Programme, $n = 67$ to Control) Group assignment by school → To examine remediating effects of intervention on children's functioning and symptomatology [Analysis of programme effects] Comparisons pre-, post-programme, and 6-month follow-up (*CBCL; RCMAS; ADIS-P*)	• smaller percentage progressed to diagnosable anxiety disorder at follow-up (16% versus 54 %)	• no significant differences found on individual ratings at post-test
Ease of Handling Social Aspects in Everyday Life-Training (LISA) University of Tübingen	RCT: $N = 324$ ($n = 200$ to Programme, $n = 147$ to Control)	• fewer symptoms among adolescents with subsyndromal depression	• no difference in automatic thoughts or social support

(*continued*)

Table 5.2.4 (*Continued*)

Name, Institute, Country[a], Reference	Design →Objectives [type of evaluation] Methods(*outcome measures*)	Significant results programme versus control	
		Positive results	Negative/unexpected results
Germany (Possel *et al.*, 2004a; Possel *et al.*, 2004b)	→To determine programme's effect on depressive symptoms and risk factors for development of depression [Analysis of programme effects] Comparisons pre-, post-programme, 3- and 6-month follow-up (*CES-D; ATQ; FESU*)	• greater network sizes at 3-month follow-up • greater decrease in percentage of adolescents with clinically relevant symptoms, subsyndromal depression	
Family Styles Project University of Michigan *USA* (Garvin Leber, and Kalter, 1991)	Within-group evaluation: $N = 53$ →To assess if children would benefit from intervention for depressive symptoms, attributional style, perceived competence [Analysis of programme effects; programme analysis] Comparison pre- and post-programme (*CDI; PCSC; N-SLCSC*)	• main effect of time for cognitive competence, general self-worth, and locus of control • interaction effect of time and grade on physical and cognitive competence • majority of children experienced change in positive direction	• no obvious pattern that would explain association between predictors and outcomes
Stress Inoculation Training for Adolescents University of Wisconsin-Milwaukee *USA* Hains *et al.*, 1992	Within-group evaluation: $N = 6$ →To examine effectiveness of programme in high school setting [Analysis of programme effects] Comparisons pre, post-programme, and 3-month follow-up (*STAXI; CSE; RADS; APES*)	• trait anxiety and trait anger improved at post-test and 3-month follow up for 84% of subjects	• 16% experienced increase in anxiety scores during programme

Prevention Programme for Anxious-withdrawn Preschoolers University of Maine, University of Sherbrooke *Canada* (LaFreniere and Capuano, 1997)	RCT: *N* = 42 preschool children (*n* = 21 to Programme, *n* = 22 to Control) →To evaluate outcome in child's behavior in preschool classroom as assessed by teacher [Analysis of programme effects] Comparisons pre- and post-programme (*SCBE; PSI; observational ratings of emotional support, appropriate control, motivation*)	• parenting stress scores of mothers showed significant decline between pre- and post-test • increase in emotional support toward child, more appropriate control • children showed increase in positive motivation	• no improvement in anxiety-withdrawal • no significant group difference for decline in parenting stress scores
FRIENDS for Children Pathways Health and Research Centre (Griffith University, Brisbane) *Australia*, USA, Germany, Canada, Netherlands, UK, Ireland, Portugal, New Zealand (Barkley et al., 2000; Lowry-Webster, Barrett, and Dadds,, 2001; Shortt et al., 2001; Barrett et al., 2001; Barrett et al., 2003; Lowry-Webster, Barrett, and Lock, 2003)	RCT: *N* = 594 (*n* = 432 to Programme, *n* = 162 to Control) →To examine effects of programme on levels of depression and anxiety [Analysis of programme effects] Comparisons pre-, post-programme, and 1-year follow-up (*SCAS; CDI; RCMAS*)	• results examined universally and for children who scored above clinical cut-off for anxiety at pretest • fewer anxiety symptoms at post-test, regardless of risk status • more children who had scored above clinical cut-off were diagnosis-free at follow-up (85% versus 31%)	

ADIS-P: Anxiety Disorders Interview Schedule-Parent version; **APES:** Adolescent Perceived Events Scale; **ATQ:** Automatic Thoughts Questionnaire; **BDI**: Beck Depression Inventory; **CASQ:** Children's Attributional Style Questionnaire; **CBCL:** Child Behavior Checklist; **CES-D:** Center for Epidemiological Studies-Depression Scale; **CSE:** Coopersmith Self-Esteem Inventory; **DAS:** Dyadic Adjustment Scale; **FESU:** Questionnaire of Social Support; **FRI:** Family Relationship Inventory; **N-SLCSC:** Nowicki-Strickland Locus of Control Scale for Children; **PCSC:** Perceived Competence Scale for Children; **PSI**: Parent Stress Index; **RADS:** Reynolds Adolescent Depression Scale; **RCDS:** Reynolds Children's Depression Scale; **RCMAS:** Revised Child Manifest Anxiety Scale; **RCT:** Randomized controlled trial; **SADS-L:** Schedule for Affective Disorders and Schizophrenia; **SCAS:** Spence Children's Anxiety Scale; SCBE: Social Competence and Behavior Evaluation; **SII:** Semistructured Interview about Disorders Impact and Intervention; **STAXI:** State-Trait Anger Expression Inventory

[a]The country in italic indicates where the programme was developed.

Table 5.2.5 Programmes targeting eating disorders – programme outline

Name, Institute, Country[a], Reference	Target population, Age, Sex	Theoretical orientation → Objectives	Description	Setting, Manual, Providers (Training)
Dissonance-based Eating Disorder Prevention Programme University of Texas at Austin *USA* (Stice *et al.*, 2001)	Selective (females with self-identified body issue concerns) 17–29 years old Females	– based on dual-pathway model and dissonance theory – internalization of thin-ideal promotes body dissatisfaction, negative affect, dieting, which in turn foster bulimic pathology – inconsistent cognitions create psychological discomfort, leading people to alter own cognitions to restore consistency →To reduce thin-ideal internalization by requiring participants to take a stance against it, through verbal, written, and behavioral exercises	Three weekly 1-h group ($N = 5$–10) sessions *Programme elements* • group collectively defines and critically discusses thin-ideal • participants instructed to compose written criticism of thin-ideal • counterattitudinal role-play: participants attempt to dissuade group leaders from pursuing thin-ideal	Clinical No manual Clinical psychologists
Everybody's Different University of Sydney *Australia* (O'Dea and Abraham, 2000; Wade, Davidson, and O'Dea, 2003)	Universal 11–14 years old Males and females	– based on educational theories of cooperative, interactive, and student-centered learning – self-esteem is a distal risk factor for weight and shape concern, which in turn influences dietary restraint and disordered eating →To improve body image, eating attitudes, and behaviors of young male and female adolescents, by improving general self-esteem	– Nine weekly 50–80 min in-class sessions *Programme elements* • lessons include: how to deal with stress; building positive sense of self; identifying societal stereotypes; how to evaluate oneself positively; how to seek positive feedback from significant others; relationship skills; communication skills	School English manual (O'Dea, 1995) Teachers (1-day training session)

Free to Be Me University of Minnesota *USA* (Neumark-Sztainer *et al.*, 2000)	Selective (females) 9–12 years old Females	– based on principles of social cognitive theory, specifically concept of reciprocal determinism – socioenvironmental, personal, and behavioral factors continually interact with each other →To promote body acceptance and prevent dieting among preadolescent girls via enhancement of media literacy and advocacy skills →To help girls develop skills for recognizing media advertising strategies and understand effect on body image of images portrayed in media	– Six biweekly 90-min sessions during girl scout meetings *Programme elements* • in-group media literacy training: exposition to historical ideal images of women, comparison of media-endorsed images with real body types • media advocacy: girls write letter to companies with positive or negative media message • take-home activities with friends and family	Community English manual (no reference) Girl-scout troop leaders (3-h training session)
Full of Ourselves: **Advancing Girl Power, Health, and Leadership** Harvard Eating Disorders Center *USA* (Steiner-Adaor et al., 2002)	Selective (females) 12-14 years old Females	– focuses on esteem-building and hands-on, experiential approach to learning – incorporates strong feminist, sociopolitical perspective; emphases on translating knowledge and awareness into personal and public action; mentoring component → To improve body image by building general self-esteem, rather than attempting to increase knowledge related to diet and nutrition → To reduce risk of disordered eating by increasing self-esteem, promoting body acceptance, providing leadership opportunities, and teaching coping strategies to resist cultural emphasis on maladaptive body preoccupation	Eight weekly 45–90 min group (N = 10–15) sessions *Programme elements* • exploring a range of topics through more than 70 activities: understanding weightism as a social justice issue; ways to identify and resist unhealthy media messages; power of positive thinking and action; how to be activist in school, at home, in world • two phases: (1) completing curriculum under guidance of two women leaders; (2) designing and delivering 1–3 programme sessions to 9–11 years old girls	School, community No manual Teachers, nurses, guidance counselors

(*continued*)

Table 5.2.5 (*Continued*)

Name, Institute, Country[a], Reference	Target population, Age, Sex	Theoretical orientation → Objectives	Description	Setting, Manual, Providers (Training)
GO GIRLS! Eating Disorder Awareness and Prevention (EDAP), Seattle *USA*, Australia (Wade, Davidson, and O'Dea, 2003)	Universal 11–14 years old Males and females	– follows findings from public health arena on drug, alcohol, and tobacco use – training students to resist social pressures is more effective in preventing unwanted behavior than a standard information approach →To reduce internalization of slender ideal →To empower students to adopt critical evaluation of media content so that they can identify, analyze, challenge, and reduce internalization of thin ideal presented in mass media	– Sixteen weekly in-class sessions (reduced to five sessions for evaluation) *Programme elements* • lesson topics include: identifying consequences of negative body image and media impact on body image; how advertisements can be altered to make up stories; how to become a critical media viewer • in small groups, students prepare media awareness presentation to determine if advertising is harmful	School English manual (Eating Disorder Awareness and Prevention, 1999) Teachers
School-based Eating Disorder Prevention Programme Oxford University *UK* (Stewart, 1998; Stewart *et al.*, 2001)	Selective (females) 13–14 years old Females	– follows CBT strategies for treating ED – normal adolescent development involves number of tasks and challenges which can be difficult to negotiate, particularly for girls – adolescent girls have additional challenge of contending with sociocultural messages linking happiness to thinness – these multiple pressures can lead to development of low self-esteem, feeling of loss of control, and dieting →To reduce dieting and concerns about shape and weight by promoting behavioral and attitudinal change as well as increasing knowledge	– Six weekly 45-min in-class sessions *Programme elements* • use of guided discovery, role play, small group discussions intended to make intervention interactive rather than didactic • girls taught how to identify and challenge automatic thoughts, self-monitor eating habits, and try "nondieting" approaches to eating	School English manual (Stewart and Carter, 1995) Psychologists, psychiatrists

CBT: Cognitive behavior therapy; **DRES:** Dutch Restrained Eating Scale; **ED:** Eating disorder
[a]The country in italic indicates where the programme was developed.

Table 5.2.6 Programmes targeted at eating disorders – programme evaluation

Name, Institute, Country[a], Reference	Design →Objectives [type of evaluation] Methods (*outcome measures*)	Significant results programme versus control	
		Positive results	Negative/unexpected results
Dissonance-based Eating Disorder Prevention Programme University of Texas at Austin *USA* (Stice *et al.*, 2001)	RCT: $N = 87$ ($n = 48$ to Programme, $n = 39$ to healthy weight management Control condition) →To evaluate effectiveness of dissonance-based intervention for high-risk populations [Analysis of programme effects] Comparisons pre-, post-programme, and 4-week follow-up (*BMI; EDE-Q; IBSS-R; SDBPS; DRES; PANS-X; F-RDHQ; PYLPAS*)	• greater decrease in thin-ideal internalization from baseline to termination and follow-up • greater decrease in body dissatisfaction from baseline to termination and follow-up • decrease in dieting at termination and follow-up for both groups • decrease in negative affect for both groups	• no difference in bulimic symptoms
Everybody's Different University of Sydney *Australia* (O'Dea and Abraham, 2000; Wade, Davidson, and O'Dea, 2003)	RCT: $N = 470$ ($n = 275$ to Programme, $n = 195$ to Control) →To examine effect of a school-based self-esteem education programme on body image, eating attitudes, and behaviors [Analysis of programme effects] Comparisons pre-, post-programme, and 12-month follow-up (*EDI; S-PPA; BDI; STAI; PAR; body image questionnaire*)	• at post-test, body dissatisfaction decreased in intervention group and increased in control group • improvement in body satisfaction, importance of social acceptance, physical appearance in high-risk students (low self-esteem, high trait anxiety at baseline) at post-test, and follow-up • social acceptance less important at post-test and follow-up	• no change in body satisfaction and physical appearance rating at follow-up • no difference for weight losing behaviors at post-test or follow-up

(*continued*)

Table 5.2.6 (*Continued*)

Name, Institute, Country[a], Reference	Design →Objectives [type of evaluation] Methods (*outcome measures*)	Significant results programme versus control	
		Positive results	Negative/unexpected results
Free to Be Me University of Minnesota *USA* (Neumark-Sztainer *et al.*, 2000)	Quasi-experimental: N = 226 from 24 girl scout troops (n= 115 from 12 troops to Programme, n = 111 from 12 troops to Control) Group assignment by troop →To evaluate community-based intervention aimed at primary prevention of disordered eating in preadolescent girls [Analysis of programme effects] Comparisons pre-, post-programme, and 3-month follow-up (*authors' self-report measures for dieting behaviors, body-related knowledge and attitudes, media-related knowledge, attitudes, and behaviors, programme satisfaction*)	• internalization of thin body ideal lower at follow-up • perceived self-efficacy to effect weight-related norms higher at post-test and follow-up	• no effect on body-related knowledge
Full of Ourselves: Advancing Girl Power, Health, and Leadership Harvard Eating disorders Center *USA* (Steiner-Adair *et al.*, 2002)	RCT: N = 411 (n = 213 to Programme, n = 198 to Control) →To evaluate effectiveness and feasibility of prevention programme for risk factors for ED in adolescent girls [Analysis of programme effects] Comparisons pre-, post-programme, and 6-month follow-up (*BES; MBSRQ-BASS; SATAQ; RSES*)	• higher body esteem at post-test and follow-up • higher Body Areas Satisfaction scores at post-test and follow-up • greater increase in knowledge about ED issues	• no differences in self-esteem, eating behaviors, weight thinking and behaviors

GO GIRLS! Eating Disorder Awareness and Prevention (EDAP) , Seattle *USA*, Australia (Wade, Davidson, and O'Dea, 2003)	Quasi-experimental: $N = 86$ ($n = 25$ Media literacy programme, $n = 43$ Alternate ED programme on self-esteem, $n = 18$ Control) Group assignment by class →To compare efficacy of media literacy programme and self-esteem programme to reduce general and specific risk factors for ED [Analysis of programme effects] Comparisons pre-, post-programme, and 3-month follow-up (*EDE-Q; SPPA; Body dissatisfaction; authors' measure of sense of self-worth*)	• media literacy group had lower levels of weight concern than self-esteem group and control group • media literacy group perceived themselves to be more competent in close friendships than did self-esteem group and control group • media literacy programme perceived as more enjoyable than self-esteem programme	
School-based Eating Disorder Prevention Programme Oxford University *UK* (Stewart, 1998; Stewart *et al*., 2001)	Quasi-experimental: $N = 845$ ($n = 459$ to Programme, $n = 386$ to Control) Group assignment by school → To evaluate effectiveness of school-based ED prevention programme designed to reduce dietary restraint and concern about shape and weight among adolescent girls [Analysis of programme effects] Comparisons pre-, post-programme, and 6-month follow-up (*EDE-Q; EAT; P-HCSCS*)	• lower dietary restraint scores at post-test and follow-up	• no significant differences in weight concern, eating concern, self-concept, or behavior characteristic of ED • increase in eating concern at follow-up for intervention group

RCT: Randomized controlled trial; **BDI:** Beck Depression Inventory; **BES:** Body Esteem Scale; **BMI:** Body Mass Index; **CBT:** Cognitive behavior therapy; **DRES:** Dutch Restrained Eating Scale; **EAT:** Eating Attitudes Test; **ED:** Eating disorder; **EDE-Q:** Eating Disorder Examination-Questionnaire**; EDI:** Eating Disorder Inventory; **F-RDHQ:** Fat-Related Diet Habits Questionnaire; **IBSS-R:** Ideal-Body Stereotype Scale-Revised; **MBRSQ-BASS:** Multidimensional Body-Self Relations Questionnaire-Body Satisfaction Scale; **PANAS-X:** Positive Affect and Negative Affect Scale-Revised; **PAR:** Physical Appearance Ratings; **P-HCSCS:** Piers-Harris Children's Self-Concept Scale; **PYLPAS:** Past Year Leisure Physical Activity Scale; **SATAQ:** Sociocultural Attitudes Towards Appearance Questionnaire; **SDBPS:** Satisfaction and Dissatisfaction with Body Parts Scale; **SPPA:** Self-Perception Profile for Adolescents; **STAI:** Stat-Trait Anxiety Inventory

[a]The country in italic indicates where the programme was developed.

Table 5.2.7 Programmes targeting behavioral / conduct problems – programme outline

Name, Institute, Country[a], Reference	Target population, Age, Sex	Theoretical Orientation → Objectives	Description	Setting, Manual, Providers (Training)
Promoting Alternative Thinking Strategies (PATHS) Conduct Problems Prevention Research Group, University of Washington *USA*, Netherlands, Belgium, Great Britain, Norway, Canada, Australia, Israel (Greenberg *et al.*, 1995; Bierman *et al.*, 1999; Bierman *et al.*, 2002)	Universal 5–10 years old Males and females	– based on ABCD model of development, hybrid model that places primary importance on Developmental integration of Affect, Behavior, and Cognitive understanding – child's coping is function of emotional awareness, affective-cognitive control, and social-cognitive understanding – during maturational process, emotional development precedes most forms of cognition – affective development is important precursor of other modes of thinking and needs to be integrated with cognitive functions for optimal maturation →To provide school-aged children with instruction regarding variety of issues involved in expression, understanding and regulation of emotions	– 131 lessons (20–30 min) 3–5 times per week in class time through elementary school *Programme elements* • self-control unit: children are told story about aggressive turtle who has interpersonal and academic difficulties, and is helped by wise old turtle to develop better self-control • feelings and relationships unit: 50 affective states, and cues to recognize these feelings in oneself and others are taught, beginning with basic emotions and leading to complex emotions • interpersonal cognitive problem-solving unit: teaching steps to use to solve problem • supplemental lessons: optional extension lessons that can be taught in subsequent years	School English and Spanish manual (www.channing-bete.com) Teachers (3-day training workshop and weekly consultation from programme staff) $15–45/student/year

Better Beginnings, Better Futures Queen's University *Canada* (Sylvestre et al., 1993; Peters *et al.*, 2000; Peters, Petrunka, and Arnold, 2003)	Universal 0–8 years old Males and females	– based on holistic view of children that includes social, emotional, behavioral, and cognitive development – programme strategies should be ecologically founded, focusing on individuals, their families, and their neighborhoods – based on concepts of inclusion (acceptance, understanding, opportunities for personal growth) and modeling – there are many pathways to health or illness that include local risk and protective factors → To prevent emotional and behavioral problems and promote general development in young children → To ensure that children have "better beginnings" in all their social environments, commencing with their family, and including their immediate neighborhood and local community	– Programme provides multiple components of service delivery built on existing services and resources, and on new models unique to the programme *Programme elements* • health integration: preconception information, prenatal education, well-baby clinics, parent/child health information • family visiting: provide social support, information on pregnancy, birth, nutrition, child development, and family issues • family support: playgroups, toy-lending, parenting workshops, employment training, ESL, information and referral, caregiver support, drop-in center • in-home support: family visitors, homemakers, home support workers • center based care and family home daycare • in-class or in-school programmes: breakfast programmes, parent training, leadership training, before/after school programmes	Community No manual Mental health providers, neighborhood residents Average cost: $1000/child/year; most effective site cost: $2000/child; yearcost with large volunteer support: $300/child/year

(*continued*)

Table 5.2.7 (*Continued*)

Name, Institute, Country[a], Reference	Target population, Age, Sex	Theoretical Orientation → Objectives	Description	Setting, Manual, Providers (Training)
Interpersonal Cognitive Problem-Solving (ICPS) Intervention Programme Hahneham Medical College and Hospital *USA* (Shure and Spivack, 1982)	Selective (African–American, low SES, living in inner-city) 4–5 years old Males and females	– cognitive ability and ability to solve interpersonal problems with peers and adults distinguish normal youngsters from those with behavioral difficulties – ICPS skills predict social adjustment and interpersonal competence – strongest predictors are abilities to offer alternative solutions to peer or authority-type problems and anticipate potential consequences to interpersonal actions → To reduce and prevent impulsive and inhibited behaviors in at-risk children by helping them learn to actively solve typical, everyday interpersonal problems, and building strength to cope with daily frustrations and conflicts	Eight weeks of daily 20-min group (n = 6–9) sessions of structured lessons *Programme elements* • variety of sequenced games, discussion, group interaction techniques • pictures, puppets, simple role-playing used to teach children to listen and observe others and to learn that others have thoughts, feelings, and motives in problem situations	School No manual Teachers

ESL: English as a second language classes; **SES**: Socioeconomic class
[a]The country in italic indicates where the programme was developed.

Table 5.2.8 Programmes targeting behavioral/conduct problems – Programme evaluation

Name, Institute, Country[a], Reference	Design →Objectives [type of evaluation] Methods (*outcome measures*)	Significant results programme versus control	
		Positive results	Negative/unexpected results
Promoting Alternative Thinking Strategies (PATHS) Conduct Problems Prevention Research Group, University of Washington *USA*, Netherlands, Belgium, Great Britain, Norway, Canada, Australia, Israel (Greenberg *et al.*, 1995; Bierman *et al.*, 1999; Bierman *et al.*, 2002)	RCT: $N = 7560$ children in 378 classrooms ($n = 198$ classrooms to Programme, $n = 180$ classrooms to Control) →To examine effectiveness of PATHS on emotional development of school-aged children [Analysis of programme effect] →To examine role of implementation quality in effectiveness of PATHS [Productivity analysis] Comparisons pre- and post-programme (*TOCA-R; SHP; CRF; authors' peer report of aggression, disruptive behavior, prosocial behavior and likeability; authors' assessment of teacher's effectiveness in implementing programme*)	• programme effective in improving children's emotional competence and reducing aggression in schools • greater change in students' ability to follow rules, express feelings appropriately • greater improvement in observer ratings of classroom atmosphere • greater improvement in peer ratings of aggression and disruptive behavior • 2 factors contribute to successful implementation: adequate support from school principal; high degree of classroom implementation	• no significant effects on teacher ratings of authority acceptance, cognitive concentration, social competence, or likeability

Table 5.2.8 (*Continued*)

Name, Institute, Country[a], Reference	Design →Objectives [type of evaluation] Methods (*outcome measures*)	Significant results programme versus control	
		Positive results	Negative/unexpected results
Better Beginnings, Better Futures Queen's University *Canada* (Sylvestre et al., 1993; Peters *et al.*, 2000; Peters, Petrunka, and Arnold, 2003)	Quasi-experimental: $N = 554$ ($n = 255$ to Programme, $n = 299$ to Control) Groups assigned by demographic region Two research plans implemented: (1) baseline-focal design, comparing 1992-93 cohort (before programme initiation) with 1997-98 cohort (after programme fully operational) ; (2) longitudinal comparison, following cohort of children who turned 4 in 1993 for 5 years →To evaluate effectiveness of programme [Analysis of programme effect] Comparisons pre-programme, 1-, 2-, 3-, 4-, and 5-year follow-up (*SSRS; ROCHS; PVT; WISC-R; WRAT; SRA; PSCS; parenting behaviors*)	Improved after 5 years: • children's and parents' social-emotional functioning (decrease in teacher-rated anxiety, increase in teacher-rated self-control, reduction of stressful life events for parents, improved marital satisfaction for parents) • child physical health (improved general health ratings; improved parent sense of control over child health) • parenting behaviors (decrease in smoking for parents) • neighborhood and school characteristics (increased satisfaction with condition of dwelling; improved relationship with teacher; more involvement in school)	

Interpersonal Cognitive Problem-Solving (ICPS) Intervention Programme Hahneham Medical College and Hospital *USA* (Shure and Spivack, 1982)	Quasi-experimental: $N = 219$ ($n = 113$ to Programme, $n = 106$ to Control) Group assignment by class →To evaluate effects of teaching problem-solving skills on healthy adaptive functioning [Analysis of programme effects, programme analysis, normative evaluation of process and structure] Comparisons pre-, post-programme, 6- and 12-month follow-up (*PIPS; WHNG; HPBS*)	• ICPS impact on behavior lasted at least 1 full year • training was effective in kindergarten and in nursery school • 1 year of intervention had same immediate impact as 2 years of intervention • greater increase in cognitive problem-solving at post-test • greater percentage of children became adjusted (71% versus 50%) at post-test • greater percentage of children who began programme as impulsive or inhibited became adjusted (50% versus 21%) at post-test	• at 6-months, problem-solving ability improved in control but not intervention group • groups did not differ in degree of improvement from post-test to 6- or 12-month follow-up

HPSB: Hahnemann Preschool Behavior Scale; **PIPS:** Preschool Interpersonal Problem-Solving Test; **PSCS:** Parental Sense of Competence Scale; **PVT:** Peabody Vocabulary Test; **RCT:** Randomized controlled trial; **ROCHS:** Revised Ontario Child Health Study; SHP: Social health profile; **SSRS:** Social Skills Rating Scales; TOCA-R: Teacher observation of classroom adaptation; **WHNG:** What Happens Next Game; **WISC-R:** Weschler Intelligence Scale for Children-Revised

[a]The country in italic indicates where the programme was developed.

Table 5.2.9 Programmes targeting post traumatic stress disorder (PTSD)

Name, Institute, Country[a], Reference	Target population, Age, Sex	Theoretical orientation → Objectives	Description	Setting, Manual, Providers (Training)
Cognitive Behavioral Intervention for Trauma in Schools (CBITS) The RAND Corporation *USA* (Stein *et al.*, 2003)	Indicated (substantial exposure to violence; screened for traumatic experiences and PTSD symptoms using LES and CPSS) 11–13 years old Males and females	– Based on concepts of CBT for PTSD →To address symptoms of PTSD, anxiety, depression related to exposure to violence →To improve psychosocial functioning and classroom behavior	– 10 weekly group (N = 5–8) sessions of one class period duration *Programme elements* • relaxation training: common reactions to stress or trauma and techniques to combat anxiety • cognitive therapy: linkage between thoughts and feelings and how to combat negative thoughts • real-life exposure: using imagination, drawing, writing to induce trauma memory • social problem solving: relapse prevention	School English manual (Jaycox, 2004) School mental health clinicians (2-day training and weekly supervision)

Trauma-Focused CBT Alleghany General Hospital Center for Traumatic Stress in Children and Adolescents *USA* (Cohen and Mannarino, 1997)	Selected (children who have experienced a traumatic life event) 3–18 years old Males and females	– Traumatized children may develop extreme fear of anything that reminds them of traumatic event, leading to avoidance of reminders and extreme emotional and physiological vigilance – Based on CBT model →To help children talk about traumatic experiences in supportive environment where they can become less fearful, less avoidant, more able to tolerate trauma-related thoughts and feelings	– 12–16 weekly individual sessions with child and one parent *Programme elements* • children taught to examine their thoughts, feelings and behaviors • children provided with tools to relax and solve problems • parents assisted to explore own thoughts and feelings about child's experience, learn effective parenting skills, provide optimal support to child	Clinical English and Spanish manual (no reference) Mental health worker (1–3 day training with manual)
Project Heartland Oklahoma Department of Mental Health and Substance Abuse Services *USA* (Call and Pfefferbaum, 1999; Pfefferbaum, Call, and Sconzo, 1999)	Universal No age range specified Males and females	– Based on four-phase model of disaster: (1) heroic phase (individual attempts to survive and help others); (2) honeymoon phase(characterized by optimism); (3) disillusionment (characterized by anger, cynicism, frustration); (4) reconstruction (people and community work to rebuild their lives) →To provide accessible and phase-appropriate crisis counseling, support groups, outreach, education for individuals affected by Oklahoma bombing	Designed for entire community, adult and child, with main goal as increasing accessibility of mental health services *Programme elements* • immediate individual and family therapy provided by mental health professionals • school-based educational and clinical services • teacher training in topics such as emotional impact of disaster, effects of trauma and grief on classroom behavior	Community No manual Mental health workers

CBT: Cognitive behavioral therapy; **CPSS:** Child-PTSD Symptom Scale; **LES:** Life events scale; **PTSD:** Post-traumatic stress-disorder
[a]The country in italic indicates where the programme was developed.

Table 5.2.10 Programmes targeting post-traumatic stress disorder – programme evaluation

Name, Institute, Country[a], Reference	Design →Objectives [type of evaluation] Methods (*outcome measures*)	Significant results programme versus control	
		Positive results	Negative/unexpected results
Cognitive Behavioral Intervention for Trauma in Schools (CBITS) The RAND Corporation *USA* (Stein *et al.*, 2003)	RCT: N = 113 (n = 53 to Programme, 60 to Control) →To evaluate effectiveness of collaboratively designed school-based intervention for reducing children's symptoms of PTSD and depression [Analysis of programme effects] Comparisons pre-programme and 3-month follow-up (*CPSS; CDI; PSCL; T-CRS*)	• at 3 months, fewer symptoms of PTSD, depression, and less psychosocial dysfunction	At follow-up, no difference in teacher-reported classroom acting out
Trauma-Focused CBT Alleghany General Hospital Center for Traumatic Stress in Children and Adolescents *USA* (Cohen *et al.*, 1997)	RCT: N = 43 (n=28 to Programme, n=15 to Control) - control condition designed to reduce isolation, loneliness, hopelessness and anxiety, by increasing support available to mother and child →To investigate effects of intervention on sexually abused preschool children [Analysis of programme effects] – comparisons pre-, post-programme, 6- and 12-month follow-up (*CBCL-PV; CSBI; WBR*)	• less acting-out behavior and fewer PTSD symptoms, greater improvement in depressive symptoms, reduction in sexually inappropriate behavior	
Project Heartland Oklahoma Department of Mental Health and Substance Abuse Services *USA* (Call and Pfefferbaum, 1999; Pfefferbaum, Call, and Sconzo, 1999)	Anecdotal clinical report →To describe and discuss development, implementation, and lessons learned from project's first 2 years [Normative evaluation of process and structure]	• programme appears to have acted as buffer for many of direct survivors of traumatic event • good acceptance of project by Oklahoma City's citizens • programmes are most effective when planned with people who will be participants	

CBCL-PV: Child Behavior Checkli st-Parent Version; **CDI:** Child Depression Inventory; **CPSS:** Child-PTSD Symptom Scale; **CSBI:** Child Sexual Behavior Inventory; **NST:** Nonspecific therapy
[a]The country in italic indicates where the programme was developed.

Table 5.2.11 Programmes targeting suicide – programme outline

Name, Institute, Country[a], Reference	Target population, Age, Sex	Theoretical orientation → Objectives	Description	Setting, Manual, Providers (Training)
Coping And Support Training (CAST) Reconnecting Youth Prevention Research Programme, University of Washington *USA* (Eggert *et al.*, 2002)	Indicated (students with poor academic performance, poor school attendance or prior school dropout, who screen at risk on Suicide Risk Screen) 14–19 years old Males and females	– access to help in youths' normal settings reduces barriers to seeking help and fosters increased self-efficacy – social support, in form of expressed empathy, meets basic human needs for acceptance and belonging, leading to adaptive growth and emotional well-being →To increase personal life skills competencies and social support resources, thereby influencing the co-occurring outcomes that increase suicidal risk (suicide-risk behavior, depression, drug use)	– Twelve 1-h group ($\underline{N}$ = 6–7) sessions over 6 weeks *Programme elements* • coping and skills training programme • counseling session and social intervention with parents and school personnel • individual assessment/ feedback, adult and peer support, skills training, to impact mediating factors (personal life skills competencies, social support resources)	School No manual Group leaders are Master-level high school teachers, counselors, or nurses with extensive school-based experience (weekly supervision with programme coordinator)
Signs of Suicide (SOS) Substance Abuse and Mental Health Services Admininstration (SAMHSA) , University of Conneticut *USA* (Aseltine, Jr. and DeMartino, 2004)	Universal 14–18 years old Males and females	– occurrence of suicide can be reduced through two components: (1) promotion of more adaptive attitudes toward depressive symptoms and suicidal behavior; (2) self-screening for depression and suicidal thoughts →To follow the ACT steps: A-*acknowledge* the signs of suicide; C-show the person you *care*; T-*tell* a responsible adult	– Two-day programme *Programme elements* • educational component: video dramatizations that depict signs of suicidality and depression, consequences of suicide, and how to react to these warning signs • self-screening: students complete CDS and score themselves using a scoring and interpretation sheet • students with high scores on CDS encouraged to seek help and provided with resources for assistance	School No manual Teachers

(*continued*)

Table 5.2.11 (*Continued*)

Name, Institute, Country[a], Reference	Target population, Age, Sex	Theoretical orientation → Objectives	Description	Setting, Manual, Providers (Training)
School-based Suicide Prevention Curriculum for Teenagers New York State Psychiatric Institute *USA* (Shaffer *et al.*, 1991; Vieland *et al.*, 1991)	Universal 14–15 years old Males and females	– suicidal students are more likely to discuss feelings and intentions with other students than with adults – students must be taught that if they are told by friend about intent to commit suicide, they must inform responsible adult →To increase awareness of adolescent suicide →To provide knowledge about "warning signs" of suicide →To make available treatment or counseling resources	– 1.5 to 4-h curriculum in classrooms *Programme elements* • mixture of didactic instruction and opportunities for discussion • emphasis on clinical features of suicidal adolescent and need to seek help from professionals	School No manual Teachers (6 to 10-h training)

CDS: Columbia Depression Scale
[a]The country in italic indicates where the programme was developed.

Table 5.2.12 Programmes targeting suicide – programme evaluation

Name, Institute, Country[a], Reference	Design →Objectives [type of evaluation] Methods (*outcome measures*)	Significant results programme versus control	
		Positive results	Negative/unexpected results
Coping And Support Training (CAST) Reconnecting Youth Prevention Research Programme, University of Washington *USA* (Eggert *et al.*, 2002)	RCT: $N = 341$ ($n = 103$ received CAST, $n = 121$ received usual care, $n = 117$ received C-CARE) – usual care: 30-min assessment interview – C-CARE: programme similar to CAST except no skills training/peer support →To evaluate post-intervention efficacy of CAST versus usual care versus C-CARE for reducing suicide risk [Analysis of programme effects] Comparisons pre-, post-programme, and 9-month follow-up (*High School Questionnaire: a Profile of Experience*)	• all three groups showed decline in depression, suicide-risk taking behaviors, and drug involvement • CAST and C-CARE produced greater reduction in depression than usual care • CAST produced more favorable reduction in alcohol use, hard drug use, and drug use problems than C-CARE and usual care	• follow-up data collection still in progress at time of publication
Signs of Suicide (SOS) Substance Abuse and Mental Health Services Admininstration (SAMHSA), University of Conneticut *USA* (Aseltine, Jr. and DeMartino, 2004)	RCT: $N = 2100$ ($n = 1027$ to Programme, $n = 1073$ to Control) →To assess short-term impact of programme on suicidal behavior, help-seeking, and knowledge of attitudes toward suicide and depression [Analysis of programme effects]	• greater knowledge of depression and suicide, and more adaptive attitudes toward these problems • fewer self-reported suicide attempts (3.6% versus 5.4%)	• nonsignificant trend for intervention group to be less likely to seek help for emotional problems than control group

(continued)

Table 5.2.12 *(Continued)*

Name, Institute, Country[a], Reference	Design →Objectives [type of evaluation] Methods (*outcome measures*)	Significant results programme versus control Positive results	 Negative/unexpected results
	Comparisons post-programme only (*Author's self report measures on suicide attempts, help-seeking behaviors, suicidal behaviors and thoughts, knowledge and attitudes toward suicide, depression, and suicidal individuals*)		
School-based Suicide Prevention Curriculum for Teenagers New York State Psychiatric Institute *USA* (Shaffer *et al.*, 1991; Vieland *et al.*, 1991)	Quasi-experimental design: *N* = 1438 students (*n* = 758 to Programme; *n* = 680 to Control) Group assignment by school (*N* = 11 schools) → To examine acquisition of suicide-related information and changes in attitudes toward suicide and help-seeking for emotional problems, after exposure to suicide curriculum [Analysis of programme effects and process] Comparisons pre-programme, 1-month and 18-month follow-up (*Authors' self-report questionnaire on attitudes to suicide, warning signs, help-seeking for emotional distress*)	• 2/3 students in intervention group rated programme as comforting; 4/5 stated programme would help them deal with friends' problems; <10% found programme upsetting or knew someone upset by programme • programme effective in increasing students' knowledge about where to get help for emotional problems	• higher proportion of students exposed to programme changed their minds to indicate that they now could see suicide as a reasonable solution • high proportion of students knew and subscribed to some of programme goals before exposure to programme • no evidence of programme effect at 18 months (suicide attempts = 2.5% versus 2.7%)

[a]The country in italic indicates where the programme was developed.

Table 5.2.13 Programmes targeting general health promotion – programme outline

Name, Institute, Country[a], Reference	Target population, Age, Sex	Theoretical orientation → Objectives	Description	Settinging, Manual, Providers (Training)
Gatehouse Project (GHP) Center for Adolescent Health, Melbourne *Australia* (Patton *et al.*, 2000; Patton *et al.*, 2003)	Universal 13–19 years old Males and females	– based on attachment theory – anxiety and depressive symptoms are more likely to arise when social and interpersonal bonds are threatened or insecure – sense of connectedness is unifying factor that can improve individual characteristics (learning, health, emotional well-being) as well as social and learning environments →To instill sense of connectedness, effective communication, perception of adults caring, to promote positive behavioral and health outcomes →To instill sense of active engagement and broader participation to lead to more supportive social environment →To prevent or delay onset of depressive symptoms through promotion of positive school social environment	– broad-based approach directed to individual students as well as school and social environment – focuses on three facets of social context -security, communication, participation- to promote sense of connectedness with school, and buffer changes in attachment to family, teachers and peers that occur in adolescence – standardized process of intervention, but programme relies on repeated reviews to provide strategies based on each school's profile of needs *Programme elements* • school social climate profile, derived from questionnaire survey of students (re: security, communication, participation, health risk behaviors, socially disruptive behavior, depression, deliberate self-harm, bullying, perceived social, and emotional support) • school-based action team, drawn from staff members, using survey information to set priorities for changes within school (health education curriculum, changing school structure) • Critical Friends: Gatehouse Project staff members, responsible for support, training and resources for implementation	School English manual: "Gatehouse Project Training Package" School-based action team (6-h teacher development programme, then weekly sessions with Gatehouse Project staff)

(*continued*)

Table 5.2.13 *(Continued)*

Name, Institute, Country[a], Reference	Target population, Age, Sex	Theoretical orientation → Objectives	Description	Setting, Manual, Providers (Training)
			• whole school strategies: guidelines based on school climate profile • promotion of positive classroom climate • early high school curriculum addressing skills relevant to social functioning and emotional adjustment	
Well-Being Therapy University of Bologna *Italy* (Fava and Ruini, 2003)	Indicated (subclinical or in remission – affective disorder, OCD, body image disorder) Age range not specified Males and females	– based on concepts of positive psychology and Ryff' (1989) model of well-being – well-being can mitigate vulnerability to stressors →To improve subject's level of psychological well being, encompassing six dimensions: autonomy, personal growth, environmental master, purpose in life, positive relations, self-acceptance	– eight individual 30–50-min therapy sessions – focuses on instances of well-being rather than distress – short-term psychotherapy that is structured, directive, problem-oriented, based on an educational model – emphasis on self-observation *Programme elements* • patient and therapist first identify episodes of well-being, and thoughts and beliefs that disrupt well-being • irrational thoughts are challenged by therapist • activities conducive to well-being are reinforced through task assignment • Ryff's dimensions of well-being are explained in a manner relevant to subject	Clinical No manual Clinicians, therapists

Kuumba Kids Progressive Life Centre, Arts and Cultural Council for Greater Rochester *USA* (Mason and Chuang, 2001)	Selective (African–American, low SES, inner-city) 7–10 years old Males and females	– based on seven Nguzo Saba principles that promote healthy African-based values within an American/Western context – formal after school programmes provide rich social experience – participation in arts programmes leads to academic success and sense of competency →To provide a vehicle for African–American artists to serve as role models by working with young people who share cultural heritage →To use arts to build constructive behavior patterns for urban children living in poor neighborhoods	– one semester: 16 weekly 2-h sessions Programme elements • culturally relevant after-school arts-based programme • key components: cultural awareness, cultural pride, cultural history • engage children in drama and dance activities, to assist in development of self-esteem, noncompetitive creativity, and creative problem solving	Community (after -school) No manual African–American artists (supervised by Arts and Cultural Council for Greater Rochester)

SES: Socio-economic class
[a]The country in italic indicates where the programme was developed.

was developed in Australia and has been adapted for use in the United States, Germany, Canada, the Netherlands, the United Kingdom, Ireland, Portugal, and New Zealand (Barrett *et al.*, 2000; Mohr *et al.*, 2001; Shortt *et al.*, 2001; Barrett *et al.*, 2003). The *Penn Prevention Programme*, later renamed *Penn Resiliency Programme* (Adaptive Learning Systems, 2000; Gillham *et al.*, 1995; Gillham and Reivich, 1999; Jaycox *et al.*, 1994), was developed in Pennsylvania and has been adapted for implementation in other parts of the United States, Canada, Australia, and China. The eating disorders prevention programme, *Go Girls* (Wade, Davidson, and O'Dea, 2003), has been implemented in both the United States and .

Target population

Most of the programmes (n = 26) are universal and appropriate for all types of youth. A number of programmes (n = 14) targeted a selective population. Examples of these at-risk youth are: those who have witnessed or experienced a traumatic event (Cohen and Mannarino, 1997; Stein *et al.*, 2003); and children of divorce (Garvin *et al.*, 1991) or of substance abusing parents (Aktan *et al.*, 1996). The remaining programmes (n = 7) targeted indicated populations displaying diverse symptoms but not regarded as having a mental disorder according to identified diagnostic criteria, such as anxious children who do not meet criteria for an anxiety disorder (Dadds *et al.*, 1997); or subjects who have screened at-risk for depression (Jaycox *et al.*, 1994; Gillham *et al.*, 1995; Gillham and Reivich, 1999). Most of the programmes are appropriate for both boys and girls (n = 43); only a small number (n = 4) are targeted for girls only. No programme is indicated for a male population alone. The programmes reviewed target age groups ranging from birth to 25 years. Most programmes (n = 38) are indicated for preadolescents/adolescents (12–19 years). A large number (n = 27) are aimed at children in middle childhood (6–11 years). Few programmes (n = 9) are designed for infants and children in early childhood (0–5 years). Some programmes span more than one age category. Two do not specify an age range but are considered appropriate for youth in general (Call and Pfefferbaum, 1999; Pfefferbaum *et al.*, 1999; Fava and Ruini, 2003).

Implementation Setting

The wide majority of programmes (n = 32) were administered in school settings. A number of programmes (n = 6) were intended either solely for a community setting or for a setting in schools as well as the community (n = 4). The remaining programmes (n = 5) were designed for clinical settings.

Availability of a Standardized Manual

Of the 47 programmes reviewed, 26 refer to a standardized manual for implementation. Nineteen programmes indicate that the manual is available in English; two programmes have both English and Spanish versions; one programme manual is available in French;

one in English, German, and Dutch; one in German; and two programmes do not specify in what language the manual is available.

Providers of the programmes

The majority of the programmes reviewed are designed for delivery by teachers (n = 23), mental health professionals or graduate students (n = 16). Other providers include school nurses and school health personnel (n = 6), police officers (n = 1), artists (n = 1), girl scout leaders (n = 1), and adult community leaders (n = 3). Four programmes employ "youth facilitators" or peer leaders to deliver some or all of the programmes. Twenty-four programmes describe some sort of training with regard to implementation of programme content, programme philosophy, or general information concerning adolescent needs and problems. Training duration ranged from 3 to 40 hours.

Estimates of cost of implementing programmes

Only three of the 47 programmes report the average cost of programme implementation. The cost of the *PATHS* programme (Greenberg *et al.*, 1995; Kam *et al.*, 2003) was reported as ranging from $15 to 45 per student per year. The average cost reported for the *Better Beginnings, Better Futures* project (Sylvestre and Brophy, 1993; Peters *et al.*, 2000; Peters *et al.*, 2003) was $1000 per child per year, the developers specify that the cost at the most effective site was $2000 per child per year, whereas, in other sites with large volunteer support, the cost could be reduced to $300 per child per year. The cost of the *FRIENDS* programme was estimated at £24–34 (approximately $ 47–67)per student per term (Barrett *et al.*, 2000; Mohr *et al.*, 2001; Shortt *et al.*, 2001; Barrett *et al.*, 2003).

Programme outcome evaluation

As a criterion for inclusion in this review, all programmes had to be assessed for efficacy, either formally or informally. If there was more than one report describing the evaluation of a programme, only one was selected for review. Although the reports often referred to the same evaluation at different time points, the most recent report was used, as it included the results in earlier reports.

The design, objectives, methods, and main findings (either expected or uncertain/negative) for all programme evaluation studies are summarized in Tables 5.2.2–5.2.14, with programmes being grouped according to the disorders targeted, as for corresponding programme outlines (Tables 5.2.1–5.2.13).

Most of the programmes were evaluated using a quasi-experimental design (n = 24), in which the group receiving the prevention programme and the control group (no intervention or alternative programme) were not randomly assigned. Seventeen programmes had RCT designs, in which subjects were randomly assigned to either the programme or a control condition. One study did not specify how the groups were assigned (Mason and Chuang, 2001). Five programmes used a within-subject pre- and post-intervention evaluation,

Table 5.2.14 Programmes targeting general health promotion – programme evaluation

Name, Institute, Country[a], Reference	Design →Objectives [type of evaluation] Methods (*outcome measures*)	Significant results programme versus control	
		Positive results	Negative/unexpected results
Gatehouse Project (GHP) Center for Adolescent Health, Melbourne *Australia* (Patton *et al.*, 2000; Patton *et al.*, 2003)	Quasi-experimental: N = 2463 students in 26 schools (12 schools to Programme, 14 to Control) →To determine programme's effectiveness and any changes to be made [Analysis of programme effects] "Social climate profile" completed by grade eight students in 1997, 1999, 2001Cohort of grade eight students in 1997 followed in high school on four occasions (*Authors' self-report measures on health risk behaviors, socially disruptive behavior, depression, deliberate self-harm, school connection, bullying, perceived social, and emotional support*)	• substantial and sustained change in behavioral profile of students (i.e., smoking, drug-use, having friends who smoke or use drugs) • prevalence of tobacco use lower both in cross-sectional and cohort sample • reduction in marijuana use	• no reduction in depressive symptoms
Well-Being Therapy University of Bologna *Italy* (Fava and Ruini, 2003)	RCT including subjects who had responded to pharmacotherapy with antidepressant: N = 20 (n = 10 to Programme, n = 10 to Control) – intervention: well-being therapy part of CBT package combined with lifestyle modification	• lower relapse rate • lower level of residual symptoms • lower level of cognitive symptoms associated with depression	• difficult to isolate specific contribution of well-being therapy to overall outcomes

	– Control: usual clinical management →To determine intervention's effect on preventing future depressive episodes after termination of drug treatment with antidepressant [Analysis of programme effects] Comparisons pre- and post-programme (*CID, Personal Growth Scale*)	
Kuumba Kids Progressive Life Centre, Arts and Cultural Council for Greater Rochester *USA* (Mason and Chuang, 2001)	Study sample include 18 parents (n = 9 with children in Programme, n = 9 in Control) and 33 children (n = 17 in Programme; n = 16 in Control) . Group assignment not specified →To evaluate programme effect on adaptive functioning and problem behaviors [Analysis of programme effects] Comparisons pre- and post-programme (*BASC -self-report, parent form, and teacher form-; authors' self-report measures on self-reliance, self-esteem, negative attitude towards school*)	• *self-report*: increase in self-esteem, social skills, leadership competencies • *parents' report*: child attention problems reduced; social skills and leadership competencies increased • *teachers' report*: lower scores for social withdrawal and attention problems, higher scores for social skills and leadership

BASC: Behavior Assessment System for Children; **CID:** Clinical Interview for Depression; **OCD:** Obsessive compulsive disorder; **RCT:** Randomized controlled trial
[a]The country in italic indicates where the programme was developed.

with no comparison group. Other methods for programme evaluation included an informal survey ($n = 1$), and an anecdotal clinical report ($n = 1$).

Regarding the types of programme evaluation [using Breton *et al.* (2002) categorization], most evaluations ($n = 44$) examined programme effects. A small number of evaluations sought to examine the programme's process ($n = 6$) or structure ($n = 3$). Four evaluations analyzed the programme's theoretical basis (programme analysis). Analyses of programme implementation ($n = 1$) and productivity ($n = 1$) were also reported. Most of the evaluations ($n = 45$) reported results supporting programme efficacy. However, twenty-seven studies reported both negative and positive results. Three studies reported only negative results, or indicated no significant programme effect (Moskowitz *et al.*, 1983; Malvin *et al.*, 1984; Clarke *et al.*, 1993).

DISCUSSION

The findings suggest that evidence-based primary prevention programmes directed to child and adolescent mental health exist and are available. Almost all the evidence we could retrieve is from the United States or other industrialized countries. However, it is quite possible that the paucity of published evidence-based preventive programmes designed and applied in other countries is partly due to a publication bias. Our literature search was limited to reports available through a regional library in either French or English, which necessarily narrowed the scope of our findings.

Many reasons can be posited to explain why substance abuse and depressive/anxiety disorders were the disorders most often targeted by the programmes retrieved. Given that most of the programmes are administered in the United States, it is not surprising that substance abuse is a common focus of prevention. The abundance of substance abuse prevention programmes in the United States is a product of need (based on epidemiological data) and feasibility (due to legislation and the availability of governmental funding and support). The prevalence of lifetime substance abuse and dependence in the United States is as high as 26.6% (Jaffe, 2000). Legislation passed in 1986 authorized the United States government to spend nearly $4 billion dollars on efforts against drugs and drug abuse. Bodies such as the Substance Abuse and Mental Health Services Administration (SAMHSA) work together to facilitate drug and alcohol abuse prevention (Jaffe, 2000).

Substance abuse and depressive/anxiety disorders have identifiable risk factors that help to focus preventive efforts. For example, a number of programmes target children and adolescents whose parents have either substance abuse problems or an affective disorder (Jaycox *et al.*, 1994; Gillham *et al.*, 1995; Aktan *et al.*, 1996; Beardslee *et al.*, 1997; Gillham and Reivich, 1999), as well as children who exhibit high-risk behavior such as dropping out of school (Eggert *et al.*, 2002; Eggert *et al.*, 1994).

Adolescence is a time when many mental health problems emerge, and this is particularly the case for substance abuse disorders. By the twelfth grade, 79.2% of students in the United States report having used alcohol (Jaffe, 2000). Although adolescent experimentation does not necessarily lead to abuse or dependency, it has been reported that the first evidence of alcohol-related problems is usually observed in the late teenage years (Jaffe, 2000). Similarly, depressive and anxiety disorders often begin at school age, making the teenage years a favorable time for prevention (Blazer, 2000).

It is not surprising that most of the programmes reviewed were implemented in school settings. Most children and adolescents in industrialized countries spend the bulk of their time at school, and schools are ideal for reaching children with a broad spectrum of mental health conditions, especially those who may be experiencing the first signs of a disorder but are not yet receiving treatment. A number of the school programmes reviewed involved a community component (Werch, 1991; Perry *et al.*, 1993; Komro *et al.*, 1994; Komro *et al.*, 1996; Perry *et al.*, 1996; Perry *et al.*, 2000; Dedobbeleer and Desjardins, 2001; Komro *et al.*, 2001; Perry *et al.*, 2002; Steiner-Adair *et al.*, 2002), endorsing the benefit of community involvement.

In light of the fact that schools are the setting of choice for the majority of prevention programmes reviewed, it follows that teachers are most often delivering these programmes. Teachers have regular contact with children and youth, and their teaching skills translate readily into counseling and administering prevention curricula. A small number of effective programmes were successfully delivered by police officers, local artists, and Girl Scout leaders, which suggests that effective prevention needs not be limited to the classroom.

The large number of school-delivered programmes explains why the vast majority of the programmes targeted school-aged children and adolescents, and are largely universally applicable to both sexes. A small number of programmes aimed specifically at girls were designed in that way because of the nature of the disorder targeted: all four programmes aimed at preventing eating disorders (Neumark-Sztainer *et al.*, 2000; Stewart *et al.*, 2001; Stice *et al.*, 2001; Steiner-Adair *et al.*, 2002), which are much more prevalent in females than in males (Fairburn and Beglin, 1990; Wolf, 1991).

Although few of the programmes reviewed recommend translation to other countries, cultures or groups, it was noted by the reviewers that most of them had potential for export. However, the school-based programmes delivered by teachers might not be directly transposable to countries where school staff is limited or school attendance is low.

RCTs are considered the most scientifically robust empirical design for demonstrating the efficacy of a therapeutic or preventive intervention. They are therefore most likely to be published in the scientific literature. However, the implementation of most of the programmes reviewed in school settings may explain why the majority were evaluated according to a quasi-experimental design. This type of evaluation is the most compatible with school populations, as groups can be assigned by school or classroom. It would be impracticable to allocate students randomly to different conditions within the one classroom or school, and there would be a danger of cross-contamination between students. It is possible that some school- or community-based prevention programmes are not documented in the scientific literature because they employed unscientific methods to evaluate their impact, and were not endorsed by the academic community.

Lacking from most published reports is an estimate of the cost of programme implementation. Only three of the 47 programmes estimated the cost of delivering the intervention. Prevention is aimed at large groups, and cost estimates are crucial if communities are to decide whether they will implement particular programmes. Cost estimates would also enable prevention researchers and policy makers to compare and contrast cost-effectiveness.

CONCLUSION

Although child and adolescent mental health is crucial for the future of individuals and societies, it has not yet received enough political and research attention. Although priorities vary from country to country, the need to prevent child and adolescent psychiatric disorders is universal. The primary prevention programmes identified in this review demonstrate that effective programmes are available and could be incorporated into the lives of young people around the world, to improve their current and future mental health. The programmes described can also be used as prototypes for future programmes that could be rigorously examined in modern empirical designs. Greater efforts are required to design and disseminate scientifically sound, evidence-based interventions, to promote healthy psychological development in children and adolescents worldwide, and to address the factors known to be linked to specific mental disorders.

REFERENCES

Adaptive Learning Systems (2000) *Penn Resiliency Project: A Depression–Prevention and Life-Skills Porgram for Children and Adolescents. Executive Summary*, Adaptive Learning Systems, King of Prussia, PA.

Aktan, G. B., Bridges, S. D., and Kumpfer, K. L. (1994) *The Safe Haven Program: Strengthening African–American Families. Parent Training Manual*, Detroit Department of Health, Bureau of Substance Abuse, Detroit.

Aktan, G. B., Kumpfer, K. L., and Turner, C. W. (1996) Effectiveness of a family skills training program for substance use prevention with inner city African–American families. *Subst Use Misuse*, **31**, 157–75.

Ambtman, R., Madak, P., Koss, D., and Strople, M. J. (1990) Evaluation of a comprehensive elementary school curriculum-based drug education program. *J Drug Ed*, **20**, 199–225.

APA (1994) *Diagnostic and Statistical Resource Book of Mental Disorders (DSM-IV)*, 4th Edition, American Psychiatric Association, Washington, DC.

Aseltine, R. H., Jr. and DeMartino, R. (2004) An outcome evaluation of the SOS Suicide Prevention Program. *Am J Public Health*, **94**, 446–51.

Ayers, T. S., Short, J. L., Gensheimer, L. K. *et al.* (1989) *The Stress Managemetn and Alcohol Awareness Program: A Preventive Intervention for Children of Problem Drinking Parents. Group Leader's Manual*, Program for Prevention Research Arizona State University, Tempe.

Bandura, A. (1977) *Social Learning Theory*, Prentice Hall, Englewood Cliffs.

Bandura, A. (1996) *Social Foundation of Thought and Actions: A Social Cognitive Theory*, Prentice Hall, Englewood Cliffs.

Barkley, R. A., Shelton, T. L., Crosswait, C. *et al.* (2000) Multi-method psycho-educational intervention for preschool children with disruptive behavior: Preliminary results at post-treatment. *J Child Psychol Psychiatry Allied Dis*, **41**, 319–32.

Barlow, J. and Coren, E. (2000) Parent-training programmes for improving maternal psychosocial health. *Cochrane Database Sys Rev*, CD002020.

Barlow, J. and Coren, E. (2001) Parent-training programmes for improving maternal psychosocial health (update of Cochrane Database Syst Rev. 2000;(4):CD002020; PMID: 11034741). *Cochrane Database Syst Rev*, CD002020 (Review) and references therein.

Barlow, J. and Coren, E. (2004) Parent-training programmes for improving maternal psychosocial health. *Cochrane Database Sys Rev*, CD002020.

Barrett, P. M., Dadds, M. R., and Holland, D. E. (1994) *The Coping Koala: Prevention Manual*, University of Queensland, Queensland.

Barrett, P. M., Moore, A. F., and Sonderegger, R. (2000) The FRIENDS program for young former Yugoslavian refugees in Australia: A pilot study. *Behav Change*, **17**, 124–33.

Barrett, P. M. and Turner, C. M. (2001) Prevention of anxiety symptoms in primary school children: Preliminary results from a universal trial. *Br J Clin Psychology*, **40**, 399–410.

Barrett, P. M., Webster, H., and Turner, C. (2003) Introduction to FRIENDS – A Program for Enhancing Life Skills. www.friendsinfo.net

Beardslee, W. R. and Gladstone, T. R. (2001) Prevention of childhood depression: Recent findings and future prospects. *Bio Psychiatry*, **49**, 1101–10 (Review) and references therein.

Beardslee, W. R., Hoke, L., Wheelock, I. *et al.* (1992) Initial findings on preventive intervention for families with parental affective disorders. *Am J Psychiatry*, **149**, 1335–40.
Beardslee, W. R., Versage, E. M., Wright, E. J. *et al.* (1997) Examination of preventive interventions for families with depression: Evidence of change. *Dev Psychopathol*, **9**, 109–30.
Bell, R. M., Ellickson, P. L., and Harrison, E. R. (1993) Do drug prevention effects persist into high school? How project ALERT did with ninth graders. *Prev Med*, **22**, 463–83 (see comments).
Bierman, K. L., Coie, J. D., Dodge, K. A. *et al.* (1999) Initial impact of the fast track prevention trial for conduct problems: II classroom effects. *J Consult Clin Psychol*, **67**, 48–657.
Bierman, K. L., Coie, J. D., Dodge, K. A. *et al.* (2002) Using the Fast Track randomized prevention trial to test the early-starter model of the development of serious conduct problems. *Dev Psychopathol*, **14**, 925–43.
Bird, H. R. (1996) Epidemiology of childhood disorders in a cross-cultural context. *J Child Psychol Psychiatry*, **37**, 35–49.
Blazer, D. G. (2000) Mood disorder: Epidemiology, in *Comprehensive Textbook of Psychiatry* (eds B. J. Sadock and V. A. Sadock), 7th Edition, Lippincott Williams & Wilkins, Philadelphia, PA, pp. 1298–307.
Breton, J. J., Boyer, R., Bilodeau, H. *et al.* (2002) Is evaluative research on youth suicide programs theory-driven? The Canadian experience. *Suicide Life Threat Behav*, **32**, 176–90.
Briar, S. and Piliavin, I. (1965) Deliquency, situational inducements and commitment to conformity. *Soc Probl*, **13**, 25–45.
Briggs, D. (1970) *Your Child's Self Esteem*, Doubleday, New York.
Buddeberg-Fischer, B., Klaghofer, R., Reed, V., and Buddeberg, C. (2000) Curriculum module for health promotion. Results of a controlled intervention study in 2 high schools. *Sozial.- und Praventivmedizin*, **45**, 191–202 (in German).
Call, J. A. and Pfefferbaum, B. (1999) Lessons from the first two years of Project Heartland, Oklahoma's mental health response to the 1995 bombing. *Psychiatr Serv*, **50**, 953–55.
Capuano, F. (1995) Evaluation d'une intervention dans le milieu familial auprès de mères dont les enfants d'age préscolaire song anxieux et isolés. *Doctoral thesis*, Université de Montreal.
Carpenter, R. A., Lyons, C. A., and Miller, W. R. (1985) Peer-managed self-control program for prevention of alcohol abuse in American Indian high school students: A pilot evaluation study. *Int J Addict*, **20**, 299–310.
Carr, A. (2002) *Prevention: What Works with Children and Adolescents.* Taylor and Francis Inc., New York.
Champagne, F., Contandriopoulos, A. P., and Pineault, R. (1986) A health care evaluation framework. *Health Manag Forum*, 57–65.
Clarke, G. N. (1991) *Adolescent depression health class curriculum*, 2nd Edition, Oregon Health Sciences University, Portland.
Clarke, G., Hawkins, W., Murphy, M., and Sheeber, L. (1993) School-based primary prevention of depressive symptomatology in adolescents: Findings from two studies. *J Adolesc Res*, **8**, 183–204.
Cohen, J. A. and Mannarino, A. P. (1997) A treatment study for sexually abused preschool children: Outcome during a one-year follow-up. *J Am Acad Child Adolesc Psychiatry*, **36**, 1228–35.
Cuijpers, P., Jonkers, R., de Weerdt, I., and de Jong, A. (2002) The effects of drug abuse prevention at school: The 'Healthy School and Drugs' project. *Addiction*, **97**, 67–73.
Dadds, M. R., Spence, S. H., Holland, D. E. *et al.* (1997). Prevention and early intervention for anxiety disorders: A controlled trial. *J Consult Clin Psychol*, **65**, 627–35.
De Vries, H., Weijts, W., and Kok, G. (1992) The utilization of qualitative and quantitative data for health education programme planning, implementation and evaluation: A spiral approach. *Health Educ Q*, **19**, 101–15.
Dedobbeleer, N. and Desjardins, S. (2001) Outcomes of an ecological and participatory approach to prevent alcohol and other drug "abuse" among multiethnic adolescents. *Sub Use Misuse*, **36**, 1959–91.
Durlak, J. A. and Wells, A. M. (1997) Primary prevention mental health programs for children and adolescents: A meta-analytic review. *Am J Community Psychol*, **25**, 115–52.
Eating Disorder Awareness and Prevention, Inc. (1999). *GO GIRLS!*™, EDAP, Seattle.
Eggert, L. L., Thompson, E. A., Herting, J. R. *et al.* (1994) Preventing adolescent drug abuse and high school dropout through an intensive school-based social network development program. *Am J Health Promot*, **8**, 202–15.

Eggert, L. L., Thompson, E. A., Randell, B. P., and Pike, K. C. (2002) Preliminary effects of brief school-based prevention approaches for reducing youth suicide-risk behaviors, depression, and drug involvement. *J Child Adolesc Psychiatr Nurs*, **15**, 48–64.

El-Hazmi, M. A. F. (1997) Early recognition and intervention for prevention of disability and its complications. *East Mediterr Health J*, **3**, 154–61.

Ellickson, P. and Bell, R. (1990) Prospects for preventing drug use among young adolescents. *ERIC Digest.*

Fairburn, C. G. and Beglin, S. J. (1990) Studies of the epidemiolgoy of bulimia nervosa. *Am.J.Psychiatry*, **147**, 401–08.

Fava, G. A. and Ruini, C. (2003) Development and characteristics of a well-being enhancing psychotherapeutic strategy: Well-being therapy. *J Behav Ther Exp Psychiatry*, **34**, 45–63.

Garvin, V., Leber, D., and Kalter, N. (1991) Children of divorce: Predictors of change following preventive intervention. *Am J Orthopsychiatry*, **61**, 438–47.

Giel, R., de Arango, M. V., Climent, C. E. *et al.* (1981) Childhood mental disorders in primary health care: Results of observations in four developing countries. A report from the WHO collaborative study on strategies for extending mental health care. *Pediatrics*, **68**, 677–83.

Gillham, J. and Reivich, K. J. (1999) Prevention of depressive symptoms in schoolchildren: A research update. *Psychol Sci*, **10**, 461–62.

Gillham, J., Reivich, K. J., Jaycox, L. H., and Seligman, M. E. (1995a) Prevention of depressive symptoms in schoolchildren: Two-year follow-up. *Psychol Sci*, **6**, 343–51.

Gordon, R. (1987). An operational classification of disease prevention, in *Preventing Mental Disorders: A Research Perspective* (eds J. Steinberg and M. Silverman), Department of Health and Human Services, National Institute of Mental Health, Bathesda, MD, pp. 20–26.

Graham, J. W., Johnson, C. A., Hansen, W. B. *et al.* (1990) Drug use prevention programs, gender, and ethnicity: Evaluation of three seventh-grade Project SMART cohorts. *Prev Med*, **19**, 305–13.

Green, J. J. and Kelley, J. M. (1989) Evaluating the effectiveness of a school drug and alcohol prevention curriculum: A new look at "Here's Looking at You, Two". *J Drug Ed*, **19**, 117–32.

Greenberg, M. T., Kusche, C., Cook, E. T., and Quamma, J. P. (1995) Promoting emotional competence in school-aged children: The effects of the PATHS curriculum. *Dev Psychopathol*, **7**, 117–36.

Hains, A. A. (1992) A stress inoculation training program for adolescents in a high school setting: a multiple baseline approach. *Journal of Adolescence*, 15 163–175.

Hains, A. A. and Szyjakowski, M. (1990) A cognitive stress-reduction intervention program for adolescents. *J Couns Psychol*, **37**, 79–84.

Hansen, W. B., Johnson, C. A., Flay, B. R. *et al.* (1988) Affective and social influences approaches to the prevention of multiple substance abuse among seventh grade students: Results from project SMART. *Prev Med*, **17**, 135–54.

Institute of Medicine (1994). *Reducing Risks for Mental Disorders: Frontiers for Preventive Intervention Research.* National Academy Press, Washington, D.C.

Jaffe, J. H. (2000). Substance-related disorders, in *Comprehensive Textbook of Psychiatry* (eds B. J. Sadock and V. A. Sadock),7th Edition, Lippincott Williams & Wilkins, Philidelphia, PA, pp. 924–1095.

Jaycox, L. H. (2004) *Cognitive-Behavioral Intervention for Trauma in Schools* (in press) West Educational Services, Longmont.

Jaycox, L. H., Reivich, K. J., Gillham, J., and Seligman, M. E. (1994). Prevention of depressive symptoms in school children. *Behav Res Therapy*, **32**, 801–16.

Kalter, N., Schaefer, M., Lesowitz, M. *et al.* (1988) School-based support groups for children of divorce: A model of brief intervention, in *Marshalling social support: Formats, processes and effects* (ed B. H.Gottlieb), Sage Publications, Newbury Park, CA, pp. 165–85.

Kam, C. M., Greenberg, M. T., and Walls, C. T. (2003) Examining the role of implementation quality in school-based prevention using the PATHS curriculum. Promoting Alternative Thinking Skills Curriculum. *Prev Sci*, **4**, 55–63.

Kaplan, H. B. (1980) Self-esteem and self-derogation theory of drug abuse, in *Theories of Drug Abuse: Selected Contemporary Perspectives, NIDA Research Monograph 30*, NIDA, Rockville, pp. 128–31.

Kim, S., McLeod, J. H., and Shantzis, C. (1990) A short-term outcome evaluation of the "I'm Special" drug abuse prevention program: A revisit using SCAT inventory. *J Drug Educ*, **20**, 127–38.

Knapp, M., McCrone, P., Fombonne, E. *et al.* (2002) The Maudsley long-term follow-up of child and adolescent depression: 3. Impact of comorbid conduct disorder on service use and costs in adulthood. *Br.J Psychiatry*, **180**, 19–23.

Kolvin, I. (1994) Prevention in psychiatric specialties: Child psychiatry, in *Prevention in Psychiatry* (eds E. S.Paykel and R. Jenkins), The Royal College of Psychiatrists, London, pp. 115–29.

Komro, K. A., Perry, C. L., Murray, D. M. *et al.* (1996) Peer-planned social activities for preventing alcohol use among young adolescents. *J Sch Health*, **66**, 328–34.

Komro, K. A., Perry, C. L., Veblen-Mortenson, S., and Williams, C. L. (1994) Peer participation in Project Northland: A community-wide alcohol use prevention project. *J Sch Health*, **64**, 318–22.

Komro, K. A., Perry, C. L., Williams, C. L. *et al.* (2001) How did Project Northland reduce alcohol use among young adolescents? Analysis of mediating variables. *Health Educ Res*, **16**, 59–70.

Kornhouser, R. R. (1978) *Social Sources of Delinquency: An Appraisal of Analytic Models*. University of Chicago Press, Chicago.

Kraus, D., Dupree, T., and Bolcskei, P. L. (2003) Parents as partners in school-based health promotion and addiction prevention: an empirical study for the example of Class2000. *Gesundheitswesen*, **65**, 371–77 (in German).

Krupka, L. F. and Knox, L. A. (1985) Enhancing the effectiveness of alcohol and substance abuse prevention programs for children. *Int J Addic*, **20**, 1435–42.

LaFreniere, P. J. and Capuano, F. (1997) Preventive intervention as means of clarifying direction of effects in socialization: Anxious-withdrawn preschoolers case. *Dev Psychopathol*, **9**, 551-564.

Lesesne, T. S. (1986) *I'm Special: A Program for Third and Fourth Graders*. The Drug Education Center Publications, Charlotte.

Lowry-Webster, H. M., Barrett, P. M., and Dadds, M. R. (2001) A universal prevention trial of anxiety and depressive symptomatology in childhood: Preliminary data from an Australian study. *Behav Change*, **18**, 36–50.

Lowry-Webster, H. M., Barrett, P. M., and Lock, S. (2003) A universal prevention trial of anxiety symptomatology during childhood: Results at one-year follow-up. *Behav Change*, **20**, 25–43.

Lynam, D. R., Milich, R., Zimmerman, R. *et al.* (1999) Project DARE: No effects at 10-year follow-up. *J Consult Clin Psychol*, **67**, 590–93.

Lyons, C. A., Carpenter, R. A., and Strelich, A. J. (1981) *The Intermountain Model: An American Indian Peer-assisted Alcohol Abuse Prevention Program*. National Institute on Alcohol Abuse and Alcoholism, Brigham City.

Malvin, J. H., Moskowitz, J. M., Schaeffer, G. A., and Schaps, E. (1984) Teacher training in affective education for the primary prevention of adolescent drug abuse. *Am J Drug Alc Abuse*, **10**, 223–35.

Manion, I. G., Davidson, S., Clark, S. *et al.* (1997a) Working with youth in the 1990s: Attitudes, behaviours, impressions, and opportunities. *CPA Bull*, 111–14.

Manion, I. G., Davidson, S., Norris, C., and Brandon, S. (1997b) Innovations in mental health promotion: Youth Net/Réseau Ado. *Ado Paediatr Child Health*, **2**, 398–99.

Maslow, A. H. (1970) *Motivation and Personality*, Harper and Row, New York.

Mason, M. and Chuang, S. (2001) Culturally-based after-school arts programming for low-income urban children: Adaptive and preventive effects. *J Pri Prev*, **22**, 45–54.

McBride, N. (2003) A systematic review of school drug education. *Health Educ Res*, **18**, 729–42 (Review) and references therein.

McGuire, W. J. (1985) Attitudes and attitude change, in *The Handbook of Social Psychology, Vol. 2. Special Fields and Application*, 3rd Edition, Knopf, New York, pp. 233–346.

Miller, Y., Kuschel, A., and Hahlweg, K. (2002) Early prevention of externalizing disorders – Basic princinples and parent-centred approaches to prevention of expansive childhood behavior disorders. *Praxis der Kinderpsychologie und Kinderpsychiatrie*, **51**, 441–53.

Mohr, C. D., Averna, S., Kenny, D. A., and Del Boca, F. K. (2001) "Getting by (or getting high) with a little help from my friends": An examination of adult alcoholics' friendships. *J Stud Alc*, **62**, 637–45.

Moskowitz, J. M., Malvin, J., Schaeffer, G. A., and Schaps, E. (1983) Evaluation of a junior high school primary prevention program. *Add Behav*, **8**, 393–401.

Neumark-Sztainer, D., Sherwood, N. E., Coller, T., and Hannan, P. J. (2000) Primary prevention of disordered eating among preadolescent girls: Feasibility and short-term effect of a community-based intervention. *J Am Diet Assoc*, **100**, 1466–73.

Nyden, A., Paananen, M., and Gillberg, C. (2000) Neuropsychiatric problems among children are signigicantly underdiagnosed. Intervention programs result in better and less expensive care. *Lakartidningen*, **97**, 5634–39 (in Swedish).

O'Dea, J. A. (1995) *Everybody's Different: A Self-esteem Program for Young Adolescents*. University of Sydney, Sydney.

O'Dea, J. A. and Abraham, S. (2000) Improving the body image, eating attitudes, and behaviors of young male and female adolescents: A new educational approach that focuses on self-esteem. *Int J Eat Disord*, **28**, 43–57.

Patton, G., Bond, L., Butler, H., and Glover, S. (2003) Changing schools, changing health? Design and implementation of the Gatehouse Project. *J Adol Health*, **33**, 231–39.

Patton, G. C., Glover, S., Bond, L. *et al.* (2000) The Gatehouse Project: A systematic approach to mental health promotion in secondary schools. *Aust NZ J Psychiatry*, **34**, 586–93.

Perry, C. L., Komro, K. A., Veblen-Mortenson, S. *et al.* (2000) The Minnesota DARE PLUS Project: Creating community partnerships to prevent drug use and violence. *J Sch Health*, 70, 84–88.

Perry, C. L., Komro, K. A., Veblen-Mortenson, S. *et al.* (2003) A randomized controlled trial of the middle and junior high school D.A.R.E. and D.A.R.E. Plus programs. *Arch Pediatr Adolesc Med*, **157**, 178–84.

Perry, C. L., Williams, C. L., Forster, J. L. *et al.* (1993) Background, conceptualization and design of a community-wide research program on adolescent alcohol use: Project Northland. *Health Educ Res*, **8**, 125–36.

Perry, C. L., Williams, C. L., Komro, K. A. *et al.* (2002) Project Northland: Long-term outcomes of community action to reduce adolescent alcohol use. *Health Educ Res*, **17**, 117–32.

Perry, C. L., Williams, C. L., Veblen-Mortenson, S. *et al.* (1996) Project Northland: Outcomes of a communitywide alcohol use prevention program during early adolescence. *Am J Pub Health*, **86**, 956–65.

Peters, R. D., Arnold, R., Petrunka, K. *et al.* (2000) Better Beginnings Better Futures project short-term findings report. Google (Online).

Peters, R. D., Petrunka, K., and Arnold, R. (2003) The Better Beginnings, Better Futures Project: A universal, comprehensive, community-based prevention approach for primary school children and their families. *J Clin Child Adolesc Psychol*, **32**, 215–27.

Pfefferbaum, B., Call, J. A., and Sconzo, G. M. (1999) Mental health services for children in the first two years after the 1995 Oklahoma City terrorist bombing. *Psychiatr Serv*, **50**, 956–58.

Possel, P., Horn, A. B., Groen, G., and Hautzinger, M. (2004a) School-based prevention of depressive symptoms in adolescents: A 6-month follow-up. *J Am Acad Child Adolesc Psychiatry*, **43**, 1003–10.

Possel, P., Horn, A. B., Seemann, S., and Hautzinger, M. (2004b) *Trainingsprogramm zur Praventation von Depressionen bei Jugendlichen. LARS & LISA: Lust An Realistischer Sicht & Leichtigkeit Im Sozialen Alltag*. Hogrefe, Gottingen.

Pratt, B. M. and Woolfenden, S. R. (2002) Interventions for preventing eating disorders in children and adolescents. *Cochrane Database Syst Rev*, CD002891 (Review), and references therein.

Reppucci, N. D., Woolard, J. L., and Fried, C. S. (1999) Social, community, and preventive interventions. *Ann Rev Psychol*, **50**, 387–418.

Roosa, M. (1989) A Preventive intervention for children in alcoholic families: Results of a pilot study. *Fam Rel*, **38**, 295–300.

Ryff, C. D. (1989) Happiness is everything, or is it? Explorations on the meaning of psychological well-being. *J Pers Soc Psychol*, **6**, 1069–81.

Sarachuk, R. and Koss, D. (1986) *Tuning Into Health: Alcohol and Other Drug Decision for Junior High Students*. Alcoholism Foundation of Manitoba, Winnepeg.

Satir, V. (1972) *Peoplemaking*, Science and Behavior Book, Inc., Palo Alto.

Scott, S., Knapp, M., Henderson, J., and Maughan, B. (2001) Financial cost of social exclusion: Follow up study of antisocial children into adulthood. *Br Med J*, **323**, 191.

Shaffer, D., Garland, A., Vieland, V. *et al.* (1991) The impact of curriculum-based suicide prevention programs for teenagers. *J Am Acad Child Adolesc Psychiatry*, **30**, 588–96.

Shatkin, J. P. and Belfer, M. L. (2004) The global absence of a child and adolescent mental health policy. *Child Adol Men Health*, **9**, 104–08.

Short, J. L., Roosa, M. W., Sandler, I. N. *et al.* (1995) Evaluation of a preventive intervention for a self-selected subpopulation of children. *Am J Commun Psychol*, **23**, 223–47.
Shortt, A. L., Barrett, P. M., and Fox, T. L. (2001) Evaluating the FRIENDS program: A cognitive-behavioral group treatment for anxious children and their parents. *J Clin Child Psychol*, **30**, 525–35.
Shure, M. B. and Spivack, G. (1982) Interpersonal problem-solving in young children: A cognitive approach to prevention. *Am J Commun Psychol*, **10**, 341–56.
Skara, S. and Sussman, S. (2003) A review of 25 long-term adolescent tobacco and other drug use prevention program evaluations. *Prev Med*, **37**, 451–74 (Review), and references therein.
Sorensen, E. (1989) [Children and disasters. Guidelines for a working model–experiences from the mental health services for children after the aircrash at Bronnoysund]. *Tidsskrift for Den Norske Laegeforening*, **109**, 3403–06 (in Norwegian).
Stein, B. D., Jaycox, L. H., Kataoka, S. H. *et al.* (2003) A mental health intervention for schoolchildren exposed to violence: A randomized controlled trial. *JAMA*, **290**, 603–11 (see comment).
Steiner-Adair, C., Sjostrom, L., Franko, D. L. *et al.* (2002) Primary prevention of risk factors for eating disorders in adolescent girls: Learning from practice. *Int J Eat Dis*, **32**, 401–11.
Stewart, A. (1998) Experience with a school-based eating disorders prevention programme, in *The Prevention of Eating Disorders* (eds W. Vandereycken and G. Noordenbos), New York University Press, New York, pp. 99–136.
Stewart, D. A. and Carter, J. C. (1995) *Eating Disorder Prevention: A Six Session Education Programme for Use in Schools*, Unpublished manual.
Stewart, D. A., Carter, J. C., Drinkwater, J. *et al.* (2001) Modification of eating attitudes and behavior in adolescent girls: A controlled study. *Int J Eat Dis*, **29**, 107–18.
Stice, E., Chase, A., Stormer, S., and Appel, A. (2001) A randomized trial of a dissonance-based eating disorder prevention program. *Int J Eat Dis*, **29**, 247–62.
Strople, M. J. and Koss, D. (1986) *Tuning Into Health: Alcohol and Other Drug Decisions, Alcoholism Foundation of Manitoba, Winnipeg.*
Struzzo, P. (1999) Prevention of alcohol-related problems. From therapy to primary health care: experience at the Udine "Healthy City". *Recenti Progressi in Medicina*, **90**, 69–72 (in Italian).
Sylvestre, J. C. and Brophy, K. (1993) *The Development of the Better Beginnings, Better Futures Integrated Model for Primary Prevention: Executive Summary.*
Verhulst, F. C. (1995) A review of community studies, in *The Epidemiology of Child and Adolescent Psychopathology* (eds F. C. Verhulst and H. M. Koot), Oxford University Press, Oxford.
Vieland, V., Whittle, B., Garland, A. *et al.* (1991) The impact of curriculum-based suicide prevention programs for teenagers: An 18-month follow-up. *J Am Acad Child Adolesc Psychiatry*, **30**, 811–15.
Wade, T. D., Davidson, S., and O'Dea, J. A. (2003) A preliminary controlled evaluation of a school-based media literacy program and self-esteem program for reducing eating disorder risk factors. *Int J Eat Dis*, **33**, 371–83.
Werch, C. (1991) Effects of a take-home drug prevention program on drug-related communication and beliefs of parents and children. *J Sch Health*, **61**, 346–50.
Werch, C. (1996) Brief nurse consultations for preventing alcohol use among urban school youth. *J Sch Health*, **66**, 335–38.
WHO (1992) *Classification of Mental and Behavioural Disorders: Clincal Descriptions and Diagnostic Guidelines (ICD-10)*, World Health Organization, Geneva.
WHO (2001a) *Mental Health: New Understanding, New Hope*, WHO, Geneva.
WHO (2001b) *The World Health Report*, World Health Organization, Geneva.
WHO (2002) *Prevention and Promotion in Mental Health*, World Health Organization, Geneva.
WHO (2003) *World Report on Violence and Health*, WHO, Geneva.
WHO (2004a) *Prevention of Mental Disorders*, World Health Organization, Geneva.
WHO (2004b) *Promoting Mental Health*, World Health Organization, Geneva.
WHO (2005). *Child and Adolescent Mental Health Policies and Plans*, World Health Organization, Geneva.
Wilhelmsen, B. U., Laberg, J. C., and Klepp, K. I. (1994) Evaluation of two student and teacher involved alcohol prevention programmes. *Addiction*, **89**, 1157–65.
Wolf, N. (1991) *The Beauty Myth*, William Morrow, New York.

CHAPTER 5.3

Violence and Trauma: Evidence-Based Assessment and Intervention in Children and Adolescents: A Systematic Review

Ernesto Caffo and Carlotta Belaise
Mother and Child Department, University of Modena and Reggio Emilia, Italy

SUMMARY

Each year millions of children are exposed to traumatic experiences. The body of literature related to children and their responses to disasters and trauma is growing. Mental health professionals are learning more about which factors are associated with increased risk (vulnerability) or decreased risk (resilience) of psychopathology after exposure to trauma. Most victims, children included, adapt whether they have experienced trauma directly or indirectly. Nonetheless, a significant proportion of children incur severe psychological distress after traumatic events, interfering with their social and family relationships and development and learning. Post-traumatic stress disorder (PTSD), anxiety and mood disorders, sleep disorders, conduct disorders, learning disorder, and attention deficit disorder (ADHD) are the most common psychiatric problems following traumatic experiences. Although several questionnaires and semistructured interviews have been designed to measure PTSD, no single instrument has been accepted as a "gold standard" for diagnosis or monitoring the course of symptoms. The diagnosis of PTSD is based primarily on clinical interview. In terms of providing treatment, CBT emerges as the best validated therapeutic approach for children and adolescents who have experienced trauma-related symptoms, particularly anxiety and mood disorders. Family support may also be necessary. Research reveals that resilience and recovery depend on basic human protective

The Mental Health of Children and Adolescents: an area of global neglect. Edited by H. Remschmidt *et al.*

systems. This finding has produced a fundamental change in the understanding and treatment of children at high risk or already in trouble, and a new conceptualization of the goals of prevention and intervention.

SEARCH STRATEGIES

A search of the literature concerning children's and adolescent's psychopathology after trauma and of intervention strategies to prevent or reduce the severity of post-traumatic symptomatology was conducted as follows:

1. We conducted a scientific literature review, searching databases most relevant to psychiatry and psychology research (i.e., Medline and PsycInfo), using as initial keywords, the terms "trauma," "natural disasters," "PTSD," "mental health," "mental disorders," "child," "adolescent," "mood and anxiety disorders," "intervention," "psychotherapy," and "cognitive behavioral therapy." Selected papers were analyzed and additional search was made based on references cited in the papers located by the initial search.
2. In order to access a wider range of intervention programmes, we conducted general Internet searches using the keywords mentioned above. The names of specific programmes derived from the Internet search were subsequently used as key words for additional searches using the scientific literature databases. This strategy was employed in order to address the uncertain reliability of Internet sources.

In recent years there has been an upsurge of interest in the field of psychological trauma. Traumatology has been defined as "the investigation and application of knowledge about the immediate and long term consequences of highly stressful events and the factors which affect those consequences" (Figley, 2002). During the 1970s, awareness of the prevalence of post-traumatic symptomatology among Vietnam veterans (Figley, 1978), battered women (Walker, 1979), and rape victims (Burgess and Holstrom, 1974) engaged the interest of researchers. Terms such as "traumatology," "post-traumatic symptomatology," and "post-traumatic stress" were not yet in widespread use at that time. In 1980, a turning point in the awareness of the prevalence and consequences of psychological trauma occurred with the publication of the third edition of the "Diagnostic and Statistical Manual of Mental Disorders" (DSM-III) (American Psychiatric Association, 1980). Although during the nineteenth and twentieth centuries, psychological trauma had been studied in psychiatry and psychology (Kardiner, 1941; Grinker and Spiegel, 1945), currently, the range of traumatic stress studies extends from random events (e.g., natural disasters and accidents, hurricanes, and tornadoes), to "man-made disasters" (e.g., transportation accidents and toxic spills), to premeditated acts that involve an interpersonal violation (e.g., physical and sexual assault, combat, genocide, physical relocation because of war or political/social upheavals).

Trauma can involve large groups of people (e.g., war, genocide, earthquakes, toxic spills), small groups (e.g., plane crashes), two people (e.g., domestic violence, rape, physical assault, homicide), or one person (e.g., animal attack). Trauma can be experienced directly or indirectly (e.g., via the mass media) or because of a close relationship to the primary victim (e.g., when family members are traumatized when they learn of the injury or death of a relative) (Courtois, 2002). Experts have provided different definitions of psychological trauma. A definition that encompasses the subjective impact of the stressor event or experience has been suggested by Saakvitne *et al.* (2000): "... an event or situation creates psychological trauma when it overwhelms the individual's perceived ability to cope, and leaves that person fearing death, annihilation, mutilation, or psychosis. The individual feels emotionally, cognitively, and physically overwhelmed. The circumstances of the event commonly include abuse of power, betrayal of trust, entrapment, helplessness, pain, confusion, or loss."

THE INCIDENCE AND PREVALENCE OF TRAUMATIC STRESS

Pfefferbaum (1998, 1999) reported that, each year in the United States, more than 5 million children are exposed to extreme traumatic stress such as natural disaster, motor vehicle accident, life-threatening illness, burn injury, painful medical procedures, physical abuse, sexual assault, witnessing domestic or community violence, kidnapping, the sudden death of a parent, and many others. Perry (1999) reported that more than 30% of these children develop PTSD, with emotional, behavioral, cognitive, social, and physical symptoms. The estimated lifetime prevalence of PTSD in the general population ranges from 1 to 14% (Helzer *et al.*, 1987; American Psychiatric Association, 1994; Kessler *et al.*, 1995). Giaconia *et al.* (1995) found that, by the age of 18 years, more than 40% of youths in a community sample had experienced at least one episode of trauma, and more than 6% met criteria for a lifetime diagnosis of PTSD. Cuffe *et al.* (1998) examined the population prevalence of PTSD in a community sample of adolescents. They found that 3% of girls and 1% of boys met DSM-IV criteria for PTSD. In this study, girls reported more traumatic events than boys. Being female, experiencing rape or sexual abuse, and witnessing an accident or medical emergency were associated with increased risk of PTSD. A review of psychiatric consequences after injuries in children and adolescents (Stoddard and Saxe, 2001) suggests that injuries have been the largest cause of morbidity and mortality among children in the United States for many years (Dershewitz and Williamson, 1977; Baker *et al.*, 1984). Approximately one fourth of children are injured, young children and adolescents being at highest risk. Sports, falls, motor vehicle traffic injuries, and burns are the commonest causes of injury. Juvenile offenders in detention or correctional institutions are also at high risk (Stoddard and Saxe, 2001). Psychiatric disorders after traumatic events and injuries are a serious public health problem and account for high rates of morbidity in children and adolescents. Adolescents are at particular risk of physical injury. As reported by the US Department of Transportation (1993), the economic costs of child injury, disability, and death are more than $16 billion each year. Despite the high rate of injury and death, the psychiatric consequences of physical injuries in children have been neglected (National Academy of Sciences, 1985; Smith and Barss, 1991). The WHO (Murray and Lopez, 1996) predicts that, by 2020, the number of deaths caused by injuries and infectious disease will be the same.

Epidemiological data on the prevalence of PTSD in victims of car accidents, cancer, witnessing violence, rape, physical and sexual abuse, burns, and natural and man-made disasters (war) will be described in the following section.

Accidents. A 1996 report from the Child Accident Prevention Trust (Heptinstall, 1996) reminds us that "every year in the United Kingdom about 700 children die, 120000 are admitted to hospital, and over 200000 attend accident and emergency departments as a result of accidents." The most common accidents are falls and traffic accidents. Overall, 9% of the children who visited three accident and emergency departments scored so highly on a screening scale for PTSD that a diagnosis of PTSD was extremely likely. Half the children involved in road traffic accidents were judged likely to have PTSD. Other studies of road traffic accidents (DiGallo *et al.*, 1997; Mirza *et al.*, 1998) found that 33% of children met criteria for a diagnosis of PTSD, whereas even more had subthreshold clusters of distressing symptoms. After 6 months, one in six of these children had full-blown PTSD.

Cancer. Thirty-five percent of a sample of adolescents in whom cancer had been diagnosed met criteria for PTSD (Pelcovitz *et al.*, 1998). Fifteen percent of children who survived cancer had moderate to severe PTSD (Stuber *et al.*, 1997).

Witnessing violence. Ninety-three percent of a sample of children who witnessed domestic violence had PTSD (Kilpatrick and Williams, 1998; Hadi and Llabre, 1998). More than 80% of Kuwaiti children exposed to the Persian Gulf crisis had PTSD (Hadi and Llabre, 1998).

Rape and physical and sexual abuse. Seventy-three percent of juvenile male rape victims develop PTSD (Ruchkin *et al.*, 1998). Thirty four percent of a sample of children who experienced sexual or physical abuse, and 58% of children who experienced both physical and sexual abuse, met criteria for PTSD (Ackerman *et al.*, 1998). Clinically significant symptoms short of the full syndrome of PTSD were observed in virtually all children and adolescents after sexual and physical abuse.

Burns. Brigham and McLoughlin (1996) report that, in the United States, burn injuries have dropped by approximately 50%, to an estimated annual rate of 1.25 million. The reduction of burn injuries is the result of legislation, education, and burn prevention devices such as sprinkler systems and smoke alarms. Deaths from burns, the fourth leading cause of accidental death, have dropped to 5500 per year. Important settings for injury are juvenile detention and correctional centers, where 3.12 injuries and 2.4 suicidal acts per 100 juveniles occurred in a 30-day survey by Parent *et al.* (1994), and the workplace, where as many as 24% of injuries to 14- to 19-year-old persons occur (Runyan and Gerken, 1989).

Stoddard and Saxe (2001) reported several studies that identified PTSD as the most common psychological reaction in children to a diverse range of injuries, included burns (Stoddard *et al.*, 1989).

Children with severe burns present specialized issues, beginning with a threat to survival, severe pain, and family stress. A child with severe facial and other burns is at high risk for body image and identity problems and social stigmatization. These children, if followed in a specialized center, commonly survive even massive burns, and interventions such as reconstructive surgery, psychiatric care, and broad support are widely employed to assist affected children to resume development and lead productive lives (Stoddard *et al.* 1989; Sheridan *et al.*, 2000).

A wider use of social skills training to help children cope with stigma and teasing is required (Robinson *et al.*, 1996).

Natural and man-made disaster. Statistics from the International Federation of Red Cross and Red Crescent Societies (1998) indicates that, worldwide, a staggering number of people are affected by disasters. For example, in 1997 alone, 5.9 million people in Africa, 1.7 million in the United States and the Americas, 24.5 million in Asia, 0.5 million in Europe, and 0.8 million in Oceania (including Australia and New Zealand) were affected by disasters, for a total of more than 33.4 million. These figures include many children and families. However, the prevalence of exposure to mass trauma is hard to estimate. One survey of US residents revealed that 13% of the entire sample had exposure to natural or human-generated disaster during their lifetime (Burkle, 1996). In the National Comorbidity Survey, 18.9% of men and 15.2% of women reported having been affected by a natural disaster (Kessler *et al.*, 1995). Some victims are able to organize themselves, adapt, and rebound in a surprising way despite their horrific and frightful experiences (Salzer and Bickman, 1999). Children's and adolescents' reaction to disasters may vary (Vogel and Vernberg, 1993), but the most frequently studied reactions are those associated with PTSD and related symptoms. Some research has focused on other disorders, such as depression, academic problems, anxiety, sleep disorders, and separation anxiety. Different studies show marked heterogeneity in outcome (Goenjian *et al.*, 2001). Using the Child PTSD Reaction Index, Shannon *et al.* (1994) found mild reaction scores (mean = 21.7) among children and adolescents 3 months after Hurricane Hugo and estimated that 5% had PTSD. Similar results have been reported by Belter *et al.* (1991) and Garrison *et al.* (1993). The latter study reported that only 5% of the adolescents examined met DSM-III-R criteria for PTSD. Vernberg *et al.* (1996) found moderate (mean = 29.6) Child PTSD Reaction Index scores in children 3 months after Hurricane Andrew (Vernberg and La Greca *et al.*, 1996). Using the Diagnostic Interview Schedule for Children in a population-based study 6 months after Hurricane Andrew, Garrison *et al.* (1995), found that 7.3% of a mixed-exposure group of adolescents met criteria for PTSD. Shaw *et al.* (1995), using the Child PTSD Reaction Index 32 weeks after Hurricane Andrew, reported that 51% of children in the high-impact area had moderate levels of PTSD and that 38% had severe or very severe levels. La Greca *et al.* (1996) reported mild to moderate scores (mean = 24.4) on the Child PTSD Reaction Index 7 months after Hurricane Andrew: 23% experienced moderate levels and 18% experienced severe to very severe symptomatology.

War. UNICEF (1996) estimated that 2 million children have been killed in war during the past decade and another 10 million were psychologically traumatized by it. Of children exposed to war trauma, a high percentage meet criteria for PTSD or experience subclinical levels of the disorder. Allwood *et al.* (2002) reviewed the literature on this subject and located several studies that found exposure to war to be a risk factor for PTSD and other adjustment problems. Kinzie *et al.* (1986), for example, found that, in 1984, 50% of Cambodian children who had been exposed to war and genocide during the Pol Pot regime (1975–1979) met diagnostic criteria for PTSD. Follow-up studies reported PTSD rates of 48% and 38% in 1987 and 1990, respectively (Sack *et al.*, 1993). Of 364 displaced children examined during the Bosnian war, 93.8% met criteria for PTSD, 6% reported sadness, and 95.5% anxiety (Goldstein *et al.*, 1997).

In summary, PTSD, anxiety disorder, and depression constitute the most common types of clinical problems in children and adolescents after traumatic events, and they may be comorbid. What is less clear from existing research is the extent to which post-traumatic symptoms interfere with children's daily functioning and represent psychopathology or whether the symptoms should be regarded as "normal" reactions to abnormal events. Given the potential effect of trauma on children and adolescents and the likelihood of comorbid symptoms, mental health professionals must be careful to assess children's pre-trauma levels of psychopathology and their level of functioning after trauma, in order to estimate biopsychosocial vulnerability (Caffo and Belaise, 2003).

PREDICTORS OF RESPONSE IN CHILD VICTIMS OF TRAUMA

A number of factors influence a child's response to trauma and recovery from it. These factors include the following: the nature of the stressor; the nature of the individuals' exposure to its age, sex, developmental level, and psychiatric history; family characteristics; and social factors (Pfefferbaum, 1997). Pine and Cohen (2002) reviewed studies of qualitatively different traumatic events (physical and sexual abuse, natural disasters, and violence). Previous reviews from cross-sectional investigations have linked the nature of traumatic events to risk for psychopathology. Acute events that produce little change in the social milieu carry lower risks than either chronic, continuing trauma or other experiences that cause long-lasting disruption in the social environment (Dohrenwend *et al.*, 1981; Terr, 1991; Steinberg and Avenevoli, 2000; Laor *et al.*, 2001). As suggested by Pine and Cohen (2002), despite these general trends, it is problematic to compare the rates of adverse psychiatric outcomes across studies and stressors. The rates of disorder vary in accordance with demography, assessment technique, and length of follow-up. Such cross-study variations cast doubt on the appropriateness of meta-analysis. From a clinical perspective, knowledge about moderating factors could assist in the identification of children or adolescents at high risk of adverse psychiatric outcome after exposure to trauma. Clinicians could observe such individuals over time or be alert to factors that predict high degrees of symptoms in order to intercept emerging psychiatric symptoms before they become chronic (Pine and Cohen, 2002).

Prior research in this area has identified three factors linked to "differential symptom trajectories" among traumatized children: (1) the nature of traumatic event; (2) the social environment; and (3) the characteristics of the individual.

The level of exposure to an acutely dangerous event predicts the risk of later psychiatric symptoms (Pine and Cohen, 2002). This association has been confirmed in all types of trauma: physical and sexual abuse (Fergusson *et al.*, 1996a, 1996b; Fergusson and Lynskey 1997; Brown *et al.*, 1999); shipping disaster (Yule *et al.*, 2000); sniper attack (Nader *et al.*, 1990); and war-related trauma (Steinberg and Avenevoli, 2000; Smith *et al.*, 2001).

Other studies have found that social support exerts a relatively strong moderating influence on acute and long-term mental health problems in children exposed to trauma. The beneficial effect of social support has been confirmed in long-term follow-up studies, for example, of children exposed to SCUD missile attacks in Israel (Laor *et al.*, 1997, 2001; Steinberg and Avenevoli, 2000), other war-related trauma (Smith *et al.*, 2001), physical abuse (Fergusson and Lynskey, 1997), and a shipping accident (Udwin *et al.*, 2000).

Beyond level of exposure and social support, the characteristics of the individual also seem to predict outcome. The level of psychopathology before or immediately after trauma constitutes an important risk factor for later psychiatric symptoms. Trauma-related anxiety symptoms are particularly strong predictors (Pine and Cohen, 2002). As with adults (Dohrenwend *et al.*, 1981; Breslau *et al.*, 1991), sex influences defensive style and coping, the availability of and willingness to use social support, and expectations of response and recovery. As reviewed by Pfefferbaum (1997), in studies with large samples, girls are more symptomatic than boys (Green *et al.*, 1991; Lonigan *et al.*, 1991; Shannon *et al.*, 1994; Giaconia *et al.*, 1995). Girls show more mood or anxiety symptoms after traumatic stress (Green *et al.*, 1991, 1994; Pynoos *et al.*, 1993), whereas boys show more behavioral symptoms (Shaw *et al.*, 1996). On the contrary, several studies have found boys to be more symptomatic than girls, and other studies have found qualitative sex differences in symptoms and recovery (Blom, 1986; Nader *et al.*, 1993; Giaconia *et al.*, 1995; Shaw *et al*, 1995). With particular reference to the expression and development of PTSD, clinical experience and recent research suggest that, after trauma, girls exhibit more internalizing symptoms (anxiety, dysphoria, dissociation, avoidance) and boys more externalizing behavior (impulsivity, aggression, inattention, hyperactivity) (Perry *et al.*, 1995; Ackerman *et al.*, 1998). In prevalence studies in the general adult population, women have higher rates of PTSD than men (Breslau *et al.*, 1999). According to Perry *et al.* (1995), there are sex differences in adaptive response after the acute event (girls are more likely to dissociate than boys). This finding may be related to the reported sex differences in the development and expression of trauma-related symptoms.

Long-lasting or extreme traumatic experiences may convey the highest risk for psychopathology when they disrupt social support networks as a result of family displacement or disruption (Pine and Cohen, 2002). For example, Laor *et al.* (2001) reported consistently higher levels of psychiatric symptoms among children whose families were displaced after having being exposed to SCUD missile attacks in Israel, compared with similarly exposed children who lived in nondisplaced families. The same authors found that parental mental health predicted changes in symptoms over time. Lynskey and Fergusson (1997) corroborated these findings in epidemiologic studies of children exposed to physical abuse. The mechanisms behind these associations are unclear.

In summary, research supports the following risk factors for the development of symptoms in children exposed to traumatic experiences: level of exposure, extent of social disruption, and pre-trauma psychopathology (Caffo and Belaise, 2003).

Age and developmental level influence the children's exposure to risk, and their perception and understanding of trauma, susceptibility to parental distress, quality of response, coping style, problem-solving skills, and memory of the event (Handford *et al.*, 1986; Terr, 1988; Realmuto *et al.*, 1992; Weisenberg *et al.*, 1993; Pfefferbaum, 1997). Age and developmental level influence the response of other people to traumatized children, younger children being more likely to be protected. Trauma and the child's response to it have the potential to disrupt normal development (Perry, 1994) by compromising adaptation and the development of cognition, attention, social skills, personality style, self-concept, self-esteem, and impulse control (Nader *et al.*, 1990). There may also be age-related differences in symptomatology. Schwarz and Kowalski (1991) found that, after a school shooting, avoidance phenomena were more common in younger children, whereas older children suffered more intrusive and hyperarousal symptoms. Compared with adults, younger children were more likely to experience spontaneous intrusive phenomena, whereas older children and adults were more likely to suffer distress following reminders of the traumatic event. Weisenberg *et al.* (1993) noticed that adolescents who were in shelters during threatened missile attacks in the Persian Gulf War relied more upon avoidant coping than younger children did. Despite the difficulty of assessing PTSD in young children, several investigators have reported that preschool children can be affected by trauma (Kiser *et al.*, 1988; Terr, 1988; Sullivan *et al.*, 1991; Scheering *et al.*, 1995; Steinberg and Avenevoli, 2000). Scheering *et al.* (1995) described the difficulty of making a diagnosis of post-traumatic symptoms in infants and young children using existing DSM-IV criteria because of their low sensitivity. Further research is needed to establish diagnostic criteria for PTSD that are more sensitive for young children.

PRACTICE PARAMETERS FOR THE ASSESSMENT AND TREATMENT OF CHILDREN AND ADOLESCENTS WITH PTSD

A literature search was conducted to evaluate existing empirical and clinical information regarding practice parameters for the assessment and treatment of PTSD in children and adolescents. The main findings of this process revealed that a wide variety of stressors can lead to the development of PTSD symptoms and that the particular PTSD symptoms manifested vary according to the development stage of the child and the nature of the stressor. For this reason, diagnostic criteria for PTSD designed for adults may not adequately describe the disorder in children and adolescents. Another finding was that several factors seem to mediate the development of childhood PTSD following a severe stressor. Most of the therapeutic interventions recommended for children with PTSD are cognitive-behavioral (Anonymous, 1998).

Diagnostic assessment

The diagnostic assessment of a potentially traumatized child encompasses several areas of investigation: (1) an interview with parents or primary caregivers; (2) an interview with the child, including a mental status examination; (3) assessing data from school (with appropriate release of information), if clinically indicated; (4) additional evaluations (e.g., IQ testing, speech and language evaluation, pediatric evaluation); and (5) standardized interviews and rating scales.

Interview the parents and the child

The assessment of PTSD in children depends first and foremost on careful, direct clinical interviews with the child and parents. If a parent is the alleged perpetrator of child abuse or domestic violence, the nonoffending parent or other primary caretaker should be interviewed. An interview of the alleged perpetrator is not required for diagnosis and treatment.

The parental interview seeks the following information:

- An account of the traumatic event with an estimation of whether it qualifies as an "extreme" stressor (i.e., the nature of the event, when it occurred, and the parents' description of the child's level of exposure to it).
- A report of preceding, concurrent, repeated, or subsequent stressors (e.g., child abuse or neglect; significant parental discord, separation, or divorce; frequent moves, school changes, or other disruptions; family deaths, illnesses, disabilities, or substance abuse; domestic or community violence; repeated or chronic stressorss, serious traumatic events in the parents' lives of which the child has knowledge).
- A report of DSM-IV PTSD symptoms in the child, with particular attention to developmental variations in clinical presentation (reexperiencing symptoms; avoidant, dissociative, and numbing symptoms; hyperarousal).
- A report of other significant current symptoms, with particular attention to disorders likely to be comorbid with PTSD (depressive symptoms and self-injurious behavior; non-PTSD anxiety symptoms, including panic attacks; ADHD and conduct problems; substance abuse).

- A report of whether the symptoms began before or after the identified traumatic event(s), and how soon before or after.
- A report of the parents' and significant others' emotional reactions to the traumatic event, verifying whether the parent or primary caregiver was directly exposed to the trauma (e.g., driving a motor vehicle at the time of an accident) or whether he/she had only vicarious exposure (e.g., child disclosed sexual abuse by a stranger).
- A report of whether the parent had PTSD symptoms after the traumatic event.
- An assessment of how much support has been available to the child after the event.
- The child's past psychiatric history (outpatient psychotherapy; partial or inpatient hospitalization; psychotropic medication; symptom course).
- Medical history (significant current or past medical problems, somatic complaints, surgery, significant injuries; current or past medications; current primary medical care provider).
- The child's developmental history, with particular attention to reactions to normative stressors (e.g., birth of a sibling, beginning school) and the child's level of functioning before the traumatic stressor.
- Educational history, with particular reference to changes in school behavior, concentration, activity level, and academic performance following the stressor.
- Family history and family members' medical/psychiatric history (PTSD symptoms or diagnosis; mood disorders; anxiety disorders; family medical conditions including physical conditions that could present with anxiety or mood disturbance).

Next the child is interviewed in order to obtain his or her report of the reason for referral and encourage him or her to describe what happened. There is lack of consensus regarding the detail to be sought and whether leading questions are helpful or harmful. It is generally agreed that it is desirable to ask the child to describe the stressor; however, highly suggestive questioning is not recommended. The child's interview is conducted in order to obtain the following information:

- A report of trauma-related attributions and perceptions (who or what the child believes was responsible for the traumatic event; whether the child thinks he/she had any responsibility for causing or perpetuating the traumatic event; whether the child considers that he/she should have behaved differently in response to the event; and whether he/she feels damaged, ostracized, or criticized by others).

  It is crucial to elicit the child's perception of how emotionally distressed parents and significant others have been since the traumatic event, and how supportive they were. If the stressor was not public knowledge, it is important to understand the child's perception of whether adults believed his or her disclosure of the traumatic event, and the child's perception of how "normal" the current symptoms are as a reaction to the stressor.
- The child's present symptoms, with developmentally appropriate questions regarding symptomatology consistent with DSM-IV criteria for PTSD.
- The child's report of symptoms frequently concomitant with PTSD, such as the following: depression, suicidal ideation, and behavior; self-injury; substance abuse; dissociative symptoms (e.g. hallucinations, fugue states, amnesia, depersonalization, or derealization in older children and adolescents); panic attacks; and other anxiety symptoms.
- A mental status examination, including behavior commonly observed in children with PTSD such as the following: startle reactions; hypervigilance; traumatic reenactments in play; changes in affect or attention that suggest intrusive reexperiencing.

Obtain information from the school with appropriate release of information, if clinically indicated

Although school reports can help to corroborate certain symptoms or post-traumatic changes, in many cases they are not required. However, it is useful to obtain information concerning the following: academic functioning, particularly to changes since the traumatic event; interaction with peers and involvement in nonacademic activities, with particular attention to changes since the traumatic event; and the timing of any inattention or distractibility (i.e., present before or only after the traumatic event).

Determine the need for additional evaluations

It may be useful to obtain intelligence testing, psychoeducational evaluation, speech and language assessment, or a pediatric examination.

Consider the usefulness of standardized interviews and rating scales

Although several questionnaires and semistructured interviews have been designed to assess PTSD, no single instrument is accepted as the "gold standard." The assessment of PTSD is complicated by the formal requirement that a certain number of symptoms from each of three categories (reexperiencing, avoidance/numbing, and hyperarousal) be present. Consequently, no single score is sufficient to diagnose PTSD categorically (as a child could have high levels of symptoms in one set of criteria but none in another). Moreover, parental reports tend to minimize the child's PTSD symptoms, and it is difficult to elicit avoidant/numbing symptoms from child, resulting in a significant risk of underdiagnosis. Teachers and other adults may not observe or be aware of many PTSD symptoms because they are not manifested at school (e.g., sleep problems, hypervigilance) or inapparent to the untrained observer. Physiological measures of hyperarousal have not been standardized for children, nor would such measures adequately assess reexperiencing and avoidance phenomena. In short, there are considerable limitations to the accuracy of diagnosing PTSD in children. On the contrary, concern has been expressed that some clinicians diagnose PTSD too readily because they ignore the specific diagnostic criteria and mistakenly believe that, following exposure to an extreme stressor, reexperiencing and anxiety symptoms alone are sufficient to diagnose the condition. This concern has led to recent attempts to educate clinicians about the disorder. Although semistructured interviews and parent/child rating scales may be helpful in following clinical course of children with PTSD, the diagnosis of PTSD is based primarily on clinical interview. Standardized interviews and scales are not essential to make this diagnosis. The semistructured interviews to be discussed next all include PTSD sections, but none has established psychometric properties for measuring DSM-IV PTSD symptoms in children:

- *Schedule for Affective Disorders and Schizophrenia for School-Age Children-Present and Lifetime version, PTSD Scale* (Kaufman *et al.*, 1997)
- *Diagnostic Interview Schedule, PTSD* (Garrison *et al.*, 1995);
- *Structured Clinical Interview for DSM-III-R; PTSD* (Hubbard *et al.*, 1995);
- *Childhood PTSD Interview – Child Form* (Fletcher, 1997).

The following parent/child rating forms may be useful for following the course of PTSD symptoms in children:

- *PTSD Reaction Index* (Frederick, 1985; Pynoos *et al.*, 1987; Goenjian *et al.*, 1995);
- *Trauma Symptom Checklist for Children* (Briere, 1995);
- *Checklist of Child Distress Symptoms–Child and Parent Report Version* (Martinez and Richters,1993);
- *Children's Impact of Traumatic Events Scale* (Wolfe *et al.*, 1989);
- *Child PTSD Symptom Scale* (Johnson *et al.*, 1996);

Differential diagnosis

A number of psychiatric disorders may be comorbid with PTSD, or confused with it, especially acute stress disorder, adjustment disorder, panic disorder, generalized anxiety disorder, MDD, ADHD, substance use disorder, dissociative disorder, conduct disorder, borderline or other personality disorder, and schizophrenia or other psychotic disorder.

Subtyping

A complete assessment of PTSD requires subtyping (*acute/chronic/with delayed onset*).

The treatment of PTSD

Although the course of PTSD in children is extremely variable, short-term, long-term, or intermittent ("pulsed") treatment may be required. Different levels of care (outpatient, partial hospitalization, an inpatient treatment) and different modalities (individual, family, group, a psychopharmacological therapy) may be required for a child at different points in the course of the disorder. The comprehensive treatment of PTSD is usually multimodal and may include any or all of the following components:

- *Psychoeducation* (education of the child, parents, teachers, and significant others about the symptoms, clinical course, and prognosis and treatment of childhood PTSD);
- *Individual therapy* (particularly Cognitive Behavior Therapy);
- *Family therapy* (exploration and resolution of the emotional impact of the traumatic event on the parent, identification and correction of inaccurate parental attributions regarding the traumatic event such as self-blame or blaming the child, implementation of supportive parenting behavior and parental reinforcement of therapeutic interventions such as teaching parents to help the child to use progressive relaxation techniques, parent training for the management of inappropriate child behavior);
- *Group therapy* (groups of children of the same developmental level who have experienced similar trauma can encourage open discussion about the event and counteract inappropriate attribution; school-based group crisis intervention can be useful after disaster);
- *Psychopharmacology* (antidepressant medication may be useful for children with marked hyperarousal who exhibit concurrent depression or refractory anxiety, psychostimulants

or alpha-adrenergic agonists such as clonidine may be useful for children with concurrent ADHD, antianxiety medication such as benzodiazepines and propranolol are not recommended for children with PTSD (Anonymous, 1998).

- *Psychotherapy for children who develop PTSD and other symptoms after psychological trauma.*

  Psychological debriefing (PD) and *cognitive behavioral therapy* (CBT) are the two main psychological therapeutic strategies that have been investigated (Caffo and Belaise, 2005; Belaise *et al.*, 2005).

There is substantial evidence that single sessions of PD after trauma are not effective in preventing or treating PTSD and trauma-related symptoms in adults and children (Bisson *et al.*, 2000; Gist and Woodal, 2000; Van Emmerik *et al.*, 2002; Rose *et al.*, 2003). PD can exacerbate symptoms (Bisson *et al.*, 1997; Bisson, 2003). During PD, participants are encouraged to ventilate a full, detailed account of the trauma, including facts, thoughts, and emotions. After ventilation, individuals are reassured that they are "reacting normally to an abnormal event." They are warned about further emotional responses and instructed how to manage them and where to ask for help (Rose *et al.*, 2003). Individuals are invited to attend debriefing sessions regardless of the severity of their symptoms or their functional impairment (Hokanson and Wirth, 2000). The central assumption of debriefing is that everyone exposed to a potentially traumatizing event is at high risk for a stress reaction, and that all can benefit from sharing their experiences and learning about trauma and its treatment (Litz *et al.*, 2002).

There have been serious criticisms of PD. By treating trauma victims at risk and not at risk of psychopathology in the same group sessions, debriefing ignores recent epidemiological findings that people are not equally vulnerable to trauma-related symptoms after exposure to a traumatic experience (Schnyder and Moergeli, 2003; Schnyder and Orner, 2003). Most victims cope and adapt whether they experienced trauma directly or indirectly (Salzer and Bickman, 1999).

Debriefing disrupts the natural alternation of intrusive thoughts and avoidant behavior associated with the processing of a traumatic event (Horowitz, 1976). It may aggravate distress after trauma and without adequate time for habituation. In this way, it might sensitize victims to trauma stimuli and retraumatize them (Kramer and Rosenthal, 1998). Furthermore, debriefing might cause victims to disregard social support from families and friends that could be sufficient alone for a complete recovery (Van Emmerik *et al.*, 2002). Cohen (2003) reached the same conclusions after a recent review of the pediatric literature on early intervention after trauma. Furthermore, recent evidence suggests that treatment should start several months after the traumatic event rather than immediately afterwards (Cohen, 2003).

CBT protocols have been shown to avert PTSD and trauma-related symptomatology (Foa and Chambless, 1978; Resick and Schnicke, 1992; Bryant *et al.*, 1998, 1999, 2003; Fecteau, 2000; Paunovic and Ost, 2001; Ehlers and Clark, 2003; Ehlers *et al.*, 2003). In particular, exposure therapy (ET), anxiety management training, stress inoculation training (specifically for rape survivors), and cognitive restructuring are the most effective methods of alleviating acute post-traumatic stress and preventing the development of PTSD.

In vivo exposure returns the victim to the site of the traumatic event in order to counteract avoidance and promote control. Imaginal exposure (Keane and Barlow, 2002), used when *in vivo* exposure is not feasible (e.g., if the subject must return to a very distant location or an earlier time in life), consists of reliving a traumatic experience in imagination, by giving an accurate description of the event including stimuli, responses, and attributed meaning. However, technical alternatives that do not deal with the central trauma (Hodgson and Rachman, 1970; Watson and Marks, 1971) have recently been discussed, confirming earlier findings that exposure to the main trauma is not essential for PTSD to improve (Belaise *et al.*, 2005). Confrontation with subtly related avoidances and enhancement of psychological well-being by means of well-being therapy, (Fava and Ruini, 2003) may be sufficient and less traumatizing (Belaise *et al.*, 2005).

Anxiety management training teaches patients to manage their emotions due to PTSD by the use of relaxation, breathing control, guided self-dialogue, trauma education, cognitive restructuring, and communication skills training (Saigh, 1986; Cohen and Mannarino, 1993; Snodgras *et al.*, 1993; Deblinger and Heflin, 1996; Saigh *et al.*, 1996; Parson, 1997). These skills provide the child with a sense of control over thoughts and feelings rather than being overwhelmed by them, and help the child undertake therapy with more confidence. Meichenbaum's stress inoculation therapy (Meichenbaum, 1985) teaches coping skills (relaxation, breathing control, guided self-dialogue, covert modeling, role play, thought stopping), starting with education about the trauma and its aftermath in order to better understand the physical, behavioral and cognitive aspects of fear. There is evidence that a combination of these treatments is effective (Solomon *et al.*, 1992; Keane *et al.*, 1994; Frueh *et al.*, 1996; Otto *et al.*, 1996; Foa *et al.*, 1999; Facteau and Nicki, 1999).

March *et al.* (1998) evaluated the efficacy of a group-administered, 18-week CBT protocol following a single-incident stressor. A peer group of children were treated in school with sessions that dealt with issues related to each participant's traumatic experience. A parallel group design, with random assignment to different treatments, was not employed. The authors found that children and adolescents treated with CBT showed clinically and statistically significant improvement on all main dependent measures and that the improvements persisted for the duration of the study. Goenjian *et al.* (1997) provided brief trauma/grief-focused psychotherapy to adolescents exposed to the 1988 Armenian earthquake. Treatment included both school-based and individual treatment, using several techniques beyond those typical of CBT. At the end of the study, adolescents who received psychotherapy showed significant improvement in the intrusion, avoidance, and arousal symptoms of PTSD. Deblinger *et al.* (1990) evaluated the efficacy of CBT for sexually abused children with PTSD. They found significant improvements in all PTSD symptoms, externalizing and internalizing behaviors, anxiety, and depression, particularly when parents and children were jointly treated. In a multisite, randomized controlled trial for children with sexual-abuse-related PTSD symptoms, Cohen *et al.* (2004) found that children randomly assigned to trauma-focused CBT (TF–CBT), compared to those assigned to nonspecific psychotherapy, demonstrated significantly more improvement with regard to PTSD, depression, behavior problems, shame, and abuse-related attributions. Similarly, parents assigned to TF–CBT showed greater improvement with respect to self-reported levels of depression, abuse-specific distress, support of the child, and effective parenting practices.

Stoddard and Saxe (2001) reported that *in vivo* exposure, imaginal exposure, and anxiety management might be effective for PTSD following injury.

To summarize, the essential components of CBT for children with PTSD are as follows:

- exposure therapy (*in vivo* and imaginal) to counteract avoidance. However, exposure to the main trauma is not essential for improvement: Exposure to subtly related avoidances

may be sufficient for a complete recovery (Hodgson and Rachman, 1970; Watson and Marks, 1971; Belaise *et al.*, 2005);
- the use of stress management techniques (anxiety management and stress inoculation);
- the exploration and correction of inaccurate attributions regarding the trauma (cognitive restructuring);
- the inclusion of parents in treatment (Deblinger *et al.*, 1990; Friedrich, 1996; Berliner, 1997).

It would be useful in future randomized controlled trials to test whether sufferers from PTSD and other stress-related anxiety disorders could be helped by the promotion of strong positive emotions (for example, through well-being therapy) rather than negative (Belaise *et al.*, 2005).

Clinicians vary in the degree to which they advocate explicit exposure techniques. Although Deblinger and Heflin (1996) and March *et al.* (1998) advocate gradual exposure to increasingly upsetting aspects of the trauma, other protocols do not include hierarchical exposure. Persistent discussion of traumatic memories with children who are very embarrassed or defensive might aggravate symptoms or provoke the family to dropout of treatment. Indirect methods of addressing traumatic issues (e.g., through play or exposure to cues of situations generalized from the trauma rather than to central trauma triggers) might be more helpful in these situations and less traumatizing for the child (Belaise *et al.*, 2005).

Children who are asymptomatic after traumatic experiences need monitoring for the emergence of delayed "sleeper" symptoms (Gomes-Schwarz *et al.*, 1990; Mannarino *et al.*, 1991; Pfeffer, 1997).

An element common to most interventions for traumatized children is the evaluation and reconsideration of the child's assumptions with regard to the traumatic events (Pynoos and Eth, 1986; Cohen and Mannarino, 1993; Joseph *et al.*, 1993; Spaccarelli, 1995; Deblinger and Heflin, 1996; Berliner, 1997). Faulty attributions regarding the trauma (e.g., "It was my fault," "Nothing is safe anymore") should be elicited and challenged.

There is a general consensus that the inclusion of parents in treatment is important for the resolution of PTSD and trauma-related symptoms. Parental emotional reaction to the traumatic event has a powerful effect on the child's response. Parents helped to resolve their own emotional distress are more perceptive of and responsive to their children's emotional needs (Burman and Allen-Meares, 1994; Rizzone *et al.*, 1994). Parents included in treatment learn behavior management techniques. Most authors recommend the inclusion of one or more parent-directed components (Blom, 1986; Galante and Foa, 1986; Rigamer, 1986; Terr, 1989; Cohen and Mannarino, 1993; Burman and Allen-Meares, 1994; Simons and Silveira, 1994; Brent *et al.*, 1995; Butler *et al.*, 1996; Deblinger and Heflin, 1996; Friedrich, 1996; Kolko, 1996; Macksoud and Aber, 1996; Berliner, 1997; Parson, 1997).

Data on the efficacy of group versus individual therapy for children with PTSD are scarce. One meta-analysis of treatment outcome studies for PTSD in adult women survivors of childhood sexual abuse demonstrated a larger effect size for individual therapy than for group treatment across a variety of therapeutic approaches (Chard, 1994). Although most treatment protocols recommend individual therapy, several authors have focused on the efficacy of crisis intervention for parents, teachers, and children in groups at school, in hospital, or in other community settings (Blom, 1986; Galante and Foa, 1986; Rigamer, 1986; Pynoos and Nader K, 1988; Yule and Udwin, 1991; Stallard and Law,

1993; Sullivan and Evans, 1994; La Greca *et al.*, 1996; Stoddard, 1996; Goenjian *et al.*, 1997). Many of these interventions used convenience samples in schools or towns exposed to a common traumatic event. Group intervention in such situations has the advantage of providing timely intervention for the largest possible number of exposed children. Intervention programmes for children and adolescents after disasters have been designed for each phase of the traumatic event: preimpact, impact and recoil, postimpact, and recovery and reconstruction (Vernberg, 2002).

There has been a paucity of research on specific treatments for victims of other traumatic events such as natural disasters or wars. There is a need for researchers to direct future randomized controlled trials to stressors other than physical or sexual abuse, such as grief, potential loss of loved ones, interpersonal conflicts with peers, separation fears, or social concerns (Pine and Cohen, 2002). There can be no "universal formula" for dealing with all regions and all types of disaster. Similarly, those delivering psychosocial support services need to take into consideration the culture and way of life of disaster affected victims (World Health Organization, 2003). According to a recent WHO report for a health emergency in South East Asia (World Health Organization, Regional Office for South East Asia, 2005), strategies should be developed to enhance the capacity of communities to provide psychosocial support in the immediate aftermath of the disaster. In the acute relief phase, it is advisable to conduct only the psychosocial *interventions that are needed to prevent* interference with responses to vital needs such as food, shelter, and the control of communicable disease.

The following guidelines should be useful in determining appropriate responses:

- Discourage the unceremonious disposal of corpses.
- Provide family tracing for unaccompanied minors, the elderly, and other vulnerable people.
- Encourage the members of field teams to participate actively in grieving.
- Provide recreational activities for children.
- Disseminate to the community uncomplicated, reassuring, empathic information on normal stress/trauma reactions. Religious leaders, teachers and other prominent community members should be actively involved.

In the acute phase service delivery for mental and neurological disorders such as schizophrenia and epilepsy, may break down. More specific mental health activities should be initiated during the third or fourth weeks, once life-saving operations are underway.

Relief workers can be assisted with self-help tips to reduce stress. Self-help groups and peer support groups are also helpful (World Health Organization, 2005).

In conclusion, post-traumatic stress symptoms and PTSD are probably best not treated with PD. They respond to exposure therapy (even without dealing with the central trauma), anxiety management, and cognitive restructuring. The therapeutic mechanisms effective for PTSD remain unclear, and there may be more than one way to reduce fear (Marks, 2000).

THE CONCEPT OF RESILIENCE

Not all children exposed to traumatic events develop symptoms. Attempts have been made to identify the mediating and moderating factors associated with increased risk (vulnerability) and decreased risk (resilience) of PTSD following traumatic stress (Kilpatrick and Williams, 1998). As discussed by Perry (1999), each mediating factor can be related to the degree to which it either prolongs or attenuates the child's stress-response. Factors that increase stress-related reactivity (e.g., family chaos, lack of support) make children more vulnerable, whereas factors that convey structure, predictability, care, and safety will decrease vulnerability. Pelcovitz *et al.* (1998) discovered that adolescents with cancer who developed PTSD rated their families as more chaotic than did those who did not develop PTSD. Furthermore, 85% of mothers in the PTSD group had PTSD related to their children's condition. The capacity to provide a consistent, predictable, and supporting environment is compromised if the family is disorganized and the child's primary caregiver has been traumatized (Perry, 1999).

The systematic study of resilience emerged from the realization that some children at high risk for problems after stress react and develop quite well. Such children were called "invulnerable," "stress resistant," or "resilient." The concept of resilience generally refers to "a class of phenomena characterized by patterns of positive adaptation in the context of significant adversity or risk" (Masten and Reed, 2002). Why do some people fare better than others in adverse circumstances? An analysis of individual and environmental factors is required. Masten and Reed (2002) have introduced concepts such as *assets, resources,* and *protective factors.* "Assets" are the opposite of risk factors; they predict better outcome in one or more of the domains of adaptation, regardless of level of risk. "Resources" are the human, social, and material advantages available for adaptation. "Protective factors" are the characteristics of individuals or situations that predict favorable outcome in high-risk or adverse circumstances. "Protective processes" explain how protective factors work when adaptation is threatened. The most common protective factors refer to differential attributes of the child, family, and other relationships, and the context in which the child develops, such as the school and neighborhood. As protective factors within the child, Masten and Reed (2002) nominate the following: good cognitive ability (e.g., problem solving and attentional skills), favorable self-perception, self-efficacy, the ability to attribute meaning to life, and personal talents valued by self and society. Protective factors within the family involve a close relationship with care-giving adults who provide an authoritative, warm, structured, well monitored, organized home environment, and who are involved in child's education. A close relationship to prosocial peers is helpful. Within the community, an effective school, a high level of public safety, good public health resources, and health care accessibility seem to protect the child against developmental hazards. The greatest threats are those unfavorable conditions that weaken basic, human, protective systems. Consequently, efforts to promote competence and resilience in children at risk should focus on strategies that prevent damage to, or repair, or compensate for threats to, these basic systems (Masten and Reed, 2002).

A novel well-being enhancing psychotherapeutic strategy, well-being therapy, will be described later together with other strategies that aim to foster resilience in children and adolescents.

THE ROAD TO POSITIVE PSYCHOLOGY

The work on resilience suggests that we need to aim for positive goals. *Promoting healthy development and competence is at least as important as preventing problems and will serve the same end* (Masten and Reed, 2002). From a developmental perspective, recent research suggests that it may be preferable to enhance the child's and family's competencies rather than to focus on their psychological and behavioral deficits.

The building of psychological strength and well-being through psychotherapy has become increasingly important in psychological research (Diener *et al.*, 1999; Gillham and Seligman, 1999). Ryan and Deci (2001) have reviewed the concept of well-being. They describe two main approaches adopted by researchers: the *hedonic* and the *eudaimonic*. Hedonic well-being consists of subjective happiness, pleasure, and pain-avoidance: well-being is associated with satisfaction and pleasant rather than distressing emotions. Eudaimonic well-being requires the realization of potential. Under this umbrella, some researchers describe "the fully functioning person," "meaningfulness," "self-actualization," and "vitality." The two approaches are quite different, but they complement each other (Ryan and Deci, 2001). In clinical psychology the eudaimonic view has received more attention because it concerns human potential and personal strength (Ryff and Singer, 1996). Ryff's model of psychological well-being encompasses autonomy, personal growth, environmental mastery, purpose in life, positive relations, and self-acceptance. It matches particular impairments in patients with affective disorder (Rafanelli *et al.*, 2000, 2002; Fava *et al.*, 2001; Ruini *et al.*, 2002).

Johnson and Roberts (1999) suggest that "looking at strengths rather than deficits, opportunities rather than risks, assets rather than liabilities is slowly becoming an increasing presence in the psychotherapy, education, and parenting literature." In positive psychology, the paramount goal is to promote competence, adaptive functioning, psychological well-being, psychosocial skills, and coping. Working with children requires a developmental perspective (Roberts and Peterson, 1984).

Maddux *et al.* (1986) consider that two elements are required for a developmental approach: A future orientation in view of its relationship to improving health status in later life; and attention to problems evident in particular phases of childhood.

In line with the developmental perspective is the idea that childhood may be the best time to enhance healthy behavior and adjustment and to avert impairments in domains such as language, social competence, and self-efficacy. As stated by Roberts (1991), "prevention is basically taking action to avoid development of a problem and/or identify problems early enough in their development to minimize potential negative outcomes."

WELL-BEING THERAPY

The improvement of psychological well-being by means of well-being therapy (Fava and Ruini, 2003) could be an effective method of dealing with child and adolescent victims of trauma (Ramirez *et al.*, 1989). Well-being therapy is a short-term well-being-enhancing psychotherapeutic strategy which has been tested in controlled trials, both alone (Fava *et al.*, 1998; Sonino and Fava, 2003) and in addition to CBT (Fava *et al.*, 1998; Fava *et al.*, 2002; Fava *et al.*, 2004; Fava *et al.*, 2005; Belaise *et al.*, 2005). There is evidence for the effectiveness of well-being therapy in the residual phase of mood and anxiety disorders, in refractory mood and anxiety disorders, and in PTSD.

Well-being therapy is based on Ryff's model of psychological well-being (PWB) (Ryff, 1989). It extends over eight sessions of 30–50 min duration and is structured, directive, and problem-oriented.

Well-being therapy might be combined with symptom-oriented CBT in a clinical setting or implemented in school as a preventive intervention. There is substantial evidence (Fava, 1992, 1996; Ryff and Singer, 1998) that psychological well-being buffers stress, has a favorable impact on the course of disease and has important immunological and endocrine concomitants (Fava and Sonino, 2000). It is conceivable that well-being therapy yields clinical benefits by enhancing quality of life, coping style and social support in depression, PTSD and anxiety disorder, as was shown for CBT (Emmelkam and Van Oppen, 1993). It is also conceivable that well-being therapy is particularly valuable in patients whose diseases cause a sense of loss. In this context, loss refers not just to body parts and functions actually lost, but also to the deprivation of significant needs and values, such as self-esteem, security, and satisfaction (Lipowski, 1969).

A WILL TO MEANING

Viktor Frankl argued that a crucial, motivating force in people's behavior is the "will to meaning" (Frankl, 1962, 1986). Nolen-Hoeksema and Davis (2002) report that an experience of loss can cause people to change how they see themselves and the world around them and to question where they are going with their lives. Losses, especially those that are sudden and unexpected, often initiate a personal evaluation or stocktaking of the meaning of life. Frankl challenged his clients who had experienced loss to create new life meanings. "It is the attitude one adopts to adversity that is critical for adjustment" (Frankl, 1962). The challenge is to find something worthwhile in a trauma by the use of positive coping strategies. Seeking something positive following a loss is not merely denial or defensiveness (Nolen-Hoeksema and Davis, 2002). Healthy coping involves the reappraisal of events, active problem solving, the search for social support, and the expression of emotion (Nolen-Hoeksema and Larson, 1999). The most consistent predictor of the capacity to derive benefit from trauma is dispositional optimism (Tedeschi and Calhoun, 1995; Affleck and Tennen, 1996; Park *et al.*, 1996; Davis *et al.*, 1998; Tennen and Affleck, 1999). Studies of treatment for children convalescing from amputation or severe injury should evaluate the importance of positive coping strategies.

OPTIMISM

There has been an upsurge of research into the benefits of optimism and the costs of pessimism.

According to Roberts *et al.* (2002), optimists have more success in college than pessimists. They perform better in sports and at work, and may even live longer (Seligman, 1991). Seligman (1991) stated that optimism has four different sources:

1. Genetics (Schulman and Seligman, 1993; Seligman *et al.*, 1995)
2. The child's parental environment (Seligman *et al.*, 1995)
3. Criticism received from parents, teachers, coaches, and other adults
4. Life experiences that promote mastery of helplessness.

Jaycox *et al.* (1994) and Gillham *et al.* (1995) have designed a preventive intervention for children at high risk for depression. The intervention addresses the child's explanatory style and social problem-solving. Children are taught to identify negative beliefs, evaluate them, and generate realistic alternatives. They are asked to identify pessimistic explanations for events and substitute more optimistic ones for them. At the end of the programme, children exposed to this therapy had fewer depressive symptoms than a control group.

HOPE

Hope has been the subject of several studies (Snyder *et al.*, 1991, 1997; Snyder, 1994). Pilot projects by Lopez (2000) and McDermott *et al.* (1996) report promising results. Research is needed to examine the experiences related to hopefulness or despair, the circumstances in which hope leads to favorable or adverse outcome, and the types of intervention that enhance hope and optimism (Roberts *et al.*, 2002).

OTHER STRATEGIES FOSTERING RESILIENCE

Masten and Reed (2002) describe three strategies for promoting resilience:

1. *Risk-focused strategies* (e.g., prenatal care to prevent premature birth, school reform to reduce adolescents' stress due to transitions, and the prevention of homelessness)
2. *Asset-focused strategies* (e.g., tutoring, the provision of recreation centers, job programmes for parents, programmes to reinforce parents' and teachers' skills)
3. *Process-focused strategies* (e.g., the fostering of secure attachment relationships, efforts to promote mastery motivation).

REFERENCES

Ackerman, P. T., Newton, J. E., McPherson, W. B., *et al.* (1998) Prevalence of post traumatic stress disorder and other psychiatric diagnoses in three groups of abused children (sexual, physical, and both). *Child Abuse Negl*, **22**, 759–74.

Affleck, G. and Tennen, H. (1996) Construing benefits from adversity: Adaptational significance and dispositional underpinnings. *J Pers*, **64**, 899–922.

Allwood, M. A., Bell-Dolan, D., and Husain, S. A. (2002) Children's trauma and adjustment reactions to violent and nonviolent war experiences. *J Am Acad Child Adolesc Psychiatry*, **41**, 450–57.

American Psychiatric Association. (1980) *Diagnostic and Statistical Manual of Mental Disorders (DSM-III)*, American Psychiatric Association, Washington, DC.

American Psychiatric Association. (1994) *Diagnostic and Statistical Manual of Mental Disorders*, 4th Edition (DSM-IV), American Psychiatric Association, Washington, DC.

Anonymous (1998.) Practice parameters for the assessment and treatment of children and adolescents with posttraumatic stress disorder. J Am Acad Child Adolesc Psychiatry, 37, 4–26.

Baker, S. P., O'Neil, B., and Karpt, R. S. (1984) The Injury Fact Book, Lexington Books, Lexington (MA).

Belaise, C., Fava, G. A., and Marks, I. M. (2005) Alternatives to debriefing and modifications to cognitive-behavior therapy for post-traumatic stress disorder. *Psychother Psychosom*, **74**, 212–17.

Belter, R. W., Dunn, S. E., and Jeney, P. (1991) The psychological impact of Hurricane Hugo on children: A needs assessment. *Adv Behav Res Ther*, **13**, 155–61.

Berliner, L. (1997) Intervention with children who experience trauma, in *The Effects of Trauma and the Developmental Process* (eds D. Cicchetti and S. Toth), John Wiley & Sons, Inc., New York, pp. 491–514.

Bisson, J. I., Jenkins, P. L., Alexander, J., and Bannister, C. (1997) Randomized controlled trial of psychological debriefing for victims of acute burn trauma. *Br J Psychiatry*, **171**, 78–81.

Bisson, J. I., McFarlane, A. C., and Rose, S (2000) Psychological debriefing, in *Effective Treatments for PTSD* (eds E. B. Foa, T. M. Keane, and M. J. Friedman), Guilford Press, New York.

Bisson, J. I. (2003) Single session early psychological interventions following traumatic events. *Clin Psychol Rev*, **23**, 481–99.

Blom, G. A. (1986) A school disaster: Intervention and research aspects. *J Am Acad Child Pychiatry*, **25**, 336–45.

Brent, D. A., Perper, J. A., Moritz, G. *et al.* (1995) Posttraumatic stress disorder in peers of adolescent suicide victims. *J Am Acad Child Adolesc Psychiatry*, **34**, 209–15.

Breslau, N., Davis, G. C., Andreski, P. *et al.* (1991) Traumatic events and posttraumatic stress disorder in an urban population of young adults. *Arch Gen Psychiatry*, **48**, 216–22.

Briere, J. (1995) *The Trauma Symptom Checklist for Children Manual (TSC-C)*, Psychological Assessment Resources, Odessa, FL.

Brigham, P. A. and McLoughlin, E. (1996) Burn incidence and medical care in the United States: Estimates, trends, and data sources. *J Burn Care Rehabil*, **17**, 95–103.

Brown, J., Cohen, P., Johnson, J. G., and Smailes, E. M. (1999) Childhood abuse and neglect: Specificity of effects on adolescent and young adult depression and suicidality. *J Am Acad Child Adolesc Psychiatry*, **38**, 1490–96.

Bryant, R. A., Harvey, A. G., Sackville, T. *et al.* (1998) Treatment of acute stress disorder: A comparison of cognitive behavioral therapy and supportive counseling. *J Consult Clin Psychol*, **66**, 862–66.

Bryant, R. A., Moulds, M., and Nixon, R. D. V. (2003) Cognitive behavior therapy of acute stress disorder: A four-year follow-up. *Behav Res Ther*, **41**, 489–94.

Bryant, R. A., Sackville, T., Dang, S. T. *et al.* (1999) Treating acute stress disorder: An evaluation of cognitive behavioral therapy and counseling techniques. *Am J Psychiatry*, **156**, 1780–86.

Burgess, A. W. and Holstrom, L. (1974) Rape trauma syndrome. *Am J Psychiatry*, **131**, 981–86.

Burman, S. and Allen-Meares, P. (1994) Neglected victims of murder: Children's witness to parental homicide. *Soc Work*, **39**, 28–34.

Burkle, F. M., Jr. (1996) Acute-phase mental health consequences of disasters: Implications for triage and emergency medical services. *Ann Emerg Med*, **28**, 119–28.

Butler, R. W., Rizzi, L. P., and Handwerger, B. A. (1996) The assessment of posttraumatic stress disorder in pediatric cancer patients and survivors. *J Pediatr Psychol*, **21**, 499–504.

Caffo, E. and Belaise, C. (2003). Psychological aspects of traumatic injury in children and adolescents. *Child Adolesc Psychiatr Clin North Am*, **12**, 493–535.

Caffo, E. and Belaise, C. (2005). Children and adolescents' psychopathology after trauma: New preventive psychotherapeutic strategies. *Psychology of Stress*, Nova Science Publisher,New York, PP. 145–1.

Chard, K. M. (1994) A meta analysis of post traumatic stress disorder treatment outcomes of women survivors. *Dissertation*, Indiana University, Bloomington.

Cohen, J. A., Deblinger, E., Mannarino, A. P., and Steer, R. A. (2004) A multisite, randomized controlled trial for children with sexual abuse-related PTSD symptoms. *J Am Acad Child Adolesc Psychiatry*, **43**, 393–402.

Cohen, J. A. and Mannarino, A. P. (1993) A treatment model for sexually abused preschoolers. *J Interpersonal Violence*, **8**, 115–31.

Cohen, J. A. (2003) Treating acute posttraumatic reactions in children and adolescents. *Biol Psychiatry*, **53**, 827–33.

Courtois, C. A. (2002) Traumatic stress studies: The need for curricula inclusion. *J Trauma Pract*, **1**, 33–57.

Cuffe, S. P., Addy, C. L., Garrison, C. Z. *et al.* (1998) Prevalence of PTSD in a community sample of older adolescents. *J Am Acad Child Adolesc Psychiatry*, **37**, 147–54.

Davis, C. G., Nolen-Hoeksema, S., and Larson, J. (1998) Making sense of loss and benefiting from the experience: Two construals of meaning. *J Pers Soc Psychol*, **75**, 561–74.

Deblinger, E. and Heflin, A. H. (1996) *Cognitive Behavioral Interventions for Treating Sexually Abused Children*, Sage, Thousand Oaks, CA.
Deblinger, E. and Heflin, A. H. (1996) *Treating Sexually Abused Children and their Non-Offending Parents: A Cognitive Behavioral Approach*, Sage, Thousand Oaks CA.
Deblinger, E., McLeer, S. V., and Henry, D. (1990) Cognitive behavioral treatment for sexually abused children suffering post-traumatic stress: Preliminary findings. *J Am Acad Child Adolesc Psychiatry*, **29**, 747–52.
Dershewitz, R. A. and Williamson, J. W. (1977) Prevention of childhood household injuries: A controlled clinical trial. *Am J Public Health*, **67**, 1148–53.
Diener, E., Suh, E. M., Lucas, R. E., and Smith, H. L. (1999) Subjective well-being: Three decades of progress. *Psychol Bull*, **125**, 276–302.
DiGallo, A., Barton, J., and Parry-Jones, W. (1997) Road traffic accidents: Early psychological consequences in children and adolescents. *Br J Psychiatry*, **170**, 358–62.
Dohrenwend, B. P., Dohrenwend, B. S., Warheit, G. J. *et al.* Stress in the community: a report to the President's commission on the accident at three mile island. *Ann N Y Acad Sci*, **365**, 159–74.
Ehlers, A., Clark, D. M., Hacmann, A. *et al.* A randomized controlled trial of cognitive therapy, self-help, and repeated assessment as early interventions for PTSD. *Arch Gen Psychiatry*, **60**, 1024–32.
Ehlers, A. and Clark, D. M. (2003) Early psychological interventions for adult survivors of trauma: A review. *Biol Psychiatry*, **53**, 817–26.
Emmelkamp, P. G. M. and Van Oppen, P. (1993) Cognitive intervention in behavioral medicine. *Psychother Psychosom*, **59**, 116–30.
Facteau, G. and Nicki, R. (1999) Cognitive behavioral treatment of posttraumatic stress disorder after motor vehicle accident. *Behav Cogn Psychother*, **27**, 201–14.
Fava, G. A., Rafanelli, C., Cazzaro, M. *et al.* (1998) Well-being therapy. *Psychol Med*, **28**, 475–80.
Fava, G. A., Rafanelli, C., Grandi, S, *et al.* (1998) Prevention of recurrent depression with cognitive behavioral therapy. *Arch Gen Psychiatry*, **55**, 816–20.
Fava, G. A., Ruini, C., Rafanelli, C. *et al.* (2004) Six-year outcome of cognitive behavior therapy for prevention of recurrent depression. *Am J Psychol*, **161**, 1872–76.
Fava, G. A., Ruini, C., Rafanelli, C. *et al.* (2005) Well-being therapy of generalized anxiety disorder. *Psychother Psychosom*, **74**, 26–30.
Fava, G. A., Ruini, C., Rafanelli, C., and Grandi, S. (2002) Cognitive behavior approach to loss of clinical effect during long-term antidepressant treatment: A pilot study. *Am J Psychiatry*, **159**, 2094–95.
Fava, G. A. and Ruini, C. (2003) Development and characteristics of a well-being enhancing psychotherapeutic strategy: Well-being therapy. *J Behav Ther Exp Psychiat*, **34**, 45–63.
Fava, G. A. and Sonino, N. (2000) Psychosomatic medicine: Emerging trends and perspectives. *Psychother Psychosom*, **69**, 184–87.
Fava, G. A. (1992) The concept of psychosomatic disorder. *Psychother Psychosom*, **58**, 1–12.
Fava, G. A. (1996) The concept of recovery in affective disorders. *Psychother Psychosom*, **65**, 2–13.
Fava, G. A., Rafanelli, C., Ottolini, F. *et al.* (2001) Psychological well-being and residual symptoms in remitted patients with panic disorder and agoraphobia. *J Affect Disord*, **31**, 899–905.
Fecteau, G. W. (2000) Treatment of posttraumatic stress reactions to traffic accidents. *Dissertation Abstracts International, Section B. The Science and Engineering*, **61**(1-B), 527, US: Univ. Microfilms International.
Fergusson, D. M., Lynskey, T. L., and Horwood, L. J. (1996a) Childhood sexual abuse and psychiatric disorder in young adulthood: I. Prevalence of sexual abuse and factors associated with sexual abuse. *J Am Acad Child Adolesc Psychiatry*, **35**, 1355–64.
Fergusson, D. M., Lynskey, T. L., and Horwood, L. J. (1996b) Childhood sexual abuse and psychiatric disorder in young adulthood: II. Psychiatric outcomes of childhood sexual abuse. *J Am Acad Child Adolesc Psychiatry*, **35**, 1365–74.
Fergusson, D. M. and Lynskey, T. L. (1997) Physical punishment/maltreatment during childhood and adjustment in young adulthood. *Child Abuse Negl*, **21**, 617–30.
Figley, C. R. (2002) Origins of traumatology and prospects for the future. *J Trauma Pract*, **1**, 17–32.
Figley, C. R. (1978) *Stress Disorders among Vietnam Veterans: Theory, Research and Treatment Implications*, Brunner/Mazel, New York.

Fletcher, K. (1997) Childhood PTSD interview-child form, in *Trauma Assessments: A Clinician's Guide* (ed E. Carlson), Guilford, New York, pp. 248–50.

Foa, E. B. and Chambless, D. L. (1978) Habituation of subjective anxiety during flooding in imagery. *Behav Res Ther*, **16**, 391–99.

Foa, E. B., Dancu, C. V., Hembree, E. A. *et al.* (1999) A comparison of exposure therapy, stress inoculation training and their combination for reducing posttraumatic stress disorder in female assault victims. *J Consult Clin Psychol*, **67**, 194–200.

Frankl, V. E. (1962) *Man's Search for Meaning: An Introduction to Logotherapy*, Beacon, Boston.

Frankl, V. E. (1986) *The Doctor and the Soul: From Psychotherapy to Logotherapy*, 3rd Edition, Vintage, New York.

Frederick, C. J. (1985) Children traumatized by catastrophic situations, in *Posttraumatic Stress Disorder in Children* (eds S. Eth and R. S. Pynoos), American Psychiatric Press, Washington, DC, pp. 71–100.

Friedrich, W. N. (1996) Clinical considerations of empirical treatment studies of abuse children. *Child Maltreat*, **1**, 343–47.

Frueh, B. C., Turner, S. M., Beidel, D. C. *et al.* (1996) Trauma management therapy: A preliminary evaluation of a multicomponent behavioral treatment for chronic combat related PTSD. *Behav Res Ther*, **34**, 533–43.

Galante, R. and Foa, D. (1986) An epidemiological study of psychic trauma and effectiveness for children after a natural disaster. *J Am Acad Child Psychiatry*, **25**, 357–63.

Garrison, C. Z., Weinrich, M. W., Hardin, S. B. *et al.* (1993) Posttraumatic stress disorder in adolescents after a hurricane. *Am J Epidemiol*, **136**, 522–30.

Garrison, C. Z., Bryant, E. S., Addy, C.L. *et al.* (1995) Posttraumatic stress disorder in adolescents after Hurricane Andrew. *J Am Acad Child Adolesc Psychiatry*, **34**, 1193–201.

Giaconia, R. M., Reinherz, H. Z., Silverman, A. B. *et al.* (1995) Traumas and posttraumatic stress disorder in a community population of older adolescents. *J Am Acad Child Adolesc Psychiatry*, **34**, 1369–80.

Gillham, J., Reivich, K. J., Jaycox, L. H., and Seligman, M. E. P. (1995) Prevention of depressive symptoms in school children: Two year follow-up. *Psychol Sci*, **6**, 343–51.

Gillham, J. E., and Seligman, M. E. P. (1999). Footstep on the road to a positive psychology. *Behav Res Ther*, **37**, 5163–73.

Gist, R. and Woodal, S. (2000) There are no simple solutions to complex problems, in *Posttraumatic Stress Intervention: Challenges, Issues and Perspectives* (eds J. M. Violanti and P. Douglas), Charles C. Thomas, Springfield, IL, pp. 81–95.

Goenjian, A. K., Karayan, I., Pynoos, R. S. *et al.* (1997) Outcome of psychotherapy among early adolescents after trauma. *Am J Psychiatry*, **154**, 536–42.

Goenjian, A. K., Pynoos, R. S., Steinberg, A. M *et al.* (1995) Psychiatric comorbidity in children after the 1988 earthquake in Armenia. *J Am Acad Child Adolesc Psychiatry*, **34**, 1174–84.

Goenjian, A. K., Molina, L., Steinberg, A. M. *et al.* (2001) Posttraumatic stress and depressive reactions among Nicaraguan adolescents after Hurricane Mitch. *Am J Psychiatry*, **158**, 788–94.

Goldstein, R. D. and Wampler, N. S. (1997) Wise PH. War experiences and distress symptoms of Bosnian children. *Pediatrics*, **100**, 873–78.

Gomes-Schwarz, B., Horowitz, J., and Cardarelli, A. (1990) *Child Sexual Abuse: The Initial Effects*, Sage, Newbury Park, CA, pp. 132–52.

Green, B., Grace, M. C. Vary M. G. *et al.* (1994) Children of disaster in the second decade: A 17-year follow-up of Buffalo Creek survivors. *J Am Acad Child Adolesc Psychiatry*, **33**, 71–79.

Green, B. L., Korol, M., Grace, M. C. *et al.* (1991) Children and disaster: Age, gender, and parental effects on PTSD symptoms. *J Am Acad Child Adolesc Psychiatry*, **30**, 945–51.

Grinker, R. R. and Spiegel, J. P. (1945) *Men Under Stress*, Irvington Press, New York.

Hadi, F. A. and Llabre, M. M. (1998) The Gulf crisis experience of Kuwaiti children: Psychological and cognitive factors. *J Trauma Stress*, **11**, 45–56.

Handford, H. A., Mayes, S. D., Mattison, R. E. *et al.* (1986) Child and parent reaction to the Three Mile Island nuclear accident. *J Am Acad Child Psychiatry*, **25**, 346–56.

Helzer, J. E., Robins, L. N., and McEvoy, L. (1987) Post-traumatic stress disorder in the general population: Findings of the Epidemiologic Catchment Area survey. *N Engl J Med*, **317**, 1630–34.

Heptinstall, E. (1996) *Healing the Hidden Hurt: The Emotional Effects of Children's Accidents*, Child Accident Prevention Trust, London.

Hokanson, M. and Wirth, B. (2000) The critical incident stress debriefing process for the Los Angeles County Fire Department: Automatic and effective. *Int J Emerg*, **2**, 249–57.

Horowitz, M. J (1976) *Stress Response Syndromes*, Aronson, New York.

Hubbard, J., Realmuto, G. M., Northwood, A. K., and Masten, A. S. (1995) Comorbidity of psychiatric diagnoses with posttraumatic stress disorder in survivors of childhood trauma. *J Am Acad Child Adolesc Psychiatry*, **34**, 1167–73.

Hodgson, R. J. and Rachman, S. (1970) An experimental investigation of the implosion technique. *Behav Res Ther*, **8**, 21–27.

International Federation of Red Cross and Red Crescent Societies. (1998) World Disaster Report. Oxford University Press, New York.

Jaycox, L. H., Reivich, K. J., Gillham, J., and Seligman, M. E. P. (1994) Prevention of depressive symptoms in school children. *Behav Res Ther*, **32**, 801–16.

Johnson, K. M., Foa, E. B., Jaycox, L. H., and Rescoda, L. (1996) A self-report diagnostic instrument for children with PTSD. Presented at the 12th Annual Meeting of the International Society for Traumatic Stress Studies, San Francisco, November 9–13.

Johnson, N. G. and Roberts, M. C. (1999) Passage on the wild river of adolescence: Arriving safetely, in *Beyond Appearances: A New Look at Adolescent Girls* (eds N. G. Johnson, M. C. Roberts, and J. Worell), American Psychological Association, Washington, DC, pp. 3–18.

Joseph, S., Brewin, C., Yule, W., and Williams, R. (1993) Causal attributions and posttraumatic stress disorder in adolescents. *J Child Psychol Psychiatry*, **34**, 274–53.

Kardiner, A. (1941) *The Traumatic Neuroses of War*, Paul B. Hoeber, New York.

Kaufman, J., Birmaher, B., Brent, D. *et al.* (1997) Schedule for affective disorders and schizophremia for school-age children-present and lifetime version (K-SADS-PL): Initial reliability and validity data. *J Am Acad Child Adolesc Psychiatry*, **36**, 980–88.

Keane, T. M. and Barlow, D. H. (2002) Posttraumatic stress disorder, in *Anxiety and its Disorders* (ed D. H. Barlow), The Guilford Press, New York, pp. 418–53.

Keane, T. M., Fisher, L. M., Krinsley, K. E., and Niles, B. L. (1994) Posttraumatic stress disorder, in *Handbook of Prescriptive Treatments for Adults* (eds M. Hersen and R. T. Ammermann), Plenum Press, New York.

Kessler, R. C., Sonnega, A., Bromet, E. *et al.* (1995) Posttraumatic stress disorder in the national comorbidity survey. *Arch Gen Psychiatry*, **52**, 1048–60.

Kilpatrick, K. L. and Williams, L. M. (1998) Potential mediators of post-traumatic stress disorder in child witnesses to domestic violence. *Child Abuse Negl*, **22**, 319–30.

Kinzie, J. D., Sack, W. H., Angell, R. H. *et al.* (1986) The psychiatric effects of massive trauma on Cambodian children I: The children. *J Am Acad Child Adolesc Psychiatry*, **25**, 370–76.

Kiser, L. J., Ackerman, B. J., Brown, E. *et al.* (1988) Post-traumatic stress disorder in young children: A reaction to purported sexual abuse. *J Am Acad Child Adolesc Psychiatry*, **27**, 645–49.

Kolko, D. (1996) Individual cognitive-behavioral treatment and family therapy for physically abused children and their offending parents: A comparison of clinical outcomes. *Child Maltreatment*, **1**, 322–42.

Kramer, S. H. and Rosenthal, R. (1998) Meta-analytic research synthesis, in *Comprehensive Clinical Psychology: Research and Methods* (A. S. Bellak, M. Hersen, and N. R. Shooler), Pergamon, Oxford, pp. 351–68.

La Greca, A., Silverman, W. K, Vernberg, E. M., and Prinstein, M. J. (1996) Symptoms of posttraumatic stress in children after Hurricane Andrew: A prospective study. *J Consult Clin Psychol*, **64**, 712–23.

La Greca, A. M., Silverman, W. K., Vernberg, E. M., and Prinstein, M. J. (1996) Symptoms of posttraumatic stress in children after Hurricane Andrew: A prospective study. *J Consult Clin Psychol*, **64**, 712–23.

Laor, N., Wolmer, L., Hayes, L. C. *et al.* (1997) Israeli preschool children under SCUDs: A 30-month follow-up. *J Am Acad Child Adolesc Psychiatry*, **36**, 349–56.

Laor, N., Wolmer, L., Cohen, D. J. *et al.* (2001) Mother's functioning and children's symptoms 5 years after a SCUD missile attack. *Am J Psychiatry*, **58**, 1020–26.

Lipowski, Z. J. (1969) Psychosocial aspects of disease. *Ann Intern Med*, **71**, 1197–296.
Litz, B. T., Gray, M. J., Byant, R. A., and Adler, A. B. (2002) Early intervention for trauma: Current status and future directions. *Clin Psychol Sci Prac*, **9**, 112–34.
Lonigan, C. J., Shannon, M. P., Finch, A. J. *et al.* (1991) Children's reactions to a natural disaster: Symptom severity and degree of exposure. *Adv Behav Res Ther*, **13**, 135–54.
Lopez, S. J. (2000) Positive psychology in the schools: Identifying and strengthening our hidden resources. Unpublished manuscript, University of Kansas, Lawrence, KS.
Macksoud, M. S. and Aber, J. L. (1996) The war experiences and psychosocial development of children in Lebanon. *Child Dev* **67**, 70–88.
Maddux, J. E., Roberts, M. C., Sledden, E. A., and Wright, L. (1986) Developmental issues in child health psychology. *Am Psychol*, **41**, 25–34.
Mannarino, A. P., Cohen, J. A., Smith, J. A., and Moore-Motily, S. (1991) Six and twelve month follow-up of sexually abused girls. *J Int Violence*, **6**, 484–511.
March, J. S., Amaya-Jackson, L., Murray, M. C., and Schulte, A. (1998) Cognitive-behavioral psychotherapy for children and adolescents with post-traumatic stress disorder after a single-incident stressor. *J Am Acad Child Adolesc Psychiatry*, **37**, 586–93.
Marks, I. M. (2000) 40 years of psychosocial treatments. *Behav Cogn Psychother*, **28**, 323–34.
Martinez, P. and Richters, J. E. (1993) The NIMH community violence project, II: Children's distress symptoms associated with violence exposure. *Psychiatry*, **59**, 22–35.
Masten, A. S. and Reed, M. G. J. (2002) Resilience in development, in *Handbook of Positive Psychology* (eds C. R. Snyder and S. J. Lopez), Oxford University Press, New York, pp. 74–88.
McDermott, D., Hastings, S., Gariglietti, K. P. *et al.* (1996) Fostering hope in the classroom. Paper presented at the meeting of the Kansas Counseling Association, Salina.
Meichenbaum, D. H. (1985) *Stress Inoculation Training*, Pergamon Press, New York.
Mirza, K. A. H., Bhadrinath, B. R., Goodyer, I., and Gilmour, C. (1998) Post-traumatic stress disorder in children and adolescents following road traffic accidents: A preliminary study. *Br J Psychiatry*, **172**, 443–47.
Murray, C. J. and Lopez, A. D. (1996) Evidence-based health policy: Lessons from the Global Burden of Disease Study. *Science*, **274**, 740–43.
Nader, K., Pynoos, R., Fairbanks, L., and Frederick, C. (1990) Children's PTSD reactions one year after a sniper attack at their school. *Am J Psychiatry*, **147**, 1526–30.
Nader, K. O., Pynoos, R. S., Fairbanks, L. A. *et al.* (1993) A preliminary study of PTSD and grief among the children of Kuwait following the Gulf crisis. *Br J Clin Psychol*, **32**, 407–16.
National Academy of Sciences Injury in America. (1985) A *Continuing Public Health Problem*, National Academy Press, Washington, DC.
Nolen-Hoeksema, S. and Davis, C. G. (2002) Positive response to loss: Perceiving benefits and growth, in *Handbook of Positive Psychology* (eds C. R. Snyder and S. J. Lopez), Oxford University Press, Oxford, pp. 598–607.
Nolen-Hoeksema, S. and Larson, J. (1999) *Coping with Loss*, Lawrence Erlbaum Associates, Mahwah (NJ).
Otto, M. W., Penava, S. J., Pollack, R. A. and Smoller, J. W. (1996) Cognitive-behavioral and pharmacologic perspectives on the treatment of posttraumatic stress disorder, in *Challenges in Clinical Practice: Pharmacological and Psychosocial Strategies* (eds R. A. Pollack, M. W. Otto, and J. F. Rosenbaum), Guilford Press, New York.
Parent, D. G., Lieter, V., Kennedy, S. *et al.* (1994) Conditions of confinement: Juvenile detention and corrections facilities (research report NCJ 145793), Office of Justice Programs, US Department of Justice; Washington, DC.
Park, C. L., Cohen, L. H., and Murch, R. L. (1996) Assessment and prediction of stress-related growth. *J Pers*, **64**, 71–105.
Parson, E. W. (1997) Posttraumatic child therapy (P-TCT). *J Interpersonal Violence*, **12**, 172–94.
Paunovic, N. and Ost, L. G. (2001) Cognitive-behavioral therapy vs Exposure Therapy in the treatment of PTSD in refugees. *Behav Res Ther*, **39**, 1183–97.
Pelcovitz, D., Libov, B. G., Mandel, F. *et al.* (1998) Posttraumatic stress disorder and family functioning in adolescent cancer. *J Trauma Stress*, **11**, 205–21.
Perry, B. (1999) Posttraumatic stress disorder in children and adolescents. *Curr Opin Pediatr*, **11**, 310–20.

Perry, B. D., Pollard, R. A., Blakley, T. L. *et al.* (1995) Childhood trauma, the neurobiology of adaptation and use-dependent development of the brain: How states become traits. *Infant Ment Health J*, **16**, 271–91.

Perry, B. D. (1994) Neurobiological sequelae of childhood trauma: PTSD in children, in *Catecholamine Function in Posttraumatic Stress Disorder: Emerging Concepts* (ed M. M. Murburg), American Psychiatric Press, Washington, DC, pp. 233–55.

Pfeffer, C. R. (1997) *Severe Stress and Mental Disturbance in Children*, American Psychiatric Association, Washington, DC.

Pfefferbaum, B. (1997) Posttraumatic stress disorder in children: A review of the past 10 years. *J Am Acad Child Adolesc Psychiatry*, **36**, 1503–11.

Pfefferbaum, B. Allen JR. Stress in children exposed to violence. Reenactment and Rage (1998). *Child Adolesc Psychiatr Clin North Am*, **7**.(1): 121–35

Pine, D. S. and Cohen, J. A. (2002) Trauma in children and adolescents: Risk and treatment of psychiatric sequelae. *Biol Psychiatry*, **51**, 519–31.

Pynoos, R. and Eth, S. (1986) Witness to violence: The child interview. *J Am Acad Child Psychiatry*, **25**, 306–19.

Pynoos, R. S., Frederick, C., Nader, K. *et al.* (1987) Life threat and posttraumatic stress in school-age children. *Arch Gen Psychiatry*, **44**, 1057–63.

Pynoos, R. S., Goenjian A., Tashtian M *et al* (1993) Post-traumatic stress reactions in children after the 1988 Armenian earthquake. *Br J Psychiatry*, **163**, 239–47.

Pynoos, R. S. and Nader, K. (1988) Psychological first aid and treatment approach to children exposed to community violence: Research implications. *J Trauma Stress*, **1**, 445–73.

Rafanelli, C., Conti, S., Mangelli, L. *et al.* (2002) Psychological well-being and residual symptoms in patients with affective disorders. II. *Rivista di Psichiatria*, **37**, 179–83.

Rafanelli, C., Park, S. K., Ruini, C. *et al.* (2000) Rating well-being and distress. *Stress Med*, **16**, 55–61.

Ramirez, A. J., Craig, T. K. J., Watson, J. P. *et al.* (1989) Stress and relapse of breast cancer. *Br Med J*, **298**, 291–94.

Realmuto, G. M., Masten, A., Carole, L. F. *et al.* (1992) Adolescent survivors of massive childhood trauma in Cambodia: Life events and current symptoms. *J Trauma Stress*, **5**, 589–99.

Resick, P. A. and Schnicke, M. K. (1992) Cognitive processing therapy for sexual assault victims. *J Consult Clin Psychol*, **60**, 748–56.

Rigamer, E. F. (1986) Psychological management of children in a national crisis. *J Am Acad Child Psychiatry*, **25**, 364–69.

Rizzone, L. P., Stoddard, F. J., Murphy, J. M., and Kruger, L. T. (1994) Posttraumatic stress disorder in mothers of children and adolescents with burns. *J Burn Care Rehabil*, **15**, 158–63.

Roberts, M. C., Brown, K. J., Johnson, R. J., and Reinke, J. (2002) Positive psychology for children: Development, Prevention, and Promotion, in *Handbook of Positive Psychology* (eds C. R. Snyder and S. J. Lopez), Oxford University Press, New York, pp. 663–75.

Roberts, M. C. and Peterson, L. (1984) Prevention models: Theoretical and practical implications, in *Prevention of Problems in Childhood: Psychological Research and Applications* (eds M. C. Roberts and L. Peterson), Wiley-Inter Science, New York, pp. 1–39.

Roberts, M. C. (1991) Overview to prevention research: Where is the cat? Where is the cradle? in *Advances in Child Health Psychology* (eds J. H. Johnson and S. B. Johnson), University of Florida Press, Gainesville, pp. 95–107.

Robinson, E., Rumsey, N., and Partridge, J. (1996) An evaluation of the impact of social interaction skills training for facially disfigured people. *Br J Plast Surg*, **49**, 281–89.

Rose, S., Bisson, J., and Wessely, S. (2003) A systematic review of single session psychological interventions ("debriefing") following trauma. *Psychother Psychosom*, **72**, 176–84.

Ruchkin, V. V., Eisemann, M., Hagglof, B. (1998) Juvenile male rape victims: Is the level of post-traumatic stress related to personality and parenting? *Child Abuse Negl*, **22**, 889–99.

Ruini, C., Rafanelli, C., Conti, S. *et al.* (2002). Psychological well-being and residual symptoms in patients with affective disorders. I. *Rivista di Psichiatria*, **37**, 171–78.

Runyan, C. W. and Gerken, E. A. (1989) Epidemiology and prevention of adolescent injury. *JAMA*, **262**, 2273–79.

Ryan, R. M. and Deci, E. L. (2001) On happiness and human potential: A review of research on hedonic and eudaimonic well-being. *Ann Rev Psychol*, **52**, 141–66.

Ryff, C. D. and Singer, B. (1998) The contours of positive human health. *Psychol Inquiry*, **9**, 1–28.

Ryff, C. D. (1989) Happiness is everything, or is it? Explorations on the meaning of psychological well being. *J Pers Soc Psychol*, **57**, 1069–81.

Ryff, C. D. and Singer, B. H. (1996) Psychological well-being: Meaning, measurement, and implications for psychotherapy research. *Psychother Psychosom*, **65**, 14–23.

Saakvitne, K. W., Gamble, S., Pearlman, L. A, and Lev, B. T. (2000) *Risking Connection: A Training Curriculum for Working with Survivors of Childhood Abuse*, Sidran Press, Lutherville, MD.

Sack, W. H., Clarke, G., Him, C. *et al.* (1993) A 6-year follow-up study of Cambodian refugee adolescents traumatized as children. *J Am Acad Child Adolesc Psychiatry*, **32**, 431–37.

Saigh, P. A., Yule, W., and Inamdar, S. C. (1996) Imaginal flooding of traumatized children and adolescents. *J Sch Psychol*, **34**, 163–83.

Saigh, P. A. (1996) In vitro flooding in one treatment of a six year-old boy's traumatic Stress Disorder Inventory. *Int J Spec Educ*, **4**, 75–84.

Salzer, M. S. and Bickman, L. (1999) The short and long term psychological impact of disasters: Implication for mental health interventions and policy, in *Response to Disaster: Psychosocial, Community and Ecological Approaches* (eds R. Gist and B. Lubin), Brunner/Mazel, Philadelphia, pp. 63–82.

Scheering, M. S., Zeanah, C. H., Drell, M. J. *et al.* (1995) Two approaches to the diagnosis of posttraumatic stress disorder in infancy and early childhood. *J Am Acad Child Adolesc Psychiatry*, **34**, 191–200.

Schnyder, U. and Moergeli, H. (2003) The course and development of early reactions to traumatic events: Baseline evidence from a non-intervention follow-up study, in *Reconstructing Early Intervention after Trauma. Innovation in the Care of Survivors* (eds R. J. Ornerand U. Schnyder), Oxford University Press, Oxford, pp. 106–17.

Schnyder, U. and Orner, R. J. (2003) Progress made towards reconstructing early intervention after trauma: Emergent themes, in *Reconstructing Early Intervention after Trauma. Innovation in the Care of Survivors* (R. J. Orner and U. Schnyder), Oxford University Press, Oxford, pp. 249–66.

Schulman, P., Keith, D., and Seligman, M. P. E. (1993) Is optimism heritable? A study of twins. *Behav Res Ther*, **31**, 569–74.

Schwarz, E. D. and Kowalski, J. M. (1991) Malignant memories: PTSD in children and adults after a school shooting. *J Am Acad Child Adolesc Psychiatry*, **30**, 936–44.

Seligman, M. P. E., Reivich. K., Jaycox, L., and Gillham, J. (1991) *The Optimistic child*, Houghton Mifflin, Boston.

Seligman, M. P. E. (1991) *Learned Optimism*, Knopf, New York.

Shannon, M. P., Lonigan, C. J., Finch, A. J., and Taylor, C. M. (1994) Children exposed to disaster. I: Epidemiology of post-traumatic symptoms and symptom profiles. *J Am Acad Child Adolesc Psychiatry*, **33**, 80–93.

Shaw, J. A., Applegate, B., Schorr, C. (1996) Twenty-one-month follow-up study of school-age children exposed to hurricane Andrew. *J Am Acad Child Adolesc Psychiatry*, **35**, 359–64.

Shaw, J. A., Applegate, B., Tanner, S. *et al.* (1995) Psychological effects of hurricane Andrew on an elementary school population. *J Am Acad Child Adolesc Psychiatry*, **34**, 1185–92.

Sheridan, R. L., Hinson, M. I., Liang, M. H. *et al.* (2000) Long-term outcome of children surviving massive burns. *JAMA*, **283**, 69–73.

Simons, D. and Silveira, W. R. (1994) Posttraumatic stress disorder in children after television programmes. *Br Med J*, **305**, 389–90.

Smith, G. S. and Barss, P. (1991) Unintentional injuries in developing countries: The epidemiology of a neglected problem. *Epidemiol Rev*, **13**, 228–66.

Smith, P., Perrin, S., Yule, W., Rabe-Hesketh, S. (2001) War exposure and maternal reactions in the psychological adjustment of children from Bosnia-Herzegovina. *J Child Psychol Psychiatry*, **42**, 395–404.

Snodgrass, L., Yamamoto, J., and Frederick, C. (1993) Vietnamese refugees with posttraumatic stress disorder symptomatology: Intervention via a coping skills model. *J Trauma Stress*, **6**, 569–74.

Snyder, C. R., Harris, C., Anderson, J. R. *et al.* (1991) The will and the ways: The development and validation of an individual differences measure of hope. *J PersSoc Psychol*, **60**, 570–85.

Snyder, C. R., Hoza, B., Pelham, W. E. *et al.* (1997) The development and validation of the Children's Hope scale. *J Pediatr Psychol*, **22**, 399–421.

Snyder, C. R. (1994) *The Psychology of Hope: You can Get There from Here*, Free Press, New York.
Solomon, S. D., Gerrity, E. T. and Muff, A. M. (1992) Efficacy for treatments for posttraumatic stress disorder. *J Am Med Assoc*, **265**, 633–37.
Sonino, N. and Fava, G. A. (2003) Tolerance to antidepressant treatment may be overcome by ketoconazole. *J Psychiat Res*, **37**, 171–73.
Spaccarelli, S. (1995) Measuring abuse stress and negative cognitive appraisals in child sexual abuse: Validity data on two new scales. *J Abnorm Child Psychol*, **23**, 703–27.
Stallard, P. and Law, F. (1993) Screening and psychological debriefing of adolescent survivors of life threatening events. *Br J Psych*, **163**, 660–65.
Steinberg, L. and Avenevoli, S. (2000) The role of context in the development of psychopathology: A conceptual framework and some speculative propositions. *Child Dev*, **71**, 66–74.
Stoddard, F. J. and Saxe, G. (2001) Ten-year research review of physical injuries. *J Am Acad Child Adolesc Psychiatry*, **40**, 1128–45.
Stoddard, F. J. (1996) Care of infants, children, and adolescents with burn injuries, in *Child and Adolescent Psychiatry* (ed M. Lewis), American Psychiatric Press, Washington, DC, pp. 1016–33.
Stoddard, F. J., Norman, D. K., Murphy, J. M., and Beardslee, W. R. (1989) Psychiatric outcome of burned children. *J Am Acad Child Adolesc Psychiatry*, **28**, 589–95.
Stuber, M. L., Kazak, A. E., Meeske, K. *et al.* (1997) Predictors of posttraumatic stress symptoms in childhood cancer survivors. *Pediatrics*, **100**, 958–64.
Sullivan, J. M. and Evans, K. (1994) Integrated treatment for the survivor of childhood trauma who is chemically dependent. *J Psychoactive Drugs*, **26**, 369–78.
Sullivan, M. A., Saylor, C. F., Foster, K. Y. (1991) Post-hurricane adjustment of preschoolers and their families. *Adv Behav Res Ther*, **13**, 163–71.
Tedeschi, R. G. and Calhoun, L. G. (1995) *Trauma and Transformation: Growing in the Aftermath of Suffering*, Sage, Thousand Oaks CA.
Tennen, H. and Affleck, G. (1999) Finding benefits in adversity, in Coping: The Psychology of What Works (ed C. R. Snyder), Oxford University Press, New York, pp. 279–304.
Terr, L. (1988) What happens to early memories of trauma? A study of twenty children under age five at the time of documented traumatic events. *J Am Acad Child Adolesc Psychiatry*, **27**, 96–104.
Terr, L. C. (1991) Childhood traumas: an outline and overview. *Am J Psychiatry*, **148**, 10–20.
Terr, L. C. (1989) Treating psychic trauma in children: a preliminary discussion. *J Trauma Stress*, **2**, 3–19.
Udwin, O., Boyle, S., Yule, W. *et al.* (2000) Risk factors for long term psychological effects of a disaster experienced in adolescence: Predictors of post traumatic stress disorder. *J Child Psychol Psychiatry*, **41**, 969–79.
UNICEF. (1996) *The State of the World's Children*, Oxford University Press, New York.
US Department of Transportation. (1993) Traffic safety facts (National Highway Traffic Safety Administration report DOTHS 808022), US Department of Transportation, Washington, DC.
Van Emmerik, A. A., Kamphuis, J. H., Hulsbosch, A. M., and Emmelkamp, P. M. (2002) Single session debriefing after psychological trauma: A meta-analysis. *Lancet*, **360**, 766–71.
Vernberg, E. M. (2002) Intervention approaches following disasters, in *Helping Children Cope with Disasters and Terrorism* (eds A. M. La Greca, W. K. Silverman, E. M. Vernberg, and M. C. Roberts), American Psychological Association, Washington, DC, pp. 55–72.
Vernberg, E. M., La Greca, A. M., Silverman, W. K., and Prinstein, M. J. (1996) Prediction of posttraumatic stress symptoms in children after Hurricane Andrew. *J Abnorm Psychol*, **105**, 237–48.
Vogel, J. M. and Vernberg, E. M. (1993) Children psychological responses to disaster. *J Clin Child Psychol*, **22**, 464–84.
Walker L. The Battered woman. New York: Harper and Row, 1979.
Watson, J. P. and Marks, I. M. (1971) Relevant and irrelevant fear in flooding – a crossover study of phobic patients. *Behav Ther*, **2**, 275–93.
Weisenberg, M., Schwarzwald, J., Waysman, M. *et al.* (1993) Coping of school-age children in the sealed room during SCUD missile bombardment and postwar stress reactions. *J Consult Clin Psychol*, **61**, 462–67.

World Health Organization. (2003) Mental Health in Emergencies: Psychological and social aspects of health of populations exposed to extreme stressors. WHO, Geneva. Available from: http://www.who.int/mental_health/media/en/244/pdf.

World Health Organization. (2005) Psychological care of Tsunami-affected populations. Caring for your own emotional well-being. Guidelines for relief workers. WHO, Geneva.

World Health Organization. (2005) Psychological support to the community: Acute emergency phase. Regional Office for South East Asia, http://w3.whosea.org/en/Section23/Section1108/Section1835_8311.htm

Wolfe, V. V., Gentile, C., and Wolfe, D. A. (1989) The impact of sexual abuse on children: A post-traumatic stress disorder formulation. *Behav Ther*, **20**, 215–28.

Yule, W., Bolton, D. *et al.* (2000) The long-term psychological effects of a disaster experienced in adolescence: I: The incidence and course of PTSD. *J Child Psychol Psychiatry*, **41**, 503–11.

Yule, W. and Udwin O. (1991) Screening child survivors for posttraumatic stress disorder: Experiences from the Jupiter: Sighting. *Br J Clin Psychol*, **30**, 131–38.

CHAPTER 5.4

School Dropout: A Systematic Worldwide Review Concerning Risk Factors and Preventive Interventions

Ana Soledade Graeff-Martins
Federal University of Rio Grande do Sul, Brazil
Tatjana Dmitrieva, Amira Seif El Din, Ernesto Caffo, Martine F. Flament, Barry Nurcombe, Per-Anders Rydelius, Helmut Remschmidt, and Luis Augusto Rohde
WPA Presidential Programme on Child Mental Health

INTRODUCTION

School dropout is a worldwide problem, particularly in developing countries. Recently, the United Nation Children's Fund (UNICEF) document, *The State of the World's Children 2005*, noted that 121 million primary-school children are out of school worldwide (United Nations Children's Fund, 2005). In Brazil, 95% of children have access to school, but only 58% complete the 8th grade (United Nations Children's Fund, 1999). In 1998, the population of Brazilian children regularly out of classroom was 1.5 million (MEC, 1999). The school dropout rate is an index of the educational condition of a country (Kominski, 1990) and a pointer to future social problems (Berg *et al.*, 1993).

School dropout is a very complex phenomenon. It must be understood in the context of socioeconomic conditions and the adequacy of educational systems. In developing countries, it is not uncommon for adolescents to leave school to work, and for school-age children to be kept home to take care of younger siblings. Furthermore, the educational system in developing countries is often not adequately prepared to meet the capabilities and needs of poorer children, provoking a significant number to drop out of school (Tramontina *et al.*, 2002). Nevertheless, schools in developing countries are potentially in a position to

The Mental Health of Children and Adolescents: an area of global neglect. Edited by H. Remschmidt *et al.*

provide a "safety net," protecting children from hazards that affect not only their learning, but also their psychological development and well-being (Kapur, 1997).

In our search of the literature, we found several reviews regarding school dropout (Svec, 1987; Wechsler and Oakland, 1990; Afolayan, 1991; Evans and Matthews, 1992; Royer *et al.*, 1993; MacLean and Janzen, 1994; Barton *et al.*, 1997; Witt *et al.*, 1999; Kearney and Hugelshofer, 2000; Doll and Hess, 2001; Dynarski and Gleason, 2002), but none was conducted systematically. The aim of this paper is to conduct a review of the school dropout literature, using a systematic method, focusing on risk factors and intervention.

METHOD

Using Medline, PsychInfo, and LILACS, we searched the scientific literature relevant to psychiatry, psychology, and community research up to October, 2004. We defined the terms of the search as *school dropout*, *risk factors*, *prevention*, and *intervention*. All bibliographic records generated by the search were downloaded and duplicate records identified and removed. After the search was completed, a review of relevant abstracts was conducted by one of the authors. The criteria adopted for inclusion of the abstract were as follows: (1) publication in a scientific journal; (2) inclusion of original data; and (3) evaluation of school dropout risk factors or intervention/prevention programmes. All eligible abstracts were reviewed, including those in languages other than English. Eligible articles were analyzed and are summarized below. We also checked all references from the papers found through this process and reviewed those that were appropriate.

RESULTS

The search strategy generated 166 records. Of these, 112 were excluded because they were not published in scientific journals (i.e., book chapters or dissertation abstracts), did not include original data, or did not address risk factors or intervention/prevention. The remaining 54 records entered the second level of assessment, which excluded 16 reports, in accordance with the same criteria as those used in the first relevance assessment. One article (Fortin and Picard, 1998) could not be found. The 37 reports retained were analyzed and are described in this paper. The 37 studies were conducted in five countries. Most studies were conducted in the United States (27), followed by Canada (4), New Zealand (3), Brazil (2), and Norway (1).

Descriptive studies

Franklin and Streeter (1995) studied 200 school dropouts who entered an experimental alternative educational programme in Texas. The children were examined for the following: reasons for leaving school (e.g., poor school and academic history), psychological/behavioral disorders, history of counseling and treatment, and levels of family functioning. They found an excess of students with histories of drug/alcohol use, mental health treatment, and family dysfunction.

Pittman (1986) interviewed 82 (44.3%) of 185 children who had dropped out of secondary school in an American rural school system. Students identified the following reasons for leaving school: lack of interest, failing grades, dissatisfaction with teachers or principal, unhappy school experiences, or the need to work.

Two other studies addressed very specific populations: pregnant adolescents (Stevenson *et al.*, 1998), and the children of migrant farm workers (Martinez and Cranston-Gingras, 1996). Stevenson *et al.* evaluated 119 pregnant adolescents in Baltimore. Their school dropout rate was 30% (16.4% reported that they had dropped out specifically because of pregnancy). Martinez and Cranston-Gingras interviewed 345 students in a Florida High School Equivalency programme. The purpose was to assess their reasons for leaving school. The reason most cited were as follows: need to work (36%), lack of interest in school (13%), need to move (11%), many absences (8%), feeling too old to study (7%), and marriage/pregnancy (7%).

All the descriptive studies had methodological problems such as refusal to participate, selection bias, and lack of a control group. Furthermore, none of the samples was truly representative of the population involved.

Case–control studies

The 12 studies that were case–control designed, aimed to explore the association between potential risk factors and dropping out from school.

Tramontina *et al.* (2001, 2002) studied all subjects ($n = 44$) who had dropped out from the third and forth elementary school grades in 64 schools in a Brazilian city. Forty-four controls were selected from the same classrooms. The students and their mothers were evaluated for psychiatric diagnosis and intelligence quotient. Associations were found between school dropout, child conduct disorder, and mental retardation. The small sample size was a limitation of this study.

Hess and Copeland (2001) compared 46 children who had dropped out with 46 controls who completed high school in the United States in regard to stressful life experiences in the previous year and coping behavior. Students who dropped out reported significantly more life change events than did students who graduated. Moreover, those who dropped out had higher weighted stressor scores than did students who graduated. There were no differences between the groups in regard to their most favored coping strategies. As per Tramontina *et al.* (2001, 2002), the sample size was small.

From a cohort of 743 United States adolescents followed from 13–16 to 19–22 years old, Achenbach *et al.* (1998) compared 97 who had dropped out with 97 controls, matched for sex, ethnicity, and age. Low scores on the ACQ School Scale strongly predicted dropping out for both sexes. Low SES, having unmarried, separated, or divorced parents, and Delinquent and Aggressive Scale scores on the TRF predicted male dropout.

Swaim *et al.* (1997) studied 774 students who had dropped out of school and 738 controls, from three different ethnic groups in the United States. They found lifetime prevalence of drug use to be substantially higher among those who had dropped out than among controls, and that those who dropped out were more exposed than controls to drug use in the previous month.

Two studies from a New Zealand birth cohort examined the relationship between cannabis use and school dropout (Fergusson *et al.*, 1996; Fergusson and Horwood, 1997). Of 927 subjects evaluated at 16 years of age, the school dropout rate was 5.3%. There was a clear association between cannabis use by the age of 15 years and school dropout between 15 and 16 years. Two years later, the dropout rate was 18.7%. Not only was there a relation between cannabis use and dropout, but the greater the frequency of cannabis use, the higher the risk of dropping out of school.

Bates *et al.* (1997) studied the association between school dropout and the lifetime prevalence of volatile solvent use in a sample of 3416 United States subjects. Those who had dropped out were compared to two other groups: students with the same academic performance as dropouts and regular students. Those who had dropped out were 2.27 (CI 95% 1.86–2.76) times more likely than regular controls to have used volatile solvents in their lifetime, whereas academically at-risk subjects were 1.72 (CI 95% 1.40–2.11) times more likely than regular controls to have used volatile solvents in their lifetime, and those who had dropped out were 1.32 (CI 95% 1.09–1.57) times more likely than academically at-risk respondents to have used volatile solvents in their lifetime.

Three studies (Obot and Anthony, 1999, 2000; Obot *et al.*, 1999), examined the relationship between school dropout and intravenous drug use in two different ethnic groups, analyzing data from the National Household Surveys on Drug Abuse conducted between 1991 and 1995. From 34 227 African Americans, 389 intravenous drug users and 2253 controls from the same neighborhood were assessed for the prevalence of school dropout. African Americans who dropped out of high school were approximately twice as likely to have injected a drug than were high school graduates. The results were very similar when the White non-Hispanic population (n = 12 643) was evaluated.

Dunham and Alpert (1987) studied 137 juvenile delinquents from Florida, 47 who remained at school and 90 who had dropped out. They were evaluated for parental, peer, and school influences, in order to test an empirically based prediction model of school dropout. The two strongest predictors of dropout were subcategories of school influences: "misbehavior in school" and "liking school." The predictor representing peer influences added the most predictive power to the model. The major limitation to this study was its retrospective design.

Cohort studies

Eleven studies used a cohort design to examine the risk factors for, and the consequences of, school dropout.

In a sample of 193 students from two towns in southwestern Ontario, Simner and Barnes (1991) investigated the relationship between first-grade marks in reading and arithmetic and school dropout at the end of high school. Despite the small size of the sample, they found an association between the first-grade marks and high school completion, suggesting a relationship between school dropout and learning difficulty.

A cohort of 5308 Norwegian junior and senior students was followed to investigate whether alcohol intoxication predicts dropout from senior high school (Wichström, 1998). Many potentially confounding factors were analyzed. The author concluded that intoxication overrode the effect of alcohol consumption and predicted dropout. The effect was confounded by parental attachment: Parental care marginally predicted change in intoxication, whereas alcohol intoxication was not predictive of change in parental care. Truancy and association with psychologically deviant peers mediated the effect of intoxication.

The National Education Longitudinal Survey collected data in 1988, 1990, 1992, and 1994 from 11 671 U.S. students, in order to examine the association between student mobility and high school completion. There was a strong relation between mobility and school dropout. High rates of absenteeism, conduct problems, and low educational expectation predicted mobility and school dropout.

Three studies examined school dropout as a potential risk factor for other conditions. Using the data from the National Education Longitudinal Survey, Manlove (1998) analyzed 8223 female students, finding 822 who became pregnant before completing high school. Family background, school and classroom characteristics, and individual characteristics were tested as potential confounding factors. It was concluded that students who receive support from their families attend schools with greater resources, and who are engaged in school are at less risk of falling pregnant.

Gest *et al.* (1999), in the Carolina Longitudinal Study, followed 475 subjects annually from seventh grade to the end of high school, and then to 20 and 24 years of age. A total of 426 subjects completed all evaluations. Adolescent parenthood status was determined for 100% of the sample, and early adult parenthood status for 94%. Early school dropout (i.e., leaving school prior to eleventh grade) and early parenthood were moderately correlated for both sexes. The configuration that predicted early parenthood (middle-school students who were aggressive, older, lower-achieving, unpopular, and from low SES families) was also strongly associated with early school dropout. In most cases, school dropout preceded pregnancy.

Crum *et al.* (1998) followed 1038 low-SES, African-American students from Chicago over 25 years, from first grade ($n = 1242$), through adolescence, to adulthood. At the last assessment, the prevalence of alcohol abuse/dependency was 13.5%; however, the relationship between school dropout and alcohol abuse/dependency was not statistically significant.

Gleason and Dynarski (2003) collected data regarding risk factors for dropout from 2672 U.S. middle school students and 2808 U.S. high school students. After 2 and 3 years of follow-up, the prevalence of dropping out was assessed. Two models were tested: a composite risk factor and a regression risk factor. The composite risk factor defined a student as at risk if he or she had a minimum particular number of single risk factors. Alternative versions of the composite risk factor were based on whether students had at least two, three, or four of eight single risk factors. The regression-risk factor model combined single factors. The authors tested a logistic model that related 40 student characteristics and risk factors to dropping out, applying the model to calculate, for each student, the predicted probability of dropping out. The authors concluded that a composite risk factor more effectively identified those at risk for dropping out.

Fergusson and Horwood (1995) followed 1265 newborns in New Zealand, at 4 months and yearly until 16 years of age ($n = 935$, 74% of the original cohort). The school dropout rate was 5.3%. The authors concluded that scales for ADHD, ODD, and conduct disorder could be used dimensionally (rather than categorically) to predict such behavior as school dropout, substance use, and juvenile offending.

Battin-Pearson *et al.* (2000) interviewed 778 and 770 students, 14 and 16 years old, respectively, from a sample of 808 students in 18 Seattle schools. The school dropout rate was 11%. Fourteen variables were evaluated at the first assessment. Statistical analysis demonstrated that general deviance, bonding to antisocial peers, and low SES were direct predictors of dropout and poor academic achievement before the end of tenth grade. Low school bonding, early sexual activity, low parental educational expectations, parents' lack of education, male sex, and ethnicity (African-American) also predicted dropout before the end of tenth grade, mediated by poor academic achievement.

The last two studies in this group (Janosz *et al.*, 1997, 2000) were derived from the same cohort and examined two samples of Canadian high school students. One was a random, stratified sample of the student population of the Isle of Montreal (n = 791) and the other, a sample from moderate and low SES families (n = 791). The dropout prevalence at 22 years of age was 22% and 42%, respectively. The authors concluded that the most important predictors of dropping out were related to school experience (grade retention, poor school grades, and poor commitment to schooling), followed by the socioeconomic status of the family and parents' level of education. In the second study, the authors described four types of dropout, defined by a statistical analysis: (1) *quiet* (no evidence of school misbehavior; moderate or high levels of commitment to education in general); (2) *disengaged* (average-low level of school misbehavior, low commitment to school, and average grade performance); (3) *low-achiever* (weak commitment to education, average-low levels of school misbehavior, very poor school performance); and (4) *maladjusted* (poor school performance and weak commitment to education).

Intervention study – without control group

One study (Dennison, 2000) described the Peer Mentoring and Tutoring ("Big Buddies") Programme. Juniors and seniors from high school were trained as peer mentors and tutors and assigned to 25 third and fourth graders ("Little Buddies") identified by teachers as at risk of dropping out of school. Mentors met their students twice a week, in the last class period. Sessions lasted 45 min and had the objectives of building a relationship, remediating on academic deficits, and capturing the at-risk student's attention. "Little Buddies" was evaluated pre- and post-intervention on three dimensions: self-esteem, school attitude, and classroom behavior. There were no statistically significant differences between the pre- and post-total scores on the three dimensions; however, 16 of the 25 subjects improved one grade level in the academic subject in which they had received tutoring in from their mentors.

Quasi-experimental intervention studies

Six quasi-experimental studies examined interventions to prevent or reduce school dropout. All studies had control groups, but without random subject assignment.

The Chicago Longitudinal Study (Reynolds *et al.*, 2001) followed a cohort of 1539 low-income minority children born in 1980. They were exposed to two types of intervention: one during preschool/kindergarten in 20 Child–Parent Centers (CPC) (n = 989) and the other in school-age programmes, conducted for at least 1 year between first and third grade (n = 850). The Child–Parent Centers Programme provided comprehensive education, family health services, and half-day preschool at ages 3–4 years, a half-day or full-day kindergarten, and school-age services in linked elementary schools between ages 6 and 9 years. The two samples were compared, as follows: 333 children who entered the CPCs in preschool and continued their participation through second or third grade (extended intervention – 4 to 6 years) and 602 children with 1–4 years of intervention. At age 20 years, of the original sample, 83.2% ($n = 1281$) provided data on educational attainment. The outcomes evaluated were educational attainment, official juvenile arrests, and school remedial services. At 20 years, preschool participants had a significantly higher rate of high school completion and a lower rate of school dropout. Preschool participants completed more years of education. School-age participation alone was not associated with improvement in educational attainment.

Hawkins *et al.* (1999) implemented an intervention combining the following: teacher training in proactive classroom management; interactive teaching and cooperative learning (5 days per year in grades 1 through 6); parent education in behavior management skills, academic support, and the promotion of skills aimed to avert drug use (parenting classes when children were in grades 1 through 3 and 5 through 6); and social-competence training for children (in grades 1 and 6) during the elementary grades in public elementary schools located in high crime areas in Seattle. They compared children who were exposed to the full intervention with two other groups, as follows: (1) children who received late intervention (in grades 5 and 6 only) and (2) a third group who received no intervention at all. The outcomes evaluated 6 years later were as follows: self-reported violent and nonviolent crime, substance use, sexual activity, pregnancy, bonding to school, school achievement, grade repetition, school dropout, suspension and/or expulsion, school misbehavior; delinquency charges from court records, grade point average. There was no significant difference between groups in regard to school dropout. It is interesting to note that only 43% of parents from the full-intervention group participated effectively in the programme.

The Teen Outreach Programme (Allen *et al.*, 1990) evaluated the effectiveness of volunteer activities (half an hour per week) (work as aides in hospitals and nursing homes, participation in walkathons, volunteer work at school, and a wide range of other types of work), together with classroom-based group discussions on issues such as understanding oneself and one's values, communication skills, dealing with family stress, and human growth and development. The Programme was conducted in 35 different sites in 30 schools in United States. The 632 students in the programme were compared with 855 controls, from seventh to twelfth grade. The outcome measures were demographic characteristics, pregnancy, school dropout, and school suspension. Teen outreach participants had significantly lower rates of suspension, school dropout, and pregnancy than comparison students. Although the procedures of the study varied between different sites, multiple regression equations were used to examine the relationships between student outcome at exit, four sets of student entry characteristics, and programme factors. Teen outreach sites were most successful when they worked with older students and when the volunteer component of the programme was more intensively implemented. Sites working with younger students were more effective when they had more, rather than less, intensive classroom components. It is important to note that, as there was no randomization, subjects less prone to dropout might have been those who were more inclined to take part in voluntary activities and classroom groups.

Comiskey (1993) implemented a counseling technique, Reality Therapy (RT), with high school students at risk for repeated academic failure and dropout. Three groups of 15 students each were formed. Group 1 received 12 sessions of RT, the main purpose of which was to promote individual responsibility and self-esteem. Group 2 received 12 sessions of RT, in addition to which the school organization was changed as follows: students were grouped together for English and Social Science classes and received special attention from a team of teachers, counselors, and administrators. The control group experienced only a twelve-session career-development group. The second group (reality therapy and change in school organization) obtained the best results in terms of school achievement, self-esteem, and school attendance. An important limitation to this study is the small sample, and a high rate of defection. The four students in each group who did not complete the programmes were not considered in the final analysis.

The Network Social Support Programme (Eggert *et al.*, 1990) studied the effectiveness of small-group (one teacher to ten students) psychoeducational counseling classes. Groups met daily for one school semester, with the goals of improving school achievement and attendance, and minimizing drug use. These objectives were clearly communicated and frequently reiterated. The groups were conducted by teachers in the school who had expressed an interest in high-risk students, and who subsequently coordinated group discussions, implemented skill training, supervised study, and arranged visits to community agencies. The sample was composed of 264 high-risk students to whom an Interpersonal Relations elective class was offered within the regular school curriculum. The experimental group was composed of the 73 students who completed the course. The control group (n = 73) was randomly selected from the 157 high-risk students who either did not choose to enter the course or could not be accommodated in it. Controls resembled experimental cases in age, sex, and grade. Fewer students from the experimental group dropped out of school and they exhibited better school achievement, decreased truancy, and less drug use. The limitations of this study were the potential selection bias (those more motivated from the at-risk group were more likely to join the intervention), and the fact that the 34 students who began the Network Social Support Programme but did not complete it were not evaluated in the final analysis.

A similar study conducted by the same investigators (Eggert *et al.*, 1994) compared 101 students in the Personal Growth Class with 158 controls. The Personal Growth Class was structured as an elective, semester-long programme within the regular school curriculum. Students met in classrooms daily, for 55 min, on 90 school days. The class was taken for credit and graded. The teacher–student ratio was no greater than 1:12. Classes were implemented by regular high school teachers who had a strong desire to work with high-risk youth. The course was composed of four units: self-esteem enhancement, decision making, personal control, and interpersonal communication. Programme effectiveness was demonstrated by a reduction of drug-related problems and an improvement in grade-point average and the quality of bonding to the school. There was no difference between the groups in school attendance.

Experimental intervention studies

Three studies in this review present data from experimental studies with control groups and random assignment.

Vitaro *et al.* (1999) studied 259 boys selected from a sample of 904 boys in Canada whose disruptiveness had been assessed by their teachers in kindergarten. All subjects had scores above the seventieth percentile on the disruptiveness scale in the Social Behavior

Questionnaire (SBQ). They were randomly assigned to one of the three groups: (1) an intervention group ($n = 75$); (2) a no-treatment control group ($n = 60$); and (3) a sensitization contact group ($n = 124$). Thirty-two, 19, and 12 parents in each of the three groups, respectively, refused to participate in the study. The control group and the sensitization contact group did not differ on any variable and were consequently collapsed for analysis. Intervention consisted in a two-year programme, implemented from ages 7 to 9 years, with two components: social skills training and parental skill promotion. The children's groups included pro-social and target boys, and received biweekly sessions. Subjects were evaluated regarding family background, verbal IQ (assessed at 13 years), SBQ scores at 9, 10, and 11 years of age, placement in other than age-appropriate regular classrooms at 12 years, and school dropout before 17 years. At 17 years of age, there was no difference between the groups in terms of school dropout.

Caliste (1984) examined the effectiveness of an American twelve-week dropout prevention programme. One hundred and fourteen at-risk students, from ninth, tenth, and eleventh grades, were randomly assigned to experimental ($n = 55$) and control ($n = 59$) groups. The programme consisted of groups of two to five students who met with a high-school teacher–tutor twice a week for one semester, and had counseling with school counselors once a week. Topics discussed in the counseling groups included motivation, the relevance of school and course assignments, academic problems, career goals, and study habits. In the tutoring groups, students were assisted with current coursework and received some remedial instruction. The results indicated that the experimental intervention had not substantially affected the attitude measures (self-concept, attitudes toward teachers and learning), but that there was a significant difference between the experimental and control groups in the reduction of absenteeism and dropout rate.

Also in the United States, Reyes and Jason (1991) evaluated a sample of 154 at-risk ninth-grade students randomly assigned to experimental and control conditions. The project instituted the following intervention: (1) redefinition of the role of the homeroom teacher; (2) reorganization of the school environment to reduce system change; and (3) the provision of parents with information on student progress. The homeroom teacher served as a primary source of information about the school and as a link between students, parents, and the other sections of the school. Additionally, the homeroom teacher provided the students with guidance for school difficulties or concerns (e.g., problems with other teachers or students, class scheduling issues). Homeroom teachers contacted parents by telephone in order to introduce themselves and address any parental questions about the programme. The reorganization of the school environment aimed to reduce the degree of change that the students encountered, by enabling them to maintain the same classmates in the three principal subjects and homeroom, thus providing students a stable peer group. Parents were contacted every 5 weeks to inform them about students' progress. Control students did not participate in any of these components. At the end of the study, there were no differences between the groups in terms of grades, overall class rank, course failures, absenteeism, or failure to attend class.

DISCUSSION

There is a paucity of well-designed studies addressing risk factors and intervention programmes for school dropout. Moreover, almost none of the studies were conducted in developing countries where school dropout is prevalent and likely to have a huge impact on society (Tramontina *et al.*, 2002). For these reasons, together with the diversity of methodology in the studies reviewed, it is impossible to articulate a unitary concept concerning risk factors or preventive interventions for school dropout.

Furthermore, very few studies addressing risk factors for school dropout took advantage of techniques that allow adjustment for potential confounders or the examination of moderators and mediators. Even so, it is possible to describe the three most often investigated risk factors as follows: (1) *individual factors* (e.g., general deviance, disruptive behavior, conduct problems, truancy, drug and alcohol use, mental retardation, affiliation with antisocial peers, early sexual activity, gender, ethnicity, and life change in the previous year); (2) *school factors* (e.g., low school grades, low first-grade marks, grade retention, poor commitment to schooling); and (3) *family factors* (low socioeconomic status, low parental level of education, low parental educational expectations, family mobility, and having single, separated, or divorced parents). The best available evidence associates school dropout with those risk factors. Furthermore, two studies documented an association between school dropout, school-age pregnancy, and early parenthood (Gest *et al.*, 1999; Manlove, 1998).

Again, there is a paucity of preventive intervention studies. However, some findings deserve close attention. First, almost all interventions gave priority to school-based programmes, focusing on at-risk students. This strategy is consistent with recent literature on preventive intervention in mental health, which suggests that targeted interventions for at-risk populations are more promising than universal primary preventive programmes. *Universal interventions often fail to reach those most in need, and expend their energy on those who do not need them* (Nurcombe, 2006). Second, investigators should give more attention to early interventions. Despite the use of a quasi-experimental design, Reynolds *et al.* (2001) demonstrated the effectiveness of a very early (preschool) intervention for school dropout in late adolescence. Third, several of the proposed interventions had difficulty to retaining subjects or their parents (e.g., Eggert *et al.*, 1990; Comiskey, 1993; Hawkins *et al.*, 1999). This finding calls attention to the fact that innovative psychoeducational techniques should be designed and tested in such a way to keep the special population motivated to accept the intervention. Furthermore, family functioning and parental mental health problems should also be addressed. Finally, it should be noted that the most scientifically designed programmes were less likely to show significant effects. In fact, only one well-designed programme was found to have a significant impact on school dropout rate (Caliste, 1984). In this intervention, the role of teachers as tutor-counselors was central. In a recent comprehensive intervention aimed to reduce school dropout, Graeff-Martins *et al.* (2006) have documented the importance of working closely with teachers in a developing country.

The current review has limitations. We were not able to retrieve one study (Fortin and Picard, 1998). For logistic reasons, we concentrated our strategy for retrieving papers on scientific journals. Thus, relevant information not published in mainstream journals might have been missed. In general, the publication bias is against studies with negative results. Thus, there is a slight possibility that we have missed one or more very successful interventions. More importantly, we did not access the ERIC database, which could have brought information about studies from the educational perspective.

CONCLUSIONS

School dropout has not been well studied. More investigations are required with better methodological designs. It is important to implement this kind of research in developing countries and to propose conceptual models that can be tested in different countries and cultures.

ACKNOWLEDGMENT

This work was supported by a research grant from The Presidential World Psychiatric Association Programme on Global Child Mental Health, partially supported by a grant from Ely-Lilly.

REFERENCES

Achenbach, T. M., Howell, C. T., McConaughy, S. H., and Stanger, C. (1998) Six-year predictors of problems in a national sample: IV. Young adult signs of disturbance. *J Am Acad Child Adolesc Psychiatry*, **37**(7), 718–27.

Afolayan, J. A. (1991) Retention policy and school dropout rate: Implications for professional educators. *High School J*, **74**(4), 220–24.

Allen, J. P., Philliber, S., and Hoggson, N. (1990) School-based prevention of teen-age pregnancy and school dropout: Process evaluation of the national replication of the Teen Outreach Program. *Am J Community Psychol*, **18**(4), 505–24.

Barton, W. H., Watkins, M., and Jarjoura, R. (1997) Youths and communities: Toward comprehensive strategies for youth development. *Soc Work*, **42**(5), 483–93.

Bates, S. C., Plemons, B. W., Jumper-Thurman, P., and Beauvais, F. (1997) Volatile solvent use: Patterns by gender and ethnicity among school attenders and dropouts. *Drugs Society*, **10**(1–2), 61–78.

Battin-Pearson, S., Newcomb, M. D, Abbott, R. D. *et al.* (2000) Predictors of early high school dropout: A test of five theories. *J Educ Psychol*, **92**(3), 568–82.

Berg, I., Butler, A., Franklin, J. *et al.* (1993) DSM-III-R disorders, social factors, and management of school attendance problems in the normal population. *J Child Psychol Psychiatry*, **34**, 1187–203.

Caliste, E. R. (1984) The effect of a twelve-week dropout intervention program. *Adolescence*, **19**(75), 649–57.

Comiskey, P. E. (1993) Using Reality Therapy group training with at-risk high school freshmen. *J Reality Ther*, **12**(2), 59–64.

Crum, R. M., Ensminger, M. E., Ro, M. J., and McCord, J. (1998) The association of educational achievement and school dropout with risk of alcoholism: A twenty-five-year prospective study of inner-city children. *J Stud Alcohol*, **59**(3), 318–26.

Dennison, S. (2000) A win-win peer mentoring and tutoring program: a collaborative model. *J Primary Prevention*, **20**(3), 161–74.

Doll, B. and Hess, R. S. (2001) Through a new lens: Contemporary psychological perspectives on school completion and dropping out of high school. *School Psychol Quar*, **16**(4), 351–56.

Dunham, R. G. and Alpert, G. P. (1987) Keeping juvenile delinquents in school: A prediction model. *Adolescence*, **22**(85), 45–57.

Dynarski, M. and Gleason, P. (2002) How can we help? What we have learned from recent federal dropout prevention evaluations. *J Ed Stud Placed Risk*, **7**(1), 43–69.

Eggert, L. L., Seyl, C. D., and Nicholas, L. J. (1990) Effects of a school-based prevention program for potential high school dropouts and drug abusers. *Int J Addic*, **25**(7), 773–801.

Eggert, L. L., Thompson, E. A., Herting, J. R. *et al.* (1994) Preventing adolescent drug abuse and high school dropout through an intensive school-based social network development program. *Am J Health Promot*, **8**(3), 202–15.

Evans, I. M. and Matthews, A. K. (1992) A behavioral approach to the prevention of school dropout: Conceptual and empirical strategies for children and youth. *Prog Behav Modif*, **28**, 219–49.

Fergusson, D. M. and Horwood, L. J. (1995) Predictive validity of categorically and dimensionally scored measures of disruptive childhood behaviors. *J Am Child Adolesc Psychiatry*, **34**(4), 477–85.

Fergusson, D. M., Lynskey, M. T., and Horwood, L. J. (1996) The short-term consequences of early onset cannabis use. *J Abnorm Child Psychol*, **24**(4), 499–512.

Fergusson, D. M. and Horwood, L. J. (1997) Early onset cannabis use and psychosocial adjustment in young adults. *Addiction*, **92**(3), 279–96.

Fortin, L. and Picard, Y. (1998) Les effets d'un programme d'intervention multidimensionnel aupres d'elèves a risque de decrochage scolaire au secondaire. *Revue Quebecoise de Psychologie*, **19**(2), 125–45.

Franklin, C. and Streeter, C. L. (1995) Assessment of middle class youth at-risk to dropout: School, psychological and family correlates. *Children Youth Ser Rev*, **17**(3), 433–48.

Gest, S. D., Mahoney, J. L., and Cairns, R. B. (1999) A developmental approach to prevention research: Configural antecedents of early parenthood. *Am J Community Psychol*, **27**(4), 543–65.

Gleason, P., Dynarski, M. (2002) Do we know whom to serve? Issues in using risk factors to identify dropouts. *J Educ Students Placed Risk*, **7**(1), 25–41.

Graeff-Martins, A. S., Oswald, S., Comassetto, J. O., Kieling, K., Gonçalves, R. R., & Rohde, L. A. (2006) A package of interventions to reduce school dropout in public schools in a developing country: A feasibility study. *European Child and Adolescent Psychiatry*, **15**, 442–49.

Hawkins, J. D., Catalano, R. F., Kosterman, R. *et al.* (1999) Preventing adolescent health-risk behaviors by strengthening protection during childhood. *Arch Pediatr Adolesc Med*, **153**(3), 226–34.

Hess, R. S. and Copeland, E. P. (2001) Students' stress, coping strategies, and school completion: A longitudinal perspective. *School Psychol Quart*, **16**(4), 389–405.

Janosz, M., LeBlanc, M., Boulerice, B., and Tremblay, R. E. (1997) Disentangling the weight of school dropout predictors: A test on two longitudinal samples. *J Youth Adolesc*, **26**(6), 733–62.

Janosz, M., LeBlanc, M., Boulerice, B., and Tremblay, R. E. (2000) Predicting different types of school dropouts: A typological approach with two longitudinal samples. *J Educ Psychol*, **92**(1), 171–90.

Kapur, M. (1997) *Mental Health in Indian Schools*, Sage publications, New Delhi.

Kearney, C. A. and Hugelshofer, D. S. (2000) Systemic and clinical strategies for preventing school refusal behavior in youth. *J Cognitive Psychother*, **14**(1), 51–65.

Kominski, R. (1990) Estimating the national high school dropout rate. *Demography*, **27**. 303–11.

MacLean, D. A. and Janzen, H. L. (1994) A framework for keeping students in school. *Can J School Psychol*, **10**(1), 54–61.

Manlove, J. (1998) The influence of high school dropout and school disengagement on the risk of school-age pregnancy. *J Res Adolesc*, **8**(2), 187–220.

Martinez, Y. G. and Cranston-Gingras, A. (1996) Migrant farmworker students and the educational process: Barriers to high school completion. *High School J*, **80**(1), 28–38.

Ministério da Educação e Cultura (MEC). (1999) Censo escolar de,. Brasília (DF).

Nurcombe, B. (2006) The principles of preventive psychiatry. The Mental Health of Children and Adolescents, 53–64.

Obot, I. S., Hubbard, S., and Anthony, J. C. (1999) Level of education and injecting drug use among African Americans. *Drug Alc Depend*, **55**(1–2), 177–82.

Obot, I. S. and Anthony, J. C. (1999) Association of school dropout with recent and past injecting drug use among African American adults. *Addict Behav*, **24**(5), 701–05.

Obot, I. S. and Anthony, J. C. (2000) School dropout and injecting drug use in a national sample of white non-Hispanic American adults. *J Drug Educ*, **30**(2), 145–55.

Pittman, R. B. (1986) Importance of personal, social factors as potential means for reducing high school dropout rate. *High School J*, **70**(1), 7–13.

Reyes, O. and Jason, L. A. (1991) An evaluation of high school dropout prevention program. *J Community Psychol*, **19**(3), 221–30.
Reynolds, A. J., Temple, J. A., Robertson, D. L., and Mann, E. A. (2001) Long-term effects of an early childhood intervention on educational achievement and juvenile arrest: A 15-year follow-up of low-income children in public schools. *JAMA*, **285**(18), 2339–46.
Royer, E., Moisan, S., Saint-Laurent, L., and Giasson, J. (1993) L'abandon scolaire et sa prevention. *Bulletin de Psychologie Scolaire et d'Orientation*, **42**(3), 131–51.
Rumberger, R. W. and Larson, K. A. (1998) Student mobility and the increased risk of high school dropout. *Am J Educ*, **107**(1), 1–35.
Simner, M. L. and Barnes, M. J. (1991) Relationship between first-grade marks and the high school dropout problem. *J School Psychol*, **29**(4), 331–35.
Stevenson, W., Maton, K. I., and Teti, D. M. (1998) School importance and dropout among pregnant adolescents. *J Adolesc Health*, **22**(5), 376–82.
Svec, H. (1987) Youth advocacy and high school dropout. *High School J*, **70**(4), 185–92.
Swaim, R. C., Beauvais, F., Chavez, E. L., and Oetting, E. R. (1997) The effect of school dropout rates on estimates of adolescent substance use among three racial/ethnic groups. *Am J Public Health*, **87**(1), 51–55.
Tramontina, S., Martins, S., Michalowski, M. B. *et al.* (2001) School dropout and conduct disorder in Brazilian elementary school students. *Can J Psychiatry*, **46**(10), 941–47.
Tramontina, S., Martins, S., Michalowski, M. B. *et al.* (2002) Estimated mental retardation and school dropout in a sample of students from state public schools in Porto Alegre, Brazil. *Rev Bras Psiquiatr*, **24**(4), 177–81.
United Nations Children's Fund. (1999) The Progress of Nations, UNICEF publications, Brasília.
United Nation Children's Fund. (2005) The State of the World's Children 2005. Full text. Access on line at: www.unicef.org
Vitaro, F., Brendgen, M., and Tremblay, R. E. (1999) Prevention of school dropout through the reduction of disruptive behaviors and school failure in elementary school. *J School Psychol*, **37**(2), 205–26.
Wechsler, S. and Oakland, T. D. (1990) Preventive strategies for promoting the education of low-income Brazilian children: Implications for school psychologists from other Third World nations. *School Psychol Int*, **11**(2), 83–90.
Wichström, L. (1998) Alcohol intoxication and school dropout. *Drug Alc Rev*, **17**(4), 413–21.
Witt, J. C., Vanderheyden, A., and Penton, C. (1999) Prevention of common mental health problems among adolescents. National and local best practices in school-based health centers. *J La State Med Soc*, **151**(12), 631–38.

CHAPTER 5.5

School Violence: Epidemiology, Background, and Prevention

Helmut Remschmidt
Philipps University, Marburg, Germany

GENERAL ASPECTS OF VIOLENCE AND SCHOOL VIOLENCE

Violence is the deliberate threat or enactment of physical force to an extent that is highly likely to cause physical injury or psychological trauma to another person or persons. The term "violence" is closely related to "aggression," a collective term for motives, thoughts, emotions, and behavior characterized by intended damage to objects or persons (Hoffmann, 1984, p. 7). Manifest aggression (e.g., angry threats and physical assaults) can be distinguished from covert aggression (e.g., hostile thoughts, fantasies, and emotions).

Violence has three main categories:

(1) Violence in reaction to threat ("reactive aggression"), which may become out of control.
(2) Violence used as a strategy to reach a goal ("instrumental aggression"). The aggressive impulses behind this kind of violence are very often authorized and are frequently used in order to defend certain positions.
(3) Structural violence (Galtung, 1975), which is inherent in institutions, organizations, societies, and groups that advocate aggressive behavior and violent acts to solve social problems, defend territory or possessions, or assert dominance over other groups.

Violence and aggression are not synonymous: aggression does not necessarily lead to violence. Violence can be regarded as a primitive response by those who have no alternative. Nevertheless, violence is avoidable, except in extreme situations.

Violence frequently occurs in schools, at all ages. It has been reported as a serious problem in all types of schools, and everywhere in the world. School violence can be subdivided into the following groups:

The Mental Health of Children and Adolescents: an area of global neglect. Edited by H. Remschmidt *et al.*

- violence by teachers against students;
- violence by students against teachers;
- violence by students against other students (bullying);
- violence by students against school buildings and inventory (vandalism).

The most frequent and most important act of violence, bullying, will be discussed in this chapter.

Bullying is "aggressive behavior or intentional harm-doing, which is carried out repeatedly over time in an interpersonal relationship characterized by an imbalance of power" (Olweus, 1994). School violence cannot be understood without considering other manifestations of violence in the family and the society. Several studies show that school violence is related to domestic violence and hate crimes in the particular society (Horton, 2001). Preventive interventions must address these connections.

According to Garbarino (1999), violence in general, and school violence in particular, can be understood in terms of an epidemiologic model. Communities, neighborhoods, and families may become troubled and act as perfect "hosts" for an epidemic of violence. The epidemic starts among the most vulnerable fragments of a population, which do not cause, but prepare the ground for, the epidemic. The same epidemic model has been applied to the extreme form of youth violence, youth homicide (Garbarino, 1999). It is apparent that the prevention of school violence must address influences outside the school itself.

What are the sequelae of violence for individuals, families, and the society? Violence can cause serious individual harm and frequently, also, psychopathological disorders such as post-traumatic stress disorder, depression, and anxiety disorder. Interpersonal violence devastates lives and families and imposes major economic costs on societies everywhere. Several countries spend up to 4% of their gross domestic product (GDP) on violence-related injuries. Low-income nations seem to be at the top (Akiba *et al.*, 2002). The WHO report "The Economic Dimension of Interpersonal Violence" states that Columbia and El Salvador spend 3.4% of their GDP on violence-related expenditures, whereas the United States spend 3.3%. There has been no research concerning the extent to which school violence contributes to these expenditures, but it can be assumed that the contribution is substantial (WHO, 2004). In summary, the costs of interpersonal violence are high, but there is evidence that preventive intervention could be cost-effective.

EPIDEMIOLOGY

Recent studies (Akiba *et al.*, 2002) demonstrate that at least one out of four grade 7 and 8 students are afraid of being attacked or have been victims of school violence at least once during the previous months before the inquiry. There are remarkable differences between countries. One international study (Akiba *et al.*, 2002), part of the Third International Math and Science Study (TIMSS), evaluated school violence in 37 countries and found that the mean percentage of students who have been victims of violence during the previous month was 28%, the highest percentage being in Hungary (75%) and the lowest in Denmark (6%). Germany and the United States range just below the mean with 22 and 26%, respectively. The percentage of teachers who reported that their teaching was affected by the need to protect themselves and other students had an international mean of 13.7% (ranging from 7% in the Netherlands to 50% in Romania).

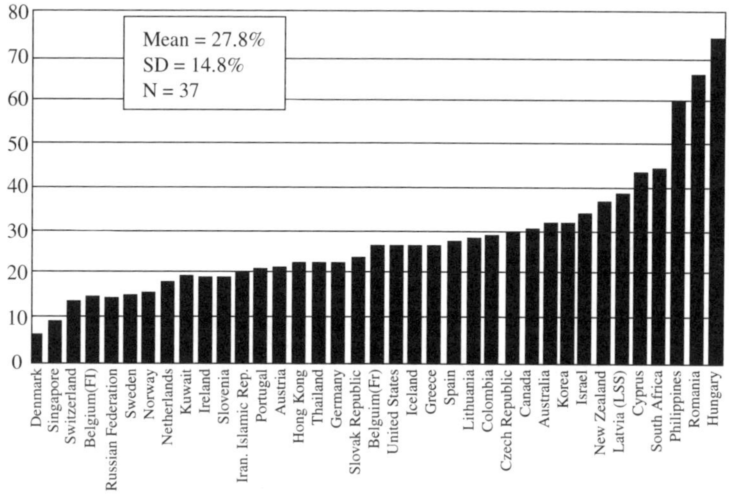

Figure 5.5.1 National rates of school violence among seventh and eighth graders in 37 nations. Student report of victimization in school (Akiba *et al.*, 2002)

These statistics are summarized in Figures 5.5.1–5.5.3. Figure 5.5.1 exemplifies the rates of school violence among seventh and eighth graders as reported by the students of 37 nations. Figure 5.5.2 demonstrates the numbers of peer victimizations accordingly, and Figure 5.5.3 demonstrates the rates of threat to teachers' and students' safety as reported by the teachers.

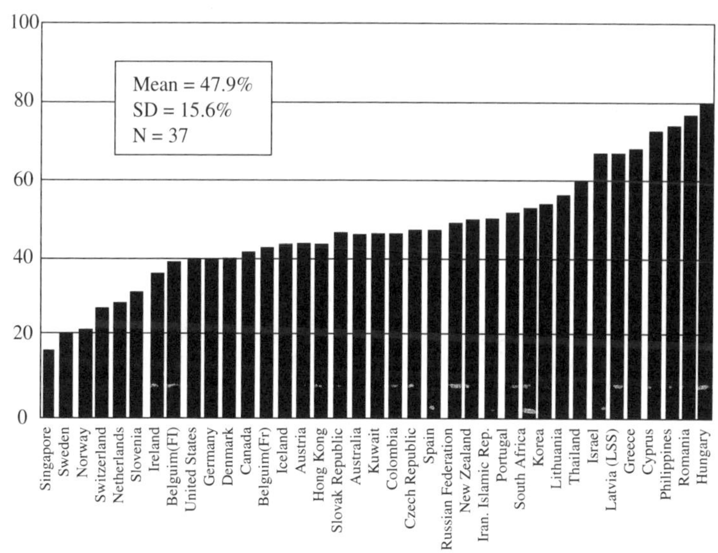

Figure 5.5.2 National rates of school violence among seventh and eighth graders in 37 nations. Student report of peer victimization in school (Akiba *et al.*, 2002)

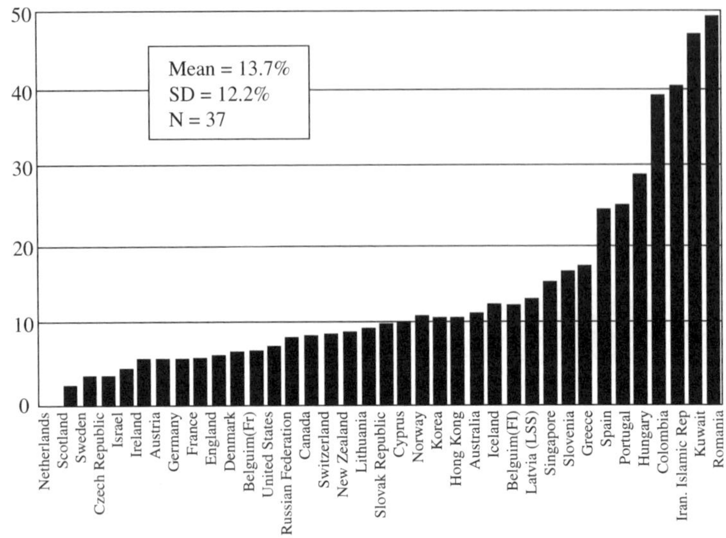

Figure 5.5.3 National rates of school violence among seventh and eighth graders in 37 nations. Teacher report of threat to teachers' and students' safety (Akiba *et al.*, 2002)

Some of the differences between the 37 nations are difficult to explain. For example, school violence rates are not related to national crime rates, to parental divorce rates, or to the percentage of linguistic minorities. They are, on the contrary, related to social indicators such as severe economic deprivation (Krahn *et al.*, 1986), age distribution (Sampson and Wooldredge, 1987), the quality of the school system, and the characteristics of the public educational system (Baker *et al.*, 2001).

"Basic national conditions (e.g. gross domestic product, GDP) and demographic conditions (size of the youth cohort) are associated with national rates of school violence. GDP is the only other major variable that is significantly associated with rates of school violence, once national characteristics of schooling have been controlled for" (Akiba *et al.*, 2002, p. 846–47).

An Israeli study has shown that nearly one third of elementary and middle school students and almost a quarter of high school students consider that violence is a big problem in their schools (Zeira *et al.*, 2003). This study was based on a national representative sample stratified by school type and Jewish/Arab ethnicity. A total of 15 916 children, grade 4 through 11, from 603 classes and 232 schools participated in the study, with a response rate of 91%. In contrast to many other studies where the bully–victim definition was used, the study used a broad definition of violence: students were asked to report if they had been victims of violent behavior of different magnitudes during the preceding month. School violence was related to school level, elementary and middle schools having higher rates than high schools.

There are many different types of school violence reaching from teasing and verbal attacks until extreme physical violence and homicide. The most frequent violent behavior, however, is bullying.

Bullying should be distinguished from teasing or playful behavior. According to Olweus (1993), bullying is characterized by an imbalance of power between bully and victim. The imbalance can be real or perceived. Tattum (1993) describes different methods of bullying: gesture bullying, verbal bullying, physical bullying, extortion bullying, and exclusion bullying. Furthermore, direct and indirect bullying can be distinguished. Direct bullying involves an open attack on the victim, whereas indirect bullying is manifest as exclusion of, or the spreading of malicious rumors about, the victim.

According to several studies (see review by McCarthy and Carr (2002)), the prevalence of being bullied once a week or more varies between 4 and 13%. Estimates of perpetrating bullying range from 1 to 7%. If one counts occasional bullying, the frequency of being a victim reaches up to 35%.

"Victims are typically anxious, insecure, cautious, sensitive, and quiet. When attacked by other students, they commonly react by crying and withdrawing. Victims have low self-esteem, look upon themselves as failures, and feel stupid, ashamed, unattractive, lonely and abandoned. They often do not have a single good friend in their class." (Olweus, 1994, p. 178)

Typical bullies are aggressive toward their peers. They are often also aggressive toward their teachers and parents. They have a more positive attitude toward violence than other students, a strong tendency to dominate others, and are impulsive. They lack empathy with the victims. If they are boys, they are likely to be physically stronger than their victims (Olweus, 1978).

ETIOLOGY: RISK AND BACKGROUND FACTORS

School violence has many precursor behaviors. Several risk factors contribute to the manifestation of violent behavior inside and outside the school.

Table 5.5.1 reviews the most important risk factors that have been identified.

Beyond these general risk factors, several specific relationships have been described. Studies acting at the macrolevel have identified national and demographic conditions

Table 5.5.1 Risk factors for violent behavior at school

Individual risk factors	Delinquent friends, substance abuse, lower intelligence, birth complications, male sex, specific temperamental characteristics such as impulsiveness, irritability, violent temper, ADHD and conduct disorder, and poor verbal intelligence
Family risk factors	History of family crime and violence, lack of expectations by parents, lax monitoring by parents, parental substance use, and child abuse and neglect. Coercive rearing attitudes characterized by (1) lack of warmth and involvement, (2) permissiveness toward or encouragement of aggressive behavior by the child, and (3) physical punishment and harsh emotional outbursts of the parents
Community risk factors	Availability of weapons and drugs, large number of broken homes/families, transient population, large youth cohort, and economic deprivation
School risk factors	Academic failure, lack of commitment to school, gang involvement, poor supervision and surveillance of students' activities, insufficient school and class rules, lack of effective instruction, and lack of a convincing value system of the school and a clear school policy

(such as GDP or the size of the youth cohort) as important factors associated with school violence. Nevertheless, the rates of school violence do not correspond with youth crime rates in the respective society (Akiba *et al.*, 2002). It is debatable whether factors outside the school are more or less important than factors inside the school. Several studies have found that the quality of a school system affects the level of violence (Akiba *et al.*, 2002). Low school achievement levels and violence go hand in hand (Kaufmann, 1997). Maguin and Loeber (1996) deduced from their meta-analysis of "academic performance and delinquency" three important relationships: poor academic performance is associated with delinquent offending; cognitive defects and attention problems are associated with poor academic performance and delinquency; the prevalence of delinquency can be reduced by improving academic performance.

INTERVENTION AND PREVENTION

Characteristics of Effective School Violence Prevention Programmes

Several reviews (Roland, 1989; Olweus, 1991, 1993, 1997; Farrington, 1993; Clarke and Kiselica, 1997; McCarthy and Carr, 2002) describe the results of intervention and prevention programmes against school violence, especially bullying. This chapter will concentrate on the distinguishing characteristics of effective programmes.

The relevant literature clearly demonstrates that interventions must extend beyond the individual victim or offender to all individuals and organizations that are school-related (students, parents, the family, teachers, and the school as a social organism). Such programmes are called "whole-school violence prevention programmes." But even whole-school approaches are sometimes insufficiently far-reaching as school violence is also affected by demographic influences, domestic violence and neighborhood violence, and social disorganization (Horton, 2001). As broader social influences cannot be changed easily, the main focus of action must be the school.

Table 5.5.2 presents an overview of the empirically based components of successful whole-school bullying prevention programmes. The table outlines the clearly defined goals and policies that are the basis of successful prevention programmes and describes the strategies of intervention at different levels of intervention (school, class, and individual) and the materials that can be used. The Olweus programme is one of the best-known and best-evaluated prevention programmes.

Table 5.5.3 summarizes seven recent preventive intervention studies, all carried out in large school populations as whole-school programmes. The chief conclusions of these studies are as follows:

(1) *Teacher level:* The teacher is the key figure. The success of the programme depends to a large extent upon his identification with and training in the programme and his engagement in its implementation (Aber *et al.*, 1998; Olweus and Kallestad 2003).
(2) *Parent level:* Domestic violence and school violence are directly related. Ethnicity plays a significant role in the correlation between domestic violence and school violence (Horton, 2001). It is essential to engage the *parents* in the programme and to keep them involved.

Table 5.5.2 Components of whole-school bullying prevention programmes

Goals	• To increase awareness and knowledge of bully–victim problems • To achieve active involvement on the part of parents and teachers • To develop clear rules against bullying • To provide support and protection for victims
Policy principles	• Parents and teachers cooperate in engaging in authoritative adult–child relationships with pupils • Firm limits to unacceptable behavior • Non-physical sanctions consistently applied for rule violations
School strategies	• Develop joint long-term action plan for the school • Regular meetings of teachers together, parents together, and parents and teachers together, to develop anti-bullying social milieu of the school • Provide supervision of children during recess and lunchtime • Teachers to be contactable by children and parents in confidence
Class strategies	• Regular class meetings • Teachers and pupils jointly establish class rules and sanctions against bullying • Teachers praise pupils for pro-social behavior • Teachers consistently apply sanctions for bullying • Teachers promote cooperative learning through group projects and activities where participation and effort are encouraged • Teachers use role-playing, rehearsal, and discussion of bullying-related videos and literature to support anti-bullying social milieu
Individual strategies	• Teachers talk with bullies and victims and their parents about bullying incidents as soon as incidents come to light • These meetings continue until the bullying is resolved • Parents and teachers cooperate in applying sanctions for bullying consistently • Parents and teachers support both victims and bullies as they move on from the bullying incident • Neutral pupils may be involved to aid this support process • Where the incident cannot be resolved within a class, the bully not the victim may be moved to another class • Assertiveness training for victims • Peer counseling where pupils run a helpline for victims • Bully courts in which peers hear both sides of the story
Materials	• Booklet for schools (37-page booklet in Olweus pack) • Booklet for parents (4-page booklet in the Olweus pack) • Bullying questionnaire • Video of bullying events for classroom discussion (25 min on events in lives of victims in the Olweus pack)

Sourse: Reproduced from McCarthy and Carr (2002) Prevention of bullying. In Carr (ed.), *Prevention*. London: Routledge.

(3) *Student level:* Important strategies at the level of the *student* are to apply consistent rules and principles to regulate behavior, promote peace-building behavior, enhance social competence, improve social skills, and intervene as soon as school conflicts occur. Peace-builder programmes, the discussion of attitudes toward weapons (guns), social skills training, the creation of opportunities for acknowledgment by others, the assigning of mentors for students at risk of violence, and teaching students, teachers,

Table 5.5.3 Recent empirical investigations on the prevention of school violence

Author(s)	Aim of the study	Methods	Results
Aber *et al.* (1998)	• Evaluation of the short-term impact of school-based violence prevention • Examination of the influence of classroom and neighborhood contexts on effectiveness of violence prevention	• Resolving Conflict Creatively Programme (RCCP): a broad intervention in violence prevention and intergroup understanding • 5053 children, grades 2–6	• Children whose teachers had a moderate amount of training from RCCP and taught many lessons showed significantly slower growth in aggression-related processes and less decrease in competence-related processes • The effect of the intervention on children's social cognition varied by context. The positive effect of many lessons was dampened in high-risk classrooms and neighborhoods.
Horton (2001)	• Identification of determinants of school violence	• Cross-sectional design with data available for all Illinois counties (102) • Multiple regression analysis including age, gender, ethnicity, social status, domestic violence, and hate crimes	• Domestic violence and school violence are directly related • Many aggressive assailants come from violent families • Ethnicity plays a significant role as to how domestic violence and hate crimes correlate with school violence
Shapiro *et al.* (2002)	• Evaluation of the violence prevention effects of The Peacemakers Programme	• The Peacemakers Programme • Almost 2000 elementary/middle school students in an urban public school system • Attitudes toward Guns and Violence Questionnaire (AGVQ) • Knowledge of psychosocial skills • Aggressive Behavior Checklist (ABC) completed by students as a self-report version (ABC-S) or completed by teachers as an observational version (ABC-T)	• Increase in acknowledgment of psychosocial skills • Decrease in ABC-S scores • Fewer disciplinary incidents involving aggressive behavior • Less involvement in the school conflict mediation service • Fewer suspensions for violent behavior • Decrease of aggression in the intervention group (tested through analysis of covariance (ANCOVA))

Flannery *et al.* (2003)	• Alteration of the climate of a school by teaching students and staff simple rules and activities aimed at improving child social competence and reducing aggressive behavior	• Peace Builders Programme • Eight elementary schools in Arizona ($n > 4000$, grades K-5)	• Consistent behavioral impact in the immediate-intervention schools • More peace-building behavior in the immediate-intervention condition • Increased social competence and decreased teacher-reported aggression
Olweus and Kallestad (2003)	• Detection and prediction of influences that affect differences in teachers' and schools' implementation of school-based intervention or prevention programmes	• Olweus Bullying Prevention Programme • Classroom intervention measures (CIM) • Individual contact (IC) • Thirty-seven schools participated ($n = 89$)	• Teachers are the key operatives of change with regard to adoption and implementation of the Olweus Bullying Prevention Programme in school • Considerable variation in the quality of implementation between teachers and schools
Rollin *et al.* (2003)	• Examination of the effectiveness of a school-based violence prevention programme for at-risk eighth graders ($n = 156$)	• Identification as being at-risk based on the presence of one or more risk factors (e.g., fighting, disciplinary problems, and high absenteeism) • Students were assigned to mentors and performed various duties at their mentors' sites • Students participated 2 h per day for 166 days (average)	• Significant reduction of number of in-school and out-of-school suspensions • Decrease of number of violations committed on school property
D'Andrea (2004)	• Building comprehensive violence prevention programmes in four elementary schools in Hawaii	• Teaching the teacher' school-based violence prevention strategies	• Twenty-one classroom-based interventions were initiated • Three new anger management counseling groups were founded • Four new counseling groups established fostering social skills, interpersonal problem-solving and coping strategies

and parents the principles of the respective violence prevention programme are all important components of an effective programme (Shapiro *et al.*, 2002; Flannery *et al.*, 2003; Olweus and Kallestad 2003; Rollin *et al.*, 2003; D'Andrea, 2004).

(4) *School level:* The school has an important influence upon students' attitudes as measured by attendance and students' reports of their attitudes toward classes and classmates (Sylva, 1994). Violence occurs in a social context. *School* is a social organism with rules, values, and principles that should be accepted by the entire school community. A clear organizational structure, good student supervision during classes and recreation periods, support for the dignity of the individual, and ethical principles reflecting a "school ideology" are important aspects of violence prevention (Rutter *et al.*, 1979; Farrington, 1993; Clarke and Kiselica, 1997).

The implementation of violence prevention programmes

Violence prevention programmes are successful only if they are fully *implemented. Full implementation* means that it is not enough to know the programme and to read the materials. Good training, continuing consultation, close supervision, and thorough monitoring are essential (Roland and Munthe, 1997). Precisely formulated implementation guidelines are helpful.

The implementation of such a programme should include the following steps:

Step 1: The decision to implement a programme.

- Define the goal of the programme (e.g., reduction of the school violence rate).
- Select the prevention programme.
- Select the school resp. school classes.
- Inform the parents, students, and school community.

Step 2: Introduction to the programme.

- Brief teachers and school personnel concerning the details of the programme.
- Explain the implementation guidelines.
- Become familiar with the assessment instruments and implementation methods (checklists, scales, questionnaires, and training packages).
- Appoint responsible staff to carry out the programme.
- Appoint consultants and supervisors.

Step 3: Pilot phase.

A pilot phase is recommended in order to test the instruments and instructions, and make sure of the applicability of all measures.

Step 4: Project phase.

- Measure the baseline of the behavior to be modified. Obtain assessment information from several informants (students, teachers, and parents).
- Implement the programme under the supervision of a programme expert.
- Conduct training and supervision sessions of staff responsible for carrying out the project.

- Inform and motivate the students in the participating classes.
- Meet regularly with the parents, teachers, and the entire school community.
- Identify "high-risk students" and implement with them special treatment and educational measures.
- Measure the behavior in question at the end of the programme; seeking information from different informants is recommended.
- Conduct a statistical analysis of the effectiveness of the programme.

Step 5: Follow-up phase.
The major aim is to ascertain whether the expected (and hopefully reached) success endures. For example, 1 or 2 years after the termination of the programme, measurements are repeated. If "high-risk students" have been identified during the project phase, analyze their data in order to check if the programme was helpful for them.

Step 6: Conclusions for school policy.
Whole-school violence prevention programmes should have a long-term impact on violent behavior. When students involved leave the school after their final examination, it is important to sustain the major principles of the prevention programme and to incorporate them in the policies of the school. The principles should be written in the form of a "constitution" for the school. Previous studies have clearly demonstrated that external factors such as buildings or administrative rules are not responsible for a low rate of violence. The decisive factors are the school's ethical principles, value system, and the key educational goals (Rutter *et al.*, 1979).

CONCLUSIONS

School violence is an immense problem in all types of school everywhere in the world. But school violence does not occur without warning; it has several precursors and is foreshadowed by predisposing and precipitating factors. Not all, but many factors can be influenced, as well as the violent behavior itself. This is the aim of school violence prevention programmes. Several programmes have reduced violence by up to 53% (compared with baseline measures) and with effect sizes of up to 1.42 (Olweus, 1997). There is evidence that the most effective interventions are whole-school in nature with school strategies, class strategies, individual strategies, involving students, teachers, parents, and families as well. An important precondition for effectiveness is that the programme be fully implemented, that implementation guidelines be followed, with supervision and consultation continuing during the entire implementation period.

It can be concluded as follows:

(1) Successful whole-school violence programmes should be routinely introduced into primary and secondary schools. School staff should be trained periodically with regard to the selected programme and have the opportunity for supervision and consultation, and to provide their opinions about the programme.
(2) As most programmes have multiple components, it is usually unclear which component or components are decisive. Further experimental analyses of the effectiveness of different components are required.

(3) Data concerning special-risk groups and at-risk individuals who respond poorly to the programme should be analyzed in order to suggest methods of modifying the programme appropriately.
(4) Programmes should be modified in the light of demographic and ethnic features, and for children from high-violence, disorganized environments.

ACKNOWLEDGMENTS

The author wants to thank Mrs Eva-Maria Schenk for her help with the literature search and Mrs Elisabeth Goy for secretarial help.

REFERENCES

Aber, J. L., Jones, S. M., Brown, J. L. *et al.* (1998) Resolving conflict creatively: Evaluating the developmental effects of a school-based violence program in neighbourhood and classroom context. *Dev Psychopathol*, **10**, 187–213.

Akiba, M., LeTendre, G. K., Baker, D. P., and Goesling, B. (2002) Student victimization: National and school system effects on school violence in 37 nations. *Am Educ Res J*, **39**, 829–53.

Baker, D. P., Akiba, M., LeTendre, G. K., and Wiseman, A. W. (2001) Worldwide shadow education: Outside-school learning, institutional quality of schooling, and gross-national mathematics achievement. *Educ Eval Policy Anal*, **23**, 1–17.

Clarke, E. A. and Kiselica, C. (1997) A systematic counselling approach to the problem of bullying. *Elem Sch Guid Couns*, **31**, 310–25.

D'Andrea, M. (2004) Comprehensive school-based violence prevention training: A developmental–ecological training model. *J Couns Dev*, **82**, 277–86.

Farrington, D. P. (1993) Understanding and preventing bullying, in *Crime and Justice: An Annual Review of Research*, Vol. 17 (eds M. Tonry and N. Morris), University of Chicago Press, Chicago, IL.

Flannery, D. J., Vaszonyi, A. T., Liau, A. K. *et al.* (2003) Initial behaviour outcomes for the Peace Builders universal school-based violence prevention program. *Dev Psychol*, **39**(2), 292–308.

Galtung, J. (1975) *Strukturelle Gewalt. Beiträge zur Friedens- und Konfliktforschung*, Reinbek, Hamburg.

Garbarino, J. (1999) *Lost Boys: Why Our Sons Turn Violent and How We Can Save Them.* Free Press, New York.

Hoffmann, S. O. (1984) Aggression, in *Handwörterbuch der Psychiatrie* (eds B. Battegay, J. Glatzel, W. Poeldinger, and U. Rauchfleisch), Enke, Stuttgart, pp. 7–11.

Horton, A. (2001) The prevention of school violence: New evidence to consider. *J Hum Behav Soc Environ*, **4**, 49–59.

Kaufmann, J. M. (1997) *Characteristics of Emotional and Behavioral Disorders of Children and Youth*, 6th Edition, Merrill, Columbus, OH.

Krahn, H., Hartnagel, T. F., and Gartrell, J. W. (1986) Income inequality and homicide rates: Gross national data and criminological theories. *Criminology*, **24**, 269–95.

Maguin, E. and Loeber, R. (1996) Academic performance and delinquency, in *Crime and Justice: A Review of Research*, Vol. 20 (ed M. Tonry), University of Chicago Press, Chicago, IL, pp. 145–264.

McCarthy, O. and Carr, A. (2002) Prevention of bullying, in *Prevention: What Works with Children and Adolescents* (ed A. Carr), Brunner-Routledge, Hove, East Sussex, pp 205–21.

Olweus, D. (1978) *Aggression in Schools: Bullies and Whipping Boys.* Hemisphere Press, Washington, DC.

Olweus, D. (1991) Bully/victim school problems among school children: Basic effects of a school-based intervention program, in *The Development and Treatment of School Aggression* (eds D. Pepler and K. Rubin), Lawrence Erlbaum Associates Inc., Hillsdale, NJ.

Olweus, D. (1993) *Bullying in Schools: What We Know and What We Can Do.* Blackwell, Oxford.

Olweus, D. (1994) Annotation: Bullying at school: Basic facts and effects of a school-based intervention program. *J Child Psychol Psychiatry Allied Disciplines*, **35**, 1171–90.

Olweus, D. (1997) Bully/victim problems in school: Knowledge base and effective intervention program. *Ir J Psychol*, **18**, 170–90.

Olweus, D. and Kallestad, J. H. (2003) Predicting teachers' and schools' implementation of the Olweus Bullying Prevention Program: A multilevel study. *Prev Treat*, **6**, 1–29.

Roland, E. (1989) A system-oriented strategy against bullying, in *Bullying: An International Perspective* (eds E. Roland and E. Munthe), David Fulton, London, pp. 143–51.

Roland E, Munthe E (1997) The 1996 Norwegian program for preventing and managing bullying in schools. *Ir J Psychology*, **18**, 233–247.

Rollin, A. S., Kaiser-Urley, C., Potts, I., and Creason, A. H. (2003) A school-based violence prevention model for at-risk eighth grade youth. *Psychol Sch*, **40**(4), 403–16.

Rutter, M., Maughan, B., Mortimore, P., Ouston, J., and Smith, A. (1979) *1500 Hours. Secondary Schools and the Effect on Children.* Open Books, London.

Sampson, J. R. and Wooldredge, J. D. (1987) Linking the micro- and the macro-level dimensions of lifestyle, routine activity, and opportunity models of predatory victimization. *J Quant Criminol*, **3**, 371–93.

Shapiro, J. P., Burgoon, J. D., Welker, C. J., and Clough, J. B. (2002) Evaluation of The Peacemakers Program: School-based violence prevention for students in grades four through eight. *Psychol Sch*, **39**(1), 87–100.

Sylva, K. (1994) School influences on children's development. *J Child Psychol Psychiatry*, **33**, 135–70.

Tattum, D. P. (1993) *Understanding and Managing Bullying*, Heinemann Educational Books, Oxford.

WHO (2004) *The Economic Dimensions of Interpersonal Violence*, World Health Organization, Geneva (www.who.int).

Zeira, A., Astor, A. R., and Benbenshty, R. (2003) School violence in Israel: Findings of a national survey. *Natl Assoc Soc Workers*, **48**, 471–83.

CHAPTER 6

Preventive Interventions in School Dropout: Three Field Studies

CHAPTER 6.1

A Comprehensive Intervention for the Prevention of School Dropout in Brazil

Ana Soledade Graeff-Martins, Sylvia Oswald, Júlia Obst Comassetto, Christian Kieling, Renata Rocha Gonçalves, and Luis Augusto Rohde
Federal University of Rio Grande do Sul, Brazil

INTRODUCTION

In developing countries, school dropout is a very complex phenomenon, which needs to be understood in the context of socioeconomic problems and inadequacies of the educational system. In Brazil, it is not uncommon for adolescents to leave school to work and for school-age children to stay home to take care of younger siblings. Furthermore, the educational system is often inadequately prepared to meet the needs of poor children, leading a significant number of these youngsters to drop out from school (Tramontina *et al.*, 2002). It is estimated that worldwide 95% of children have access to school, but only 59% of them finish the eighth grade (UNICEF, 1999).

Surprisingly, there is a lack of research in this area in Brazil, even though school dropout is problematic. In a previous paper, we documented that at least two mental disorders (conduct disorder and mental retardation) were significantly associated with school dropout in public elementary school (Tramontina *et al.*, 2002).

The aim of this chapter is to describe an intervention designed to reduce school dropout in a public school in Porto Alegre, Brazil, and developed during 2004. More detailed results of this project are described elsewhere (Graeff-Martins *et al.*, 2006).

INTERVENTION

Porto Alegre, the capital of Brazil's southernmost state, has a population of 1 800 000. The school year begins on the first day of March and ends by mid-December.

The Mental Health of Children and Adolescents: an area of global neglect. Edited by H. Remschmidt *et al.*

Based on records from the State Department of Education for 2003, one state school was randomly selected from the list of 10 schools in the city with the highest dropout rates. A package of universal interventions was implemented as follows:

Workshops with teachers: Two meetings with the teachers from all grades were conducted. The first (1 week before the beginning of the school year) addressed children's normal development. The second (during the first trimester) presented information on how to recognize and manage the most common emotional and behavioral disorders in childhood and adolescence in the school environment. These workshops were conducted by a research team at the school, each for one school day. The research team was composed of two child psychiatrists, one psychologist, one social worker, and two research assistants.

Informative letters: During the school year, five letters addressing school dropout were sent to the families of all students. The content of these letters was as follows: (1) the prevalence of school dropout in Brazil and a brief description of the project (first letter); (2) the reasons for school dropout and its outcome (second letter); (3) how to know if your child is really attending school and where to seek help to keep your child at school (third letter); (4) how to improve communication and relationship within the family and with school personnel (fourth letter); and (5) topics designed to keep parents motivated, preliminary findings on dropout in the school, and closing statements (fifth letter).

School meetings ("talking with parents"): We conducted three meetings with parents at school addressing school dropout and other topics of interest. These meetings occurred during the school year (one in the first semester and two in the second semester) on 3 days when parents were expected to attend the school in order to receive their children's evaluations. The children's grades were handed out after these meetings. In the first meeting, the purpose of the project was introduced, along with information concerning school dropout and the benefits of keeping children at school. In the same meeting, a famous former soccer player reinforced with parents the desirability of keeping their children at school – even those who planned a future in occupations requiring no formal study. A topic of parental interest was selected for the second meeting ("How to set limits for children"). In the second meeting, preliminary findings on dropout in the school during the first semester were presented. The topic chosen by the parents was negotiated with them by a child psychiatrist. A topic of parental interest was selected for the third meeting ("sexuality") (at the end of the school year) and was delivered jointly by a gynecologist specializing in the care of adolescents and a child psychiatrist.

Modifications of the school environment: A music contest was promoted in the first semester to stimulate adolescents to compose songs about problems related to school dropout and the advantages of staying at school. Parents were invited to take part on 2 days in activities (small repairs) to improve the school environment.

Telephone helpline connecting the school to the team: Throughout the year (on 1 day per week for 2 h), a member of the team was available to talk with the parents of any student about emotional and behavioral problems of students or their families. The aim was to assess the situation quickly and refer the child and family to the best available resource in the health or educational systems.

Implementation of the programme – "The Junior Achievement – Brazil Programme". The Advantages of Staying at School was implemented with seventh grade students. Junior Achievement is a nonprofit organization established originally in the United States to contribute to the development of youth in the world. Supported by companies, foundations, and individuals, it is active in more than 100 countries. *The Advantages of Staying at*

School is a structured, cognitive intervention aiming to keep students at school, combining the concepts of employability, qualifications, and education (Junior Achievement, 2003). Manuals are provided for the applicant and each participant. The programme is implemented by trained volunteers, in the classroom, and lasts one school day. It is divided into five sections: (a) personal success and qualifications; (b) statistics showing the advantages of staying at school; (c) elaborating one's personal budget; (d) anticipating one's future; and (e) debate on the "pros and contras" of staying at school. At the end of this section, students are required to write a letter to a friend explaining the importance of staying at school. Although never formally tested, the intervention had already been implemented by Junior Achievement at public schools in Porto Alegre during the previous 3 years ($n = 30$ schools each year). We selected the seventh grade because records indicated that the rate of dropping out peaks at this grade.

In addition to the universal interventions mentioned above, we provided an intervention for at-risk children (those who had stayed at least 10 consecutive days out of school). The 10-day cutoff point was chosen because previous data suggested that these children are at the highest risk of dropping out of school (Tramontina *et al.*, 2001). The target intervention included the following components:

Mental health assessment: Students absent for at least 10 consecutive school days without legitimate reasons (e.g., physical illness or trip) were visited at home on two occasions by our mental health team (social worker with training in family therapy, psychologist, and child psychiatrist) to assess both child and family mental health status.

The following instruments were administered:

- The Schedule for Affective Disorders and Schizophrenia for School-Age Children, Epidemiological Version (K-SADS-E) (Orvaschel, 1985), supplemented with questions to allow DSM-IV diagnoses to be made.
- The Self-Report Questionnaire, 20-item version (SRQ-20) (Mari and Williams, 1986), to assess maternal psychopathology. The SRQ-20 is composed of 20 questions calling for dichotomous answers (yes/no). Higher scores are associated with more severe psychopathology. The SRQ-20 has previously been validated in Brazil. A score ≥ 8 was found to be an adequate cutoff point for the detection of nonpsychotic mental disorder (sensitivity = 83%; specificity = 80%; both positive and negative predictive values = 82%) (Mari and Williams, 1986).
- The vocabulary and block design subtests of the Wechsler Intelligence Scale for Children – Third Edition (WISC-III) to estimate overall IQ (Sattler, 1988; Wechsler, 1991).
- The Family System Test (FAST) (Gehring, 1998) and the Family Identification Test (FIT) (Remschmidt and Mattejat, 1999) to assess family functioning. The FAST employs standardized figures to assess family structure (cohesion and hierarchy) through the individual perception of family members. Family identification processes were assessed with the FIT, which allows the investigation of different aspects of self-concept: real self, ideal self, and "should-be self". The correlation between real self and ideal self allows for a measure of self-congruence. The FIT also measures the degree to which a family member identifies with family members, friends, and teachers. For the purpose of this investigation, we used two variables from the FAST (family cohesion and family hierarchy, as perceived by the child) and three from the FIT (student's self-congruency, identification between student's real self and preferred teacher, and identification between student's ideal self and preferred teacher).

Connection to available resources: If a mental health problem was detected, the family was referred to resources available in the community. If the child stayed out of school for a second period of 10 consecutive days after the assessment/intervention had been offered, no other intervention was implemented.

RESULTS

During the year 2004, 40 students (7%of those registered) stayed at least 10 consecutive days out of school. Thirty-eight of them were extensively evaluated. Two students could not be assessed because their families could not be located in the addresses provided by the school. Eighteen students returned to school after receiving the intervention (45%). Twenty-two students did not respond to our interventions, staying out of school despite all efforts to reengage them in the school system. They reached the formal definition of dropout by the State Department of Education (60 consecutive days out of school). Their characteristics can be seen in Table 6.1.1.

Despite the fact that we were able to reengage in the school system 45% of the students who had been absent for 10 consecutive days, we considered that the intervention was

Table 6.1.1 Characteristics of dropouters

Characteristics[a]	Dropouters[b] (n = 22)	
Age (years)	15.6	(1.8)
Gender (male)	17	(77.3)
Grade	5.9	(1.9)
Ethnicity: African Brazilian	13	(59.1)
European Brazilian	8	(36.4)
Estimated IQ	81.8	(15.0)
Family socioeconomic status[c]		
C	6	(27.3)
D + E	15	(68.1)
Family chief's level of instruction (analphabet or incomplete elementary school)	10	(45.5)
Mental disorder (positive)[d]	18	(81.8)
Mother's SRQ (positive)[e]	10	(45.5)
Family cohesion (FAST)[f]	10.0	(0.8)
Family hierarchy (FAST)	1.2	(0.5)
Student's self-congruence (FIT)	0.5	(0.5)
Real self – preferred teacher identification (FIT)	0.4	(0.4)
Ideal self – preferred teacher identification (FIT)	0.8	(0.4)

[a]Mean and standard deviation (in parentheses) are reported for continuous variables; *n* and percent (in parentheses) are reported for categorical variables.
[b]One student was not localized.
[c]No families in classes A or B. SES was assessed with the Socioeconomic Scale of the Brazilian Association of Market Research Institutes (ABEP, 2003).
[d]Main diagnosis: ODD, ADHD, GAD, social phobia, nicotine use, and conduct disorder.
[e]Score in the Self-Report Questionnaire ≥8.
[f]As seen by the student; varies from 0.7 to 11.

only moderately well accepted by the school community. The main barriers to the implementation of the programme were

(1) low accuracy of the registration of the dropout rate;
(2) discrepancies in the manner of counting the number of dropouts between the State Department of Education and the school;
(3) a tendency for lower participation of families at-risk in the universal preventive programme;
(4) delays by school staff in quickly reporting children who stayed 10 days out of school (sometimes, the school staff referred a case to investigators only after the student had already been 1 month or more out of school);
(5) the practical difficulty of referring students for mental health intervention;
(6) lack of motivation by teachers to retain those students who had decided to return after 10 days out of school. Statements such as "The year is already lost" were not uncommon.

DISCUSSION

The effects of the intervention could be explained considering the two levels of action. The universal interventions, including the presence of the investigators in the school, mobilized the school community and might have prepared it for targeted interventions. On the contrary, targeted interventions for at-risk students had a protective or buffering effect for dropout, as 45% of the students out of school for 10 days or more returned to classes.

The characteristics of those who dropped out (mostly non-European-Brazilian male adolescents with low IQs and mental disorders who are members of families with low socioeconomic level) are consistent with other findings in the literature (Tramontina *et al.*, 2001). These findings support the idea that the school could be the most advantageous venue for prevention and early assessment in developing countries (Kapur, 1997), particularly because this special population does not have access to mental health centers and is very difficult to trace in the community by health care agents.

The intervention was innovative in that universal and targeted interventions were combined. The mixed results suggest that intensive preparation and support of school staff are required before an intervention is delivered in a school environment and that an intervention that targets family functioning should be a part of any strategy. The model could be implemented in other developing countries. For example, mental health professionals could serve as consultants to designated schools with high rates of dropout, promoting universal strategies at school and linking families and school staff with health and social facilities.

ACKNOWLEDGMENTS

We acknowledge Liliane Diefenthaeler Herter, Maria Helena Ferreira, and Paulo Roberto Falcão for their participation in the meetings with the parents; the staff from the State Department of Education and the state school Nações Unidas, especially Leila Schaan

Salis, Rosane Dorneles, and Iara Maria dos Santos Teixeira for their continuous support; Junior Achievement – Brazil for allowing us to use their manuals; and Goldzstein S.A. for their support to conduct activities with the parents at school.

REFERENCES

Associação Brasileira de Empresas de Pesquisa (2003) Critério de classificação econômica Brasil. Available at http://www.anep.org.br/codigosguias/CCEB.pdf. Accessed April 18, 2005.

Gehring, T. M. (1998) *Family System Test (FAST)*, Hogrefe & Huber Publishers, Seattle, WA.

Graeff-Martins, A. S., Oswald, S., Comassetto, J. O., Kieling, K., Goncalves, R. R., & Rohde, L. A. (2006) A package of interventions to reduce school dropout in public schools in a developing country: A feasibility study. *European Child and Adolescent Psychiatry*, **15**, 442–49.

Junior Achievement (2003) *As vantagens de permanecer na escola – manual do orientador*, Associação Junior Achievement do Brasil, Porto Alegre.

Kapur, M. (1997) *Mental Health in Indian Schools*, Sage Publications, New Delhi.

Mari, J. J. and Williams, P. (1986) A validity study of a psychiatric screening questionnaire (SRQ-20) in primary care in the city of São Paulo. *Br J Psychiatry*, **148**, 23–26.

Orvaschel, H. (1985) Psychiatric interviews suitable for use in research with children and adolescents. *Psychopharmacol Bull*, **21**, 737–44.

Remschmidt, H. and Mattejat, F. (1999) *Der Familien-Identifikations-Test (FIT): Manual*, Hogrefe, Göttingen.

Sattler, J. (1988) *Assessment of Children*, Sattler, San Diego, CA.

Tramontina, S., Martins, S., Michalowski, M. B. *et al.* (2001) School dropout and conduct disorder in Brazilian elementary school students. *Can J Psychiatry*, **46**, 941–47.

Tramontina, S., Martins, S., Michalowski, M. B. *et al.* (2002) Estimated mental retardation and school dropout in a sample of students from state public schools in Porto Alegre, Brazil. *Rev Bras Psiquiatr*, **24**, 177–81.

United Nations Children's Fund (1999) *The Progress of Nations, 1999*, UNICEF Publications, Brasília.

Wechsler, D. (1991) *WISC-III/Manual*, Psychological Corporation, New York.

CHAPTER 6.2

A Comprehensive Programme for the Prevention of Dropout in an Egyptian Public School

Amira Seif El Din, Mary Azzer, and Doa Habib
Alexandria University and the Egyptian Child Mental Health Association, Egypt

INTRODUCTION

The most favorable and convenient place to intervene with child and adolescent mental health problems is the school (Remschmidt *et al.*, 2004). In order to prevent school refusal and dropout, community-based, school-based, and family-based strategies require professional collaboration. Clinical strategies that have been implemented to reduce school dropout include structured activities outside the home, booster sessions, and change of school (Kearneg and Hugelschofer, 2000).

Janosz *et al.* (2000) found that grade retention and school achievement are the best screening variables for children at risk of dropping out. Other psychosocial variables, though significant, did not greatly improve upon educational achievement in predicting dropping out. Oill *et al.* (1986) concluded that improving school performance is a means of reducing delinquent behavior and dropping out. Giancola (1999) examined the causes, risk factors, and protective factors in relation to adolescent misbehavior. He found that the influence of deviant peers was an important predictor during high school. Although many researchers have linked school size to student behavior, Giancola did not find that large schools necessarily increased the risk of dropping out. The tendency to drop out was found to be related more to recent school failure. Schools and communities designing prevention programmes could use workplace activities and extracurricular experiences to counteract dropping out.

Olweus (1990) and Hawkins *et al.* (1999) examined the effect on health risk behavior and school dropout of intervention programmes combining teacher training, parent education and social skills training for elementary school children. The results were consistent with the theoretical model. These studies were confirmed by Eggert *et al.* (1994) and Reynolds *et al.* (2001) who stressed the use of life skills training. Other intervention

The Mental Health of Children and Adolescents: an area of global neglect. Edited by H. Remschmidt *et al.*

programmes have focused on improving the school environment through teachers as a means of preventing school dropout and enhancing school performance (Pittman, 1986; Blechman, 1996). Although school dropout is prevalent in developing countries, there is a lack of research on its causation and prevention.

SUBJECTS

This study was conducted in two public primary schools in Alexandria, Egypt. The average school dropout rate in Egypt for the academic year 2003/2004 was 9%. The school selected for the implementation of the intervention programme had Alexandria's highest school dropout rate (13.1%) during the academic year 2003/2004. The total number of students in the experimental school was 1054. The school dropout rate for the control school during the academic year 2003/2004 was 1.9% where the total number of students was 1100.

Project approval was obtained from the Ministry of Education and the ethical committee of the Egyptian Child Mental Health Association. During a preliminary visit to the target school, the aim of the programme was explained to school staff and families, and their approval sought. A formal letter was sent to parents of all students about to be promoted to the sixth grade ($n = 254$). Students absent without legitimate reason for more than four continuous weeks were regarded as having dropped out.

METHOD

Phase I

School staff awareness

At the start of the academic year 2004/2005, school staff was oriented concerning the programme. At a workshop with school staff, the following matters were discussed: problems faced by students; the causes of dropping out; ways to improve the school environment; and how teachers can manage child mental health problems and promote mental health. Information was obtained from teachers about the reasons they thought children drop out.

Teachers reported that children who drop out are affected by poverty, ill health, illiteracy, a lack of respect for education, and lack of communication between school and family. Poverty was regarded as the leading cause of dropping out, followed by disruptive family relations and lack of awareness of the importance of education. An academic curriculum with few recreational activities makes the school an unpleasant environment. Teachers conceded that verbal and physical punishment at school was associated with dropping out; however, they contended that punishment is required to cope with the large student–teacher ratio (average 50 students per class).

As defined by Sikorski (1996), academic underachievers are individuals whose academic performance is at a level below expectation. The Egyptian Ministry of Education defines an academic underachiever as a student whose total score is less than 60% at the final examination, or who has failed two subjects in the previous academic year. Those who underachieve usually drop out in the following year. In 2003/2004, 29 fifth-grade experimental school students (11.5%) were designated as underachievers.

Teacher training

In a 3-day programme, teachers were trained in communication skills, the psychosocial development of children and adolescents, and life-skills education.

Enhancing the school environment

During the 2004 summer vacation, a summer camp was conducted at which students were trained in sports, tutored in handicrafts and gardening, and encouraged to use the school library.

Parents' opinions concerning the reasons why children dropout

Two hundred and fifty-four students had been promoted to the sixth grade at the end of the academic year 2003/2004. At the beginning of 2004/2005, 219 students entered the sixth grade. Four weeks later, the number had dropped to 205. The dropout rate had, thus, increased from 13.1% in 2003/2004 to 19.3% early in 2004/2005. The families of children who had dropped out were invited to a party at the school; but of 49 invited families, only 7 attended. We could convince only two families to return their children to school, even when special coaching was offered. A further approach through local mosques and churches also failed. The team then attempted to reach the families in their homes but could contact only 6 of the 14 families whose children had dropped out in the previous 4 weeks.

Families and students cited the expense of keeping children in school (despite the fact that basic education in Egypt is free) as the main reason for dropping out. The families of most of the children who dropped out were large. Parents described teachers, as physically and verbally abusive and supportive only to those students who took private lessons. Parents considered that education did not provide enough to allow a person to live a comfortable life. Many students who dropped out were unable to read or write properly, as a result, sixth grade is arduous for them (see Appendixes 6.2.1 and 6.2.2).

Measures

The Arabic versions of the Student and Teacher Forms of the Strength and Difficulties Questionnaire (SDQ; Goodman, 1997) were adopted as measures of the psychological status of students before and at the end of the intervention programme. A socio-demographic questionnaire was distributed to sixth-grade students in the experimental (n = 205) and control (n = 120 students) schools.

The cognitive behavioral therapy programme

In the experimental school, 49 students (23.4%) had scores above the clinical level on both student and teacher forms of the SDQ. Consequently, all 49 were involved in a Cognitive Behavior Therapy (CBT) programme developed by Jensen *et al.* (2004), in addition to the school-dropout prevention programme. The goal of the CBT programme was to ameliorate externalizing and internalizing problems. The manual for the CBT programme is organized in two levels: the first level is addressed to children and families who could benefit from psycho-education and psychological support alone; the second level involves direct treatment for children in need of clinical services.

Therapy was conducted in group sessions, once per week for 75 min at a time: eight sessions for externalizing problems and six for internalizing problems. Parents attended 10–12 sessions. Six groups were held for externalizing problems ($n = 35$) and three for internalizing problems ($n = 14$). Group size ranged from five to six students. The Alexandria Mental Health Team facilitated all group sessions.

During the implementation of the CBT programme, classmates of the students involved in CBT reported that they became friendlier, controlled their temper better, and ceased to harass their colleagues verbally.

Phase II

Class activities

A member of the Alexandria University Mental Health Team coached the sixth grade classes. Most of the boys preferred to play soccer. Other activities such as gardening, drawing, handicraft, singing, and drama were provided according to students' interests. Students were encouraged to express their emotions and describe their problems. A class teacher was trained by the mental health team to manage different problems. Students discussed and approved class rules. Students elected by the class were nominated for a weekly honor board. Every class had its own garden, and competed for the award of "Best Garden."

The mental health team provided psycho-education for all sixth-grade students concerning the recognition of emotions, relaxation techniques, problem solving, and coping skills. The mental health team gave a lecture on psychosocial development and emotional feelings toward the opposite sex, in classes divided into same-sex groups, each coached by a team member of the same sex.

All these activities aimed to increase the bond between the students and the school, and to encourage students to pursue the activities of their choice and improve their academic performance, with the purpose of encouraging them to attend school regularly.

Data analysis

SDQ (student/teacher) data were collected from all sixth-grade students in the experimental and control schools. Pretest and posttest SDQ data were available for the experimental school, but only pretest data for the control school. Socio-demographic data were collected

Table 6.2.1 SDQ (teacher and student) pretest scores in the two schools

	Mean	Standard deviation	*t*	*p*
SDQ Teacher Form				
Experimental school	13.40	4.00	2.22	<0.027
Control school	12.52	3.04		
SDQ Student Form				
Experimental school	10.99	4.80	2.21	<0.027
Control school	9.99	3.29		

concerning experimental school subjects. Chi-square and *t*-tests were calculated. A 5% level of significance was adopted.

RESULTS

The total sixth-grade dropout rate for the first 2 months of 2004/2005 was 10.2% in the experimental school and 7.2% in the control school. The dropout rate for students at the experimental school was 19.3% compared to 9.1% at the control school. The sex ratio of all sixth-grade dropouts in the two schools was 5:3 and 4:3, respectively, in favor of boys.

Table 6.2.1 portrays the mean total score on the SDQ (pretest) in the experimental and control schools. There were significantly more total psychological problems among students in the experimental school than in the control school.

By the end of the year, the additional dropout rate at the experimental school was zero compared to the control school where the rate was 8%.

Forty-nine students scored in the clinical range on both teacher and student SDQ rating scales. They were designated as being at high risk of dropping out. Table 6.2.2 portrays the age distribution of subjects according to risk level. The older the age, the greater the proportion of high-risk students, but the differences were statistically insignificant ($\chi^2 = 2.636$; $df = 1$; $p = 0.10$).

Table 6.2.3 reveals that there were significantly more boys than girls in the high-risk group ($\chi^2 = 4.05$; $df = 1$; $p = 0.04$).

Table 6.2.2 Age distribution of high-risk experimental school students

	High risk	
Age in years	*N*	%
11–12	19	19.4
12–13	16	25.4
13–14	11	31.4
14–15	3	33.3
Total	49	23.9

Table 6.2.3 Distribution of students by sex at high risk of dropping out

Sex	High risk *N*	High risk %
Boys	31	29.8
Girls	18	17.8
Total	49	23.9

Table 6.2.4 portrays the socio-demographic characteristics of the two groups: high scorers on the SDQ (student and teacher) compared to low scorers on SDQ. High-risk students were more likely to have parents who had separated and parents with low levels of education, and to have experienced stressful life events, family conflict, and corporal

Table 6.2.4 Distribution of socio-demographic data according to total score on SDQ ($n = 205$)

Characteristics	SDQ high score ($n = 49$)	SDQ low score ($n = 156$)	Statistics
Parents' marital status			
Married	36 (73%)	125 (80%)	$\chi^2 = 3.41$; $df = 1$; $p = 0.18$
Widowed	4 (8%)	17 (11%)	
Separated	9 (19%)	14 (9%)	
Maternal education			
Illiterate	32 (65%)	67 (43%)	$\chi^2 = 7.47$; $df = 1$; $p = 0.02$
High school education	16 (33%)	83 (53%)	
University education	1 (2%)	6 (4%)	
Paternal education			
Illiterate	27 (55%)	71 (46%)	$\chi^2 = 1.468$; $df = 4$; $p = 0.48$
High school education	20 (33%)	79 (51%)	
University education	2 (4%)	6 (4%)	
Life events (previous 6 months)			
Family conflicts and lack of communication	45 (92%)	83 (45%)	$\chi^2 = 37.45$; $df = 2$; $p < 0.01$
Death of a parent	1 (2%)	7 (4%)	
No serious life events	3 (6%)	66 (42%)	
Parental punishment			
Corporal punishment	38 (78%)	56 (36%)	$\chi^2 = 30.62$; $df = 1$; $p = 0.00$
Verbal abuse	11(22%)	52 (33%)	
No punishment	–	48 (31%)	

Table 6.2.5 Distribution of SDQ scores (students and teacher forms) before and after the intervention programme

	Pretest mean	Posttest mean	*t*	*p** (**df* = 1)
Student SDQ	10.98 ± 4.81	9.05 ± 3.35	9.46	<0.001
Teacher SDQ	13.38 ± 3.99	11.38 ± 3.48	9.821	<0.001

punishment. Stressful life events in the sixth month prior to the programme were more prevalent among the high-risk group (92%) compared to the low-risk group (54%). (χ^2 = 37.45; $df = 2$; $p < 0.01$).

Table 5.2.5 shows the means of student and teacher SDQ scores at pretest and at the end of the programme in the experimental school. Significant differences were found between pretest and posttest. SDQ posttest data were not available from the control school due to a lack of cooperation.

Although the school dropout between the selected school and the control school was not statistically significant, but the percent differences show some differences as presented in Figure 6.2.1.

To evaluate the success of the supporting programme in respect of school dropout, we compare the dropout rates of the sixth-grade students in the experimental school before and after implementing the supporting programme.

The number of students in the experimental school that did not dropout since the start of the programme till the end of the academic year is highly supporting that this programme was effective in the experimental school.

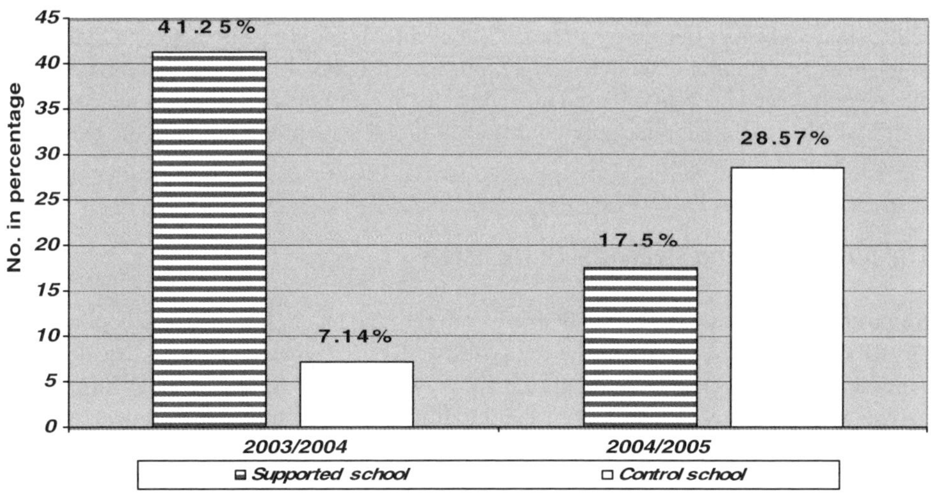

Figure 6.2.1 School dropout rates before and after the intervention programme in the experimental school compared to the rates in the control school during the academic years (2003/2004–2004/2005).

DISCUSSION

Chiland and Young (1990) have emphasized the magnitude of school refusal and failure to complete schooling and reviewed the phenomena in accordance with contemporary experience in several countries. In Japan, maternal over-involvement with the child, inadequate paternal involvement, undue pressure from peers and authority figures, and bullying are related to school dropout (Murase, 1990). In a developing country such as Brazil, where the vast majority of the population is poor, there are limited opportunities for economic advancement. Only 27% of Brazilian children remain in school as far as the fourth grade, and only 6.4% complete the third year of secondary education (Celia, 1990). In the present study, the school dropout rate in the sixth grade was 19.3%, predominantly for economic reasons.

Most studies have focused on student factors associated with dropping out; rarely have environmental factors such as family inadequacy and teacher effectiveness been examined (Rumbergers, 1987). Bryk and Thum (1989) suggest that dropout rates are lower in schools characterized by an academic emphasis, orderly environments, active staff–student interaction with students, and less differentiation of students by demographic and academic background. The present study found significant differences in student psychopathology before and after a preventive programme. Following changes in the school environment, students' attitudes toward school became more favorable, results consistent with the findings of Rutter *et al.* (1979).

DeBaryshe *et al.* (1993) found that family risk factors such as low parental academic achievement and aspirations adversely affect children's academic achievement. An inconsistent, punitive style of discipline, frequently utilized by low-achieving parents, correlates with diminished student engagement in the educational process, lower academic achievement, and a higher rate of dropping out. In the present study, compared to low-risk students, high-risk students had less well-educated parents who were more likely to use physical discipline to control their children.

The results of the present study are consistent with the recommendation of Haynes (2002) that students affected by stressful life events should be assisted to deal with their problems, in an attempt to reduce school failure and dropout. Prominent among the strategies recommended are school-based mental health programmes delivered by mental health teams which seek to address individual student problems while improving the emotional environment of the school.

The limitations and strengths of the study

No posttest SDQ measures were obtained from the students in the control school because the school staff refused to complete the posttest SDQ. They were offended, because they were not offered a supportive programme. We were unable to obtain SDQ forms from parents because many of them were illiterate. It was almost impossible to induce students who had already dropped out to return to school.

Economic problems were a barrier to a programme directed to students who had already dropped out. For this reason, we were forced to focus on high-risk students.

Finally, a lack of understanding of mental health problems among school staff sometimes hindered the programme. At the beginning of the study, the staff was reluctant to be involved in the mental health component of the programme, particularly the extracurricular school activities. Teachers' and parents' attitudes were difficult to change in the short time available. Many parents were illiterate and had little communication with the school. Parents were reluctant to discuss their children's health problems because they had little confidence that the staff would support their children.

On the contrary, participants improved in self-esteem, self-care, and in sporting, gardening and handicraft skills. They became more respectful of each other. Bullying decreased in frequency, according to teachers. By the end of the academic year, the school attendance rate of participants was very high. No sixth-grade student in the experimental school dropped out after the intervention had begun. In contrast, in the control school, attendance rates were poorer and the dropout rate higher (8%). (This is explained from the table showing the differences between the supporting school and the control one.)

Recommendations

The intervention programme should be implemented continuously for a longer duration to obtain a better and more sustained outcome. In-service training is required for school staff to promote mental health. More comprehensive school health services are required, and the academic curriculum should be modified to include practical and recreational skills attractive for children.

APPENDIX 6.2.1

Case vignette

H, a boy aged 13 years, is the third of six siblings. His two older brothers left school in the fifth grade to work with their father. H reported that his mother respects his working brothers more than her other children. H failed to attend school at the start of the academic year. He decided to leave school, because, if he did so, would no long be punished or obliged to study boring things. Now, he is more respected by his parents and earns money.

APPENDIX 6.2.2

Case vignette

M, a girl aged 12 years, in the sixth grade, is the third of three children. Her two older sisters are married. M's parents report that M is doing poorly in her studies. They say that private tutoring is expensive, and there is no benefit in educating girls who will only get married. Thus, it is preferable for her to stay at home and help her mother, particularly since her older sister married.

ACKNOWLEDGMENTS

The authors would like to thank the taskforce on Prevention of the Presidential WPA Programme on Global Child Mental Health: Prof. A. Okasha (President of WPA),

B. Nurcombe (Australia) for his support in editing the paper, E. Caffo (Italy), T. Dmitrieva (Russia), M. Flament (Canada), H. Remschmidt (Germany), P. A. Rydelius (Sweden), and L. A. Rohde (Brazil). This initiative was supported by an unrestricted grant from Eli-Lilly. Thanks also go to the Alexandria University Mental Health Team who conducted the CBT and the preventive activities at the school: W. M. Saad and I. Farouk (psychologists), D. M. ElSaid and M. O. Ebrahim (social workers); to all the staff of Gheit El Enab primary school, Alexandria; to the staff of the State Department of Education; and to all the students who participated in this study.

REFERENCES

Blechman, A. (1996) Coping, competence, and aggression prevention: Universal school-based prevention. *Appl Prevent Psychol*, **5**(1), 19–35.

Bryk, A. and Thum, Y. M. (1989) The effect of high school organization on dropping out. An exploratory investigation. *Am Educ Res J*, **26**, 353–83.

Celia, S. (1990) School refusal and school problems in Brazil, in *Why Children Reject School: Views from Seven Countries* (eds C. Chiland and J. G. Young), Yale University Press, New Haven, pp. 152–59.

Chiland, C. and Young, J. G. (eds) (1990) *Why Children Reject School: Views from Seven Countries*, Yale University Press, New Haven.

DeBaryshe, B. D., Patterson, G. R., and Kapaldi, D. M. (1993) A performance model for academic achievement in early adolescent boys. *Dev Psychol*, **29**(5), 795–804.

Eggert, L., Thompson, E., Herting, J., Nicholos L., and Dicker B. (1994) Preventing adolescent drug abuse and high school dropout through an intensive school-based social network development program. *Am J Health Promot*, **8**(3), 202–15.

Giancola, S. (1999) Student misbehavior: An exploratory study of individual, familial, social, and institutional influence. *Humanit Soc Sci*, **59**(11-A), 40–53.

Goodman, R. (1997) The strength and difficulties questionnaire: Research note. *J Child Psychcol Psychiatry*, **38**(5), 581–86.

Haynes, M. (2002) Addressing student's social and emotional needs: The role of mental health teams in schools. *J Health Soc Policy*, **16**(1–2), 109–23.

Hawkins, J., Catalano, R., Kosterman, R., *et al.* (1999) Preventing adolescent health-risk behavior by strengthening protection during childhood. *Arch Pediatr Adolesc Med*, **153**(3), 226–34.

Janosz, M., Le Blanc, M., Boulerice B., and Richard, E. (1997) Disentangling the weight of school dropout predictors: A test on two longitudinal samples. *J Youth Adolesc*, **26**(6), 733–62.

Jensen, P., Bauermeister, J., So, C., *et al.* (2004) *Helping Children and Youth with Behavioral and Emotional Problems. Treatment Manuals*, Task Force on Prevention of the Presidential WPA Program on Global Child Mental Health.

Kearneg, C. and Hugelschofer, D. (2000) Systemic and clinical strategies for preventing school refusal behavior in youth. *J Cogn Psychother*, **14**(1), 51–65.

Murase, K. (1990) School refusal and family pathology: A multifactorial approach, in *Why children reject school: Views from seven countries* (eds C. Chiland and J. G. Young), Yale University Press, New Haven, pp. 73–77.

Olweus D. (1990) Victimization among schoolchildren: Intervention and prevention, in *Improving Children's Lives: Global Preventives on Prevention* (eds G. W. Ablee, C. A. Bond, and T. V. C. Manses), Sage Publications, Newburg Park, pp. 275–97.

Pittman, R. (1986) Importance of personal, social factors as potential means for reducing high school dropout rate. *High School J*, **70**(1), 7–13.

Remschmidt, H., Belfer, M., and Goodyer, I. (2004) Prevention and intervention in school setting, in *Facilitating Pathways: Care, Treatment and Prevention in Child and Adolescent Mental Health*, Springer, Berlin, pp. 326–34.

Reynolds, A. J., Temple, J. A., Robertson, D. L., and Mann, E. A. (2001) Long term effects of an early childhood intervention on educational achievement and juvenile arrest: A 15 year follow up of low income children in public schools. *JAMA*, **285**(18), 2378–80.

Rumberger, R. W. (1987) High school dropouts: A review of issues and evidence. *Rev Educ Res J*, **32**, 583–25.

Rutter, M., Maughan, B., Mottimore, P., and Ouston, J. (1979) *Fifteen Thousand Hours. Secondary Schools and Their Effect on Children*, Harvard University, Cambridge, MA.

Sikorski, J. B. (1996) Academic underachievement and school refusal, in *Handbook of Adolescent Health Risk Behavior* (eds R. Diclemente, W. Hansen, and L. Ponton), Plenum Press, New York, London, pp. 393–411.

CHAPTER 6.3

A Comprehensive Intervention to Prevent School Dropout and Reduce School Absenteeism in a Public School in a Russian Industrial City

Valeriya Andreyuk, Andrey Zanozin, and Tatjana Dmitrieva
City Center for the Mental Health of Children and Adolescents, Nizhny Novgorod, Russia

INTRODUCTION

School dropout is a widespread phenomenon, and a precursor of family, legal, and psychiatric problems. Over 100 000 000 primary-school-age children are out of school worldwide (United Nation Children's Fund, 2005), particularly in developing countries. In Brazil, 95% of children have access to school, but only 59% complete the eight grade (United Nation Children's Fund, 1999). The school dropout rate reflects the educational status of a country. If the educational system is not adequately prepared, a significant number of disadvantaged youngsters will drop out of school (Tramontina *et al*., 2002).

The effectiveness of prevention programmes depends on the timely, accurate identification of students likely to drop out of school. The best way to confront school dropout is to address its antecedents (Ripple, 1996). Numerous variables have been found to be related to school dropout, and methods for identifying students at risk should be applicable to intervention programmes (Svec, 1987; Oakland, 1992; Trusty, Dooley-Dickey, 1993).

Previous studies have documented the fact that environmental stressors, low socioeconomic status, minority-group status, single parents, inadequate health

The Mental Health of Children and Adolescents: an area of global neglect. Edited by H. Remschmidt *et al.*

care, child abuse and neglect, substance abuse, family disruption, dissatisfaction with school, chaotic school atmosphere, low parental education, high parental psychopathology, and adolescent pregnancy are all associated with school dropout (Ekstrom *et al.*, 1987; Bryk and Thum, 1989; Maton, 1990; Srebnik and Elias, 1993; Astone and McLanahan, 1994; Center for Disease Control, 1994). On the contrary, constitutional vulnerability, developmental disability, low IQ, leading to low academic achievement and grade retention, and mental disorders such as ADHD, conduct disorder, depression, anxiety, and substance abuse disorders also contribute to dropping out of school (Kortering *et al.*, 1992; Bechtold *et al.*, 1994; Jackson *et al.*,1995; Fergusson and Horwood, 1995; Kessler *et al.*, 1995; Achenbach *et al.*, 1998; Fergusson and Horwood, 1998; Hill *et al.*,1999; Tramontina *et al.*, 2002; Barilnik and Pushkareva, 2003).

Gleason and Dynarski (2002) found that most risk factors are not effective predictors of dropping out. Dropout prevention programmes often serve students who would not have dropped out, and fail to reach those who do. Recent preventive interventions for school dropout have had inconsistent results. Some (e.g., Allen *et al.*, 1990; Eggert *et al.*, 1990; Reynolds *et al.*, 2001) have significantly reduced the level of school dropout and absenteeism, whereas others have found no significant effect (e.g., Reyes and Jason, 1991; Vitaro *et al.*, 1999; Hawkins *et al.*, 1999).

METHOD

This study was conducted in two public schools in Nizhny Novgorod, Russia, a city with a population of 1 341 000. The Russian school year begins on the first day of September and ends in late May. The project was approved by both the City Department of Education and the Ethical Committee of the City Medical Department. Verbal informed consent was asked of parents.

We selected two schools with similarly high rates of dropout and school absenteeism. All 11–15-year-old students in these schools (N = 1062, 536 boys, 526 girls) were examined during the 4 months from March to June 2004. There were 620 students in the experimental school and 442 people in the control school. The mean age of students was 13.0 (±1.4) in the experimental school and 13.6 (±1.0) in the control school. The prevention programme was implemented in the experimental school between September 2004 and March 2005.

Universal intervention

Workshops with teachers

Three one-day workshops were held with teachers in the first semester of the school year. The first, at the beginning of the school year, addressed children's normal development. The second and third presented information on how to recognize and manage emotional and behavioral disorders in childhood and adolescence.

Informative letters

During the school year, six letters were sent to the families. The content of these letters was as follows: (1) the prevalence of school maladjustment in Russia and a brief description of the project; (2) the reasons for school absenteeism and school dropout; (3) the outcome of school dropout; (4) how to know if a child is really attending school and where to seek help to keep the child at school; (5) improving communication and relationship inside the family and with school personnel; and (6) the preliminary findings of the programme and closing statements.

Meetings with parents at school

We conducted three meetings with the parents at school, addressing topics related to school absenteeism and school dropout (two in the first semester, and one in the second semester). We selected 3 days when parents were scheduled to receive their children's evaluations. The first meeting presented an introduction to the project, information about school absenteeism, and reasons for keeping children in school. A topic of the parents' choice was selected for the second meeting ("how to set limits"). Actual cases were discussed, followed by recommendations concerning possible management. In the third meeting, behavioral regulation was discussed. At the end of the school year, all parents were informed about the results of the programme.

Modifications of the school environment

Sport and other activities were promoted to stimulate adolescents to talk about the advantages of staying at school. Parents were invited to take part in activities to improve the school environment.

Telephone line connecting the school to the team

Each Wednesday, from 10 to 12 a.m., a member of the team was available to talk with parents about the emotional problems of students or family problems, for rapid assessment and referral.

Targeted intervention

At-risk children were defined as those who had been out of school without legitimate reason for seven or more consecutive days during 2004/2005, despite the universal interventions. Targeted intervention included a clinical diagnostic evaluation and 20 h of cognitive–behavioral therapy appropriate to the diagnostic formulation. The mental health status of at-risk students was assessed by structured interview. The clinical diagnostic formulation was conducted by a trained child psychiatrist. If a mental health problem was detected, the family was connected to resources in the community. Brief psychoeducational intervention and support were provided during the 20 visits.

Measures

The following instruments were used: the Strengths and Difficulties Questionnaire (SDQ, Russian Version) for children, parents, and teachers (Goodman, 1997), and the Questionnaire for Assessment of the Family and School Situation (QAFSS) for children and teachers (Dmitieva and Seif El Din, 2003). The SDQ is widely used and has demonstrated satisfactory reliability and validity (Mathai *et al.*, 2002). The QAFSS includes questions about school attainment, school performance, and socio-demographic characteristics (family composition, parental occupation, and educational status of parents, number of children in the family). The QAFSS was administered by a trained psychologist.

Variables

The outcome variables were the comparative rates of school dropout and absenteeism at the end of the school years 2003/2004 and 2004/2005, in both schools. School dropout was operationally defined as *absence from school for four consecutive weeks without legitimate reason*. Other variables recorded were age, sex, family composition, the occupational and educational status of parents, number of children in the family, school attainment, school performance, and child mental disorder (assessed in those who had been out of school for seven consecutive days without legitimate reason).

Data analysis

Comparison among categorical variables was performed using cross-tabulation and chi-square tests. Kolmogorov–Smirnov tests were performed to determine whether the quantitative variables have a normal distribution. As the test revealed that they do not have a normal distribution, comparisons among quantitative variables were analyzed using nonparametric tests (Mann–Whitney U-tests). All tests were two-tailed. Due to the explorative character of this investigation, p-values are cited nominally and there is no correction for multiple testing that was conducted.

RESULTS

There were no significant differences between the schools in regard to parents' educational level, family composition (Table 6.3.1), or the number of children in families (Figure 6.3.1). In the control school, fewer parents were unemployed or handicapped, but more worked in less qualified jobs ($p < 0.05$). Forty-three (68.3%) of the dropout and absent students in the experimental school were diagnosed as having psychiatric disorders such as ADHD, organic mental disorder, or conduct, anxiety, somatoform and posttraumatic stress disorder (Table 6.3.2).

During 2003/2004, 101 (64 boys, 37 girls) (mean age 13.23, SD = 1.3) were regularly absent in both schools. The mean days of absence in the 2003/2004 school year were 22.67 (SD = 16.70). At baseline, 63 students (10.16%) in the experimental school had been absent from school for seven or more consecutive days and 38 (8.60%) had been absent for similar time in the control school. In the experimental school, three children (0.48%) had dropped out, whereas, in the control school, four students (0.91%) had done so. The rates of

Table 6.3.1 Family background

		Control school (%)	Test school (%)
Mothers' education	Secondary	53.5	51.8
	Tertiary	46.5	48.2
Mothers' occupation	Employees	50.8	55.4
	Workers	35.3	23.1*
	Business	2.6	4.3
	Unemployed or disabled	11.3	17.2*
Fathers' education	Secondary	50.6	52.9
	Tertiary	49.4	47.1
Fathers' occupation	Employees	37.1	42.3
	Workers	52.2	41.4*
	Business	8.5	10.4
	Unemployed or disabled	2.2	5.9*
Family situation	Intact family	78.1	80.1
	Sole parent mother	20.8	18.6
	Sole parent father	0.6	1.1
	Living with carers other than parents	0.7	0.2

*$p < 0.05$.

absenteeism in the 2003/2004 school year were similar: experimental school mean = 6.82 days per student (SD = 10.7) and control school mean = 6.00 days per student (SD = 9.8).

During the 2003/2004 school year, the total sum of school absentee days among dropouts and absentees was 1527 (mean = 24.24 days/student) in the experimental school

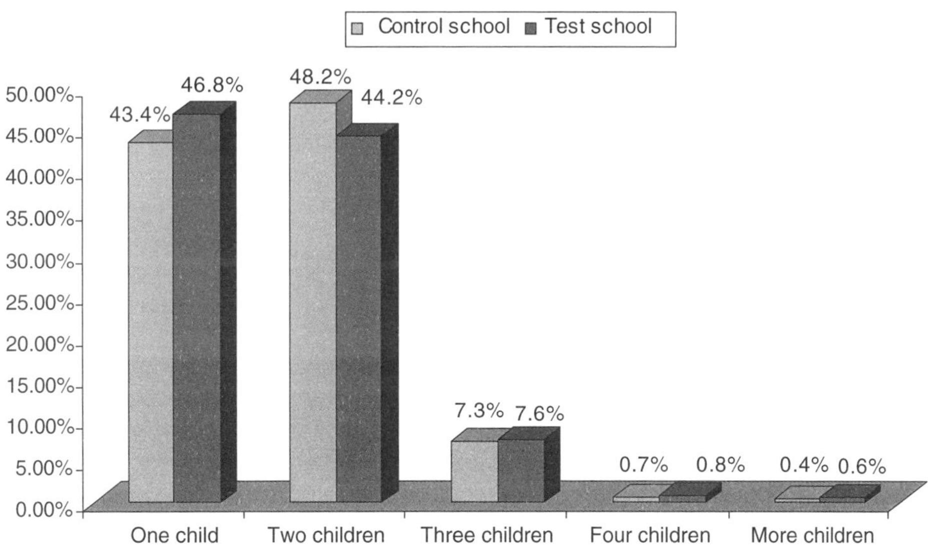

Figure 6.3.1 The number of children in the family

Table 6.3.2 Diagnosis of dropouts (ICD-10)

	The number of students		
Diagnosis	Boys	Girls	Total
F 90 ADHD	13	1	14 (22.2%)
F 06 Organic Mental Disorders	9	3	12 (19.0%)
F 92 Combined CD and Emotional Disorders	5	6	11 (17.5%)
F 91 Conduct Disorders	6	1	7 (11.1%)
F 43 Adjustment Disorders	—	7	7 (11.1%)
F 45 Somatoform Disorders	1	4	5 (7.9%)
F 94 Other Childhood Disorders Of Social functioning	—	2	2 (3.2)
Total	36	25	61[a]

[a]The number of students with psychiatric disorders is less (43) then the total number of disorders (61) because many students had comorbid disorders.

and 763 days (mean = 20.08 days/student) in the control school. The perception of the school situation by the children was similar in the two schools (Figure 6.3.2): there were no significant differences in students' relation to teachers ($\chi^2 = 0.24$, $p < 0.05$), peers ($\chi^2 = 0.08$, $p > 0.05$), or the school situation in general ($\chi^2 = 0.59$, $p > 0.05$).

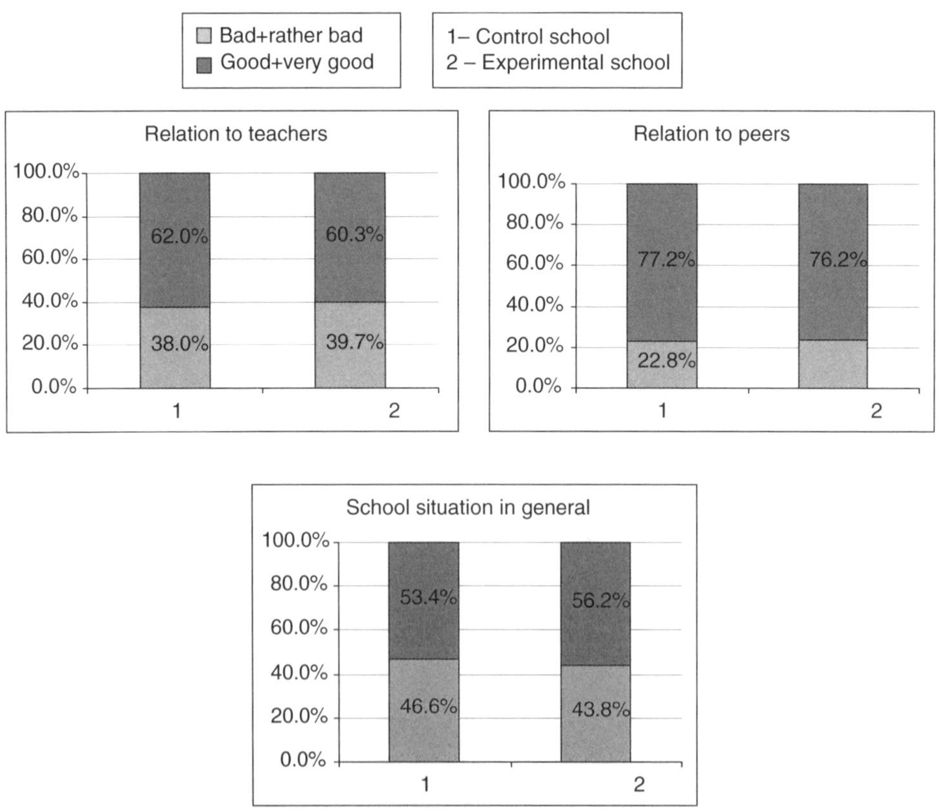

Figure 6.3.2 Assessment of the situation by children

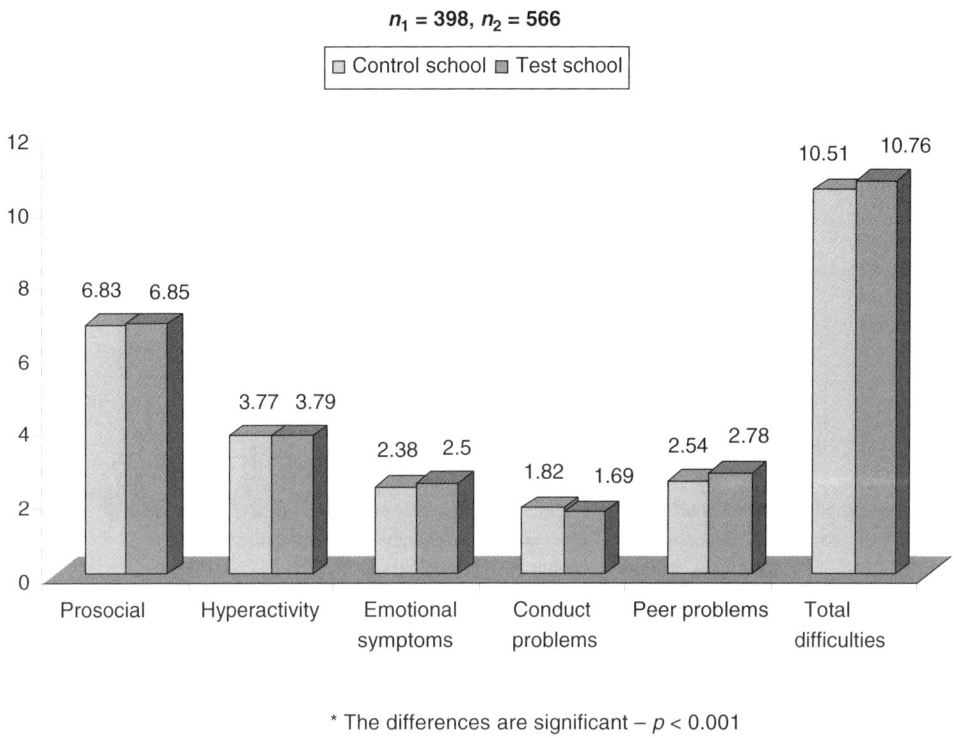

Figure 6.3.3 SDQ score teachers

There were two differences in the teachers SDQ pre-assessment: the experimental school demonstrated a significantly higher level of emotional symptoms (Mann–Whitney U-test: $z = -2.26$, $p > 0.05$) and peer problems (Mann–Whitney U-test: $z = -1.976$, $p > 0.05$) (see Figure 6.3.3). Four scales were different in parents pre-assessment: the Prosocial Scale (Mann–Whitney U-test: $z = -5.51$, $p < 0.0005$), the Hyperactivity Scale (Mann–Whitney U-test: $z = 2.04$, $p < 0.05$), the Peer Problems Scale (Mann–Whitney U-test: $z = -2.377$, $p < 0.02$), and the Total Difficulties scores (Mann–Whitney U-test: $z = -4.237$, $p < 0.0005$) were higher in the control school (Figure 6.3.4). There was one difference on the Peer Problems Scale in the students assessment (Figure 6.3.5): the test school showed significantly higher level of peer problems (Mann–Whitney U-test: $z = -3.65$, $p < 0.0005$).

Outcome assessment

The total sum of absentee days among all students in the experimental school decreased after the intervention programme from 4229 (mean = 6.82 days/student [SD = 9.97]) to 2272 (mean = 3.81 days/student [SD = 8.11]); $t = 5.79$, $p < 0.001$). The number of students regularly absent from school dropped (Figure 6.3.6) from 63 (10.16%) to 30 (5.03%) ($\chi^2 = 10.63$; $p < 0.01$). The total sum of absentee days dropped from 1527 (mean = 24.24 days/student [SD = 13.53]) in 2003/2004 to 831 (mean = 27.70 days/student [SD = 16.24] in 2004/2005 ($t = 1.02$; $p > 0.05$).

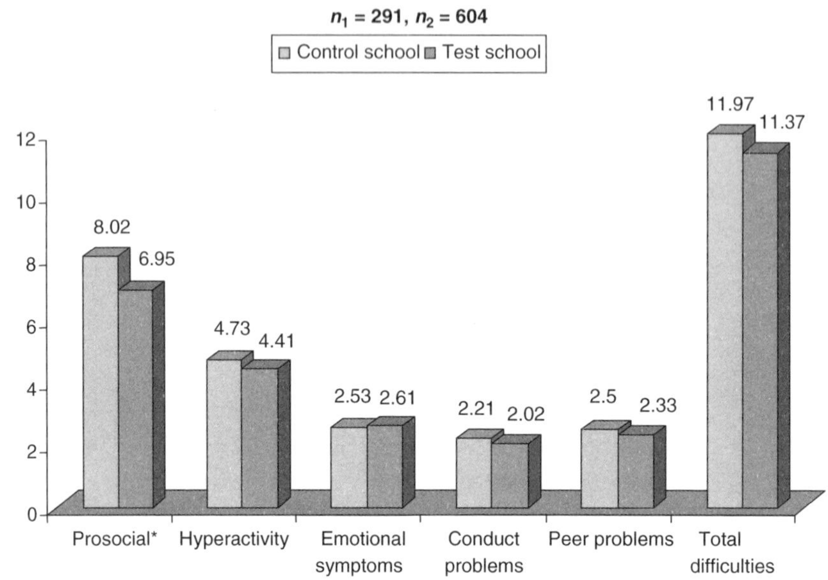

* The differences are significant – $p < 0.001$

Figure 6.3.4 SDQ score parents

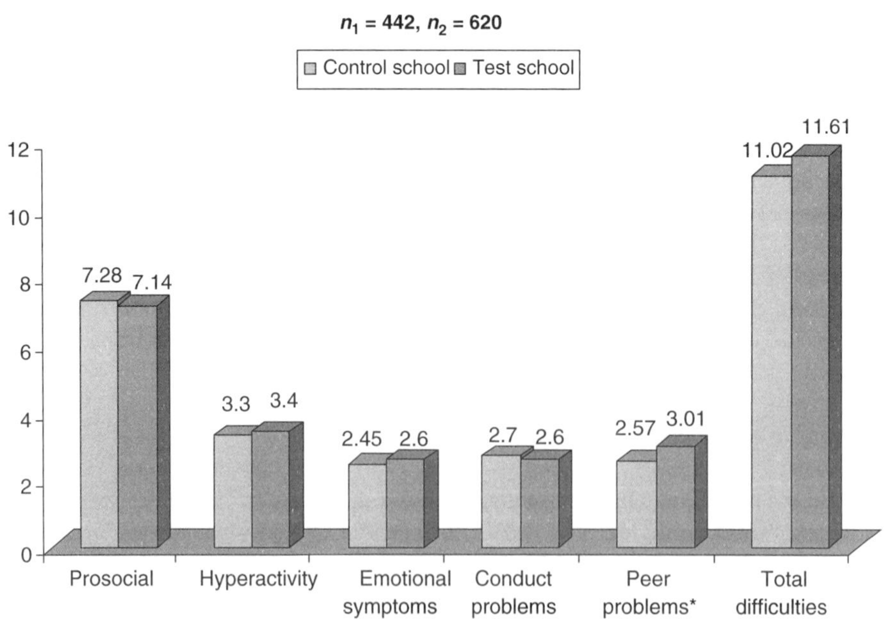

*The differences are significant – $p < 0.001$

Figure 6.3.5 SDQ score students

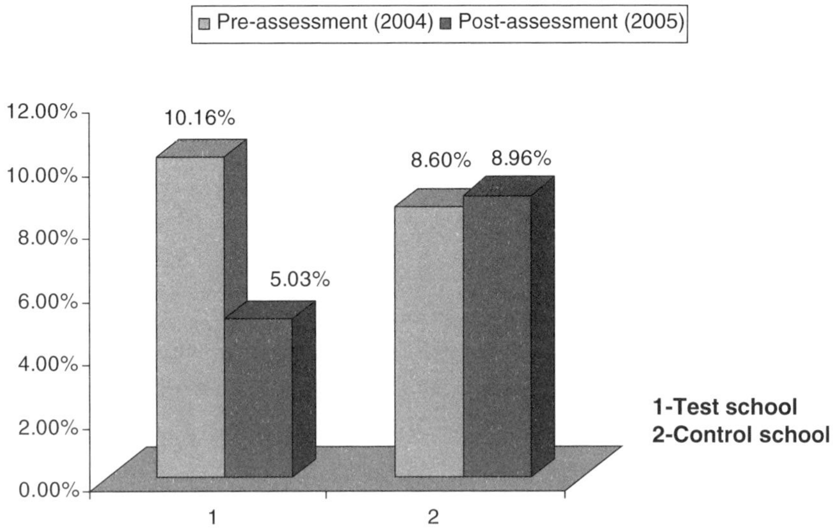

Figure 6.3.6 School absenteeism rate

In the control school, the total sum of absentee days among all students was 2651 (mean = 6.0 days/student [SD = 8.66]) in 2003/2004 and 2029 (mean = 5.05 days/student [SD = 9.81]) in 2004/2005 school year ($t = 1.48$; $p > 0.05$). The number of students regularly absent from school did not change significantly: 38 (8.60%) during the 2003/2004 and 36 (8.96%) during the 2004/2005 (Figure 6.3.6). The total sum of absentee days in the control school was 763 (mean = 20.08 days/student [SD = 16.1] in 2003/2004 and 719 (mean = 19.97 days/student [SD = 22.6]) in 2004/2005 ($t = 0.31$; $p > 0.05$).

After the intervention (i.e., at the end of 2004/2005), the dropout rate in the experimental school fell from 0.48 to 0.34%: three dropouts were out of school for 4 weeks or longer during 2003/2004, and two during 2004/2005 (both in very disturbed families without fathers). In the control school, the dropout rate remained the same (0.91 and 1.00%): four students were out of school for 4 weeks or longer during both 2003/2004 and 2004/2005 (Figure 6.3.7). In the school year 2004/2005, there was a significantly lower rate of absenteeism in the experimental school compared to the control school ($z = 5.67$, $p < 0.0005$), whereas during 2003/2004, the rate of absenteeism was higher in the experimental school. During 2004/2005, the number of students regularly absent from school was 30 (5.03%) in the experimental school and 36 (8.96%) in the control ($\chi^2 = 5.39$; $p < 0.05$).

In the experimental school, there were differences between students' pre-assessment and post-assessment SDQ scores (Figure 6.3.8): Emotional Symptoms, Conduct Problems, Peer Problems, and Total Difficulties. In the control school, there were decreases in SDQ Conduct Problems and Total Difficulties (Figure 6.3.9). In general, students' pre- and post-SDQ scores changed much more favorably in the experimental school.

There were differences between teachers' SDQ pre- and post-assessments in the experimental school (Figure 6.3.10): Prosocial Behavior, Emotional Symptoms, Peer Problems, and Total Difficulties. In the control school, there were differences between the teachers' pre-assessments and post-assessments on only Emotional Symptoms and Total Difficulties (Figure 6.3.11).

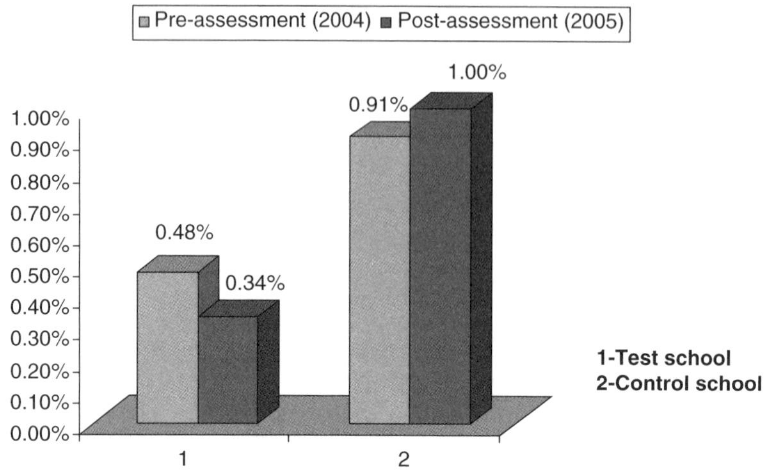

Figure 6.3.7 School dropout rate

In the experimental school, significant improvements were found in parents' pre-SDQ and post-SDQ scores in regard to Prosocial Behavior, Hyperactivity, Emotional Symptoms, and Total Difficulties (Figure 6.3.12). In the control school, there were improvements in Hyperactivity, Conduct Problems, Peer Problems, and Total Difficulties (Fig 6.3.13).

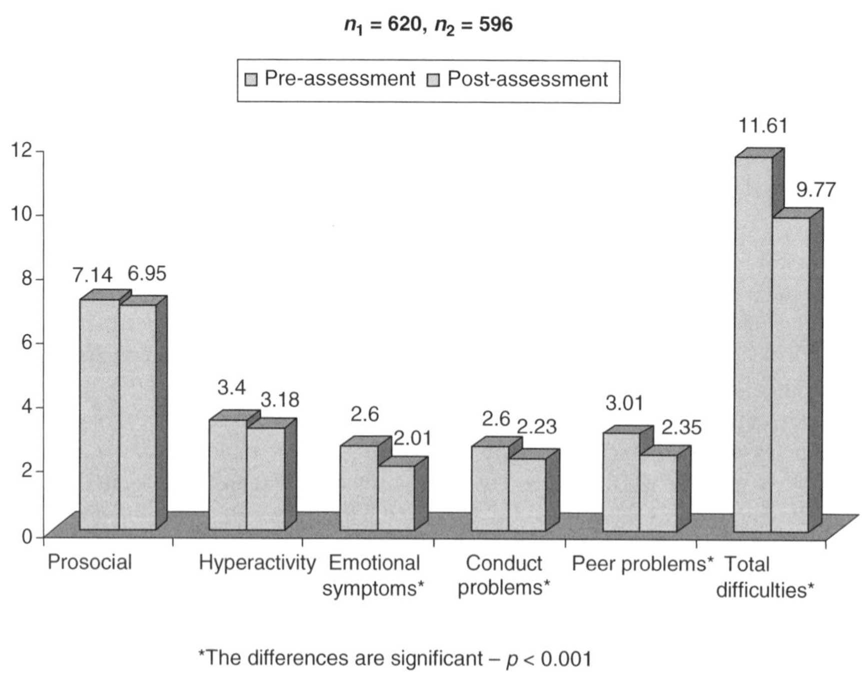

Figure 6.3.8 SDQ score experimental school (students)

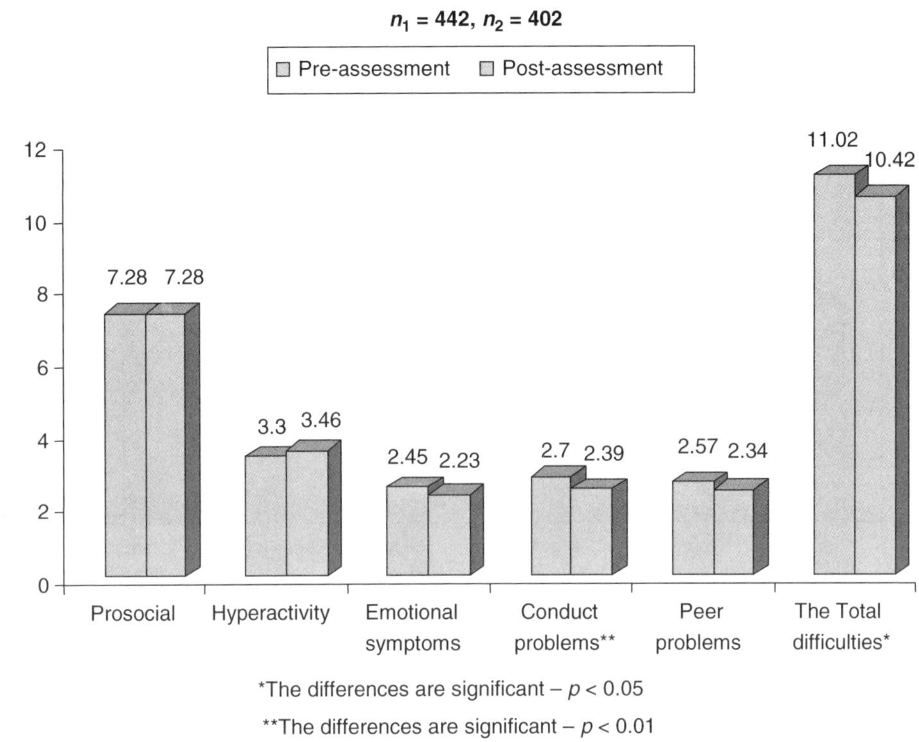

Figure 6.3.9 SDQ score control school (students)

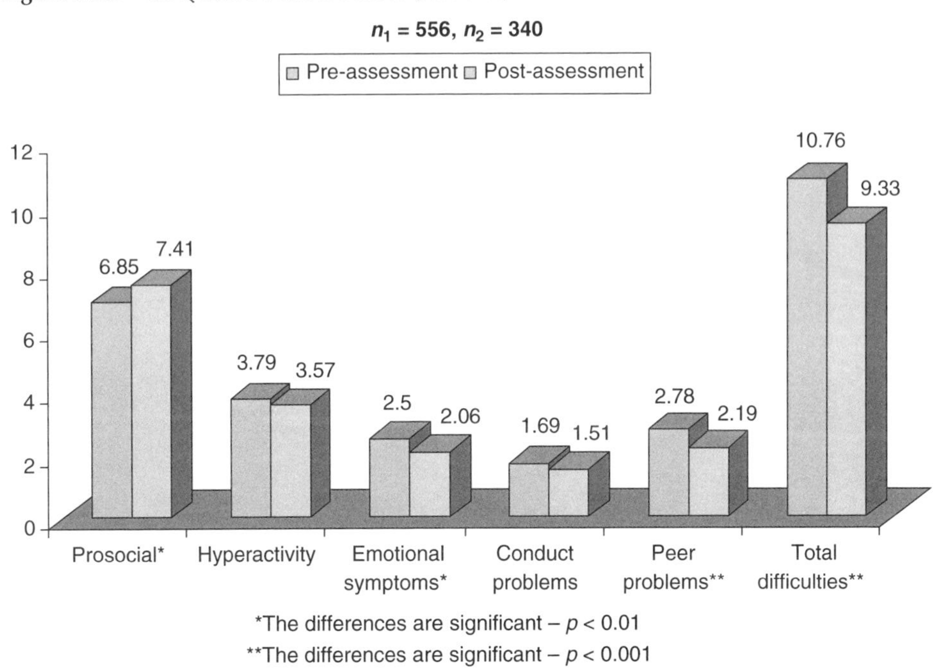

Figure 6.3.10 SDQ score experimental school (teachers)

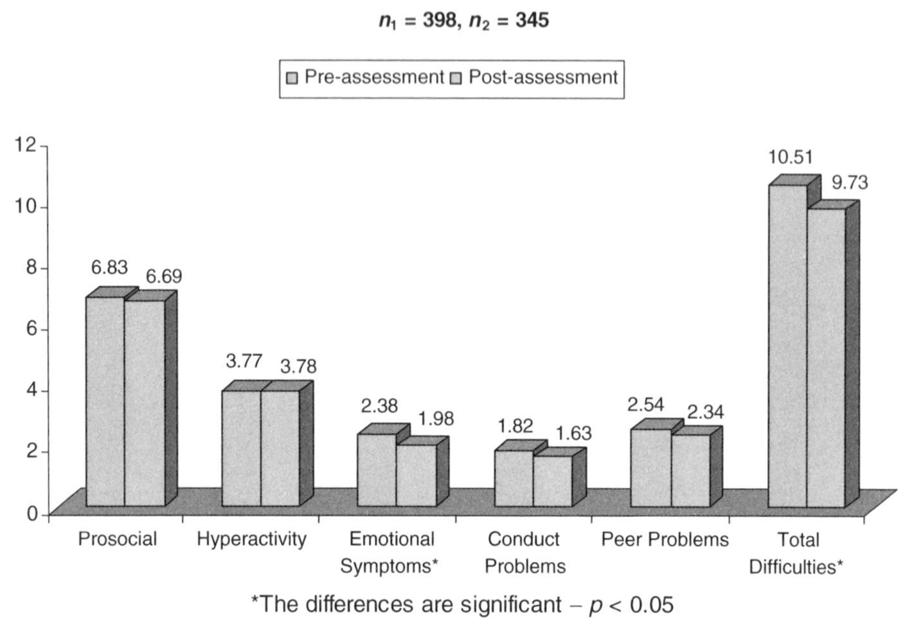

Figure 6.3.11 SDQ score control school (teachers)

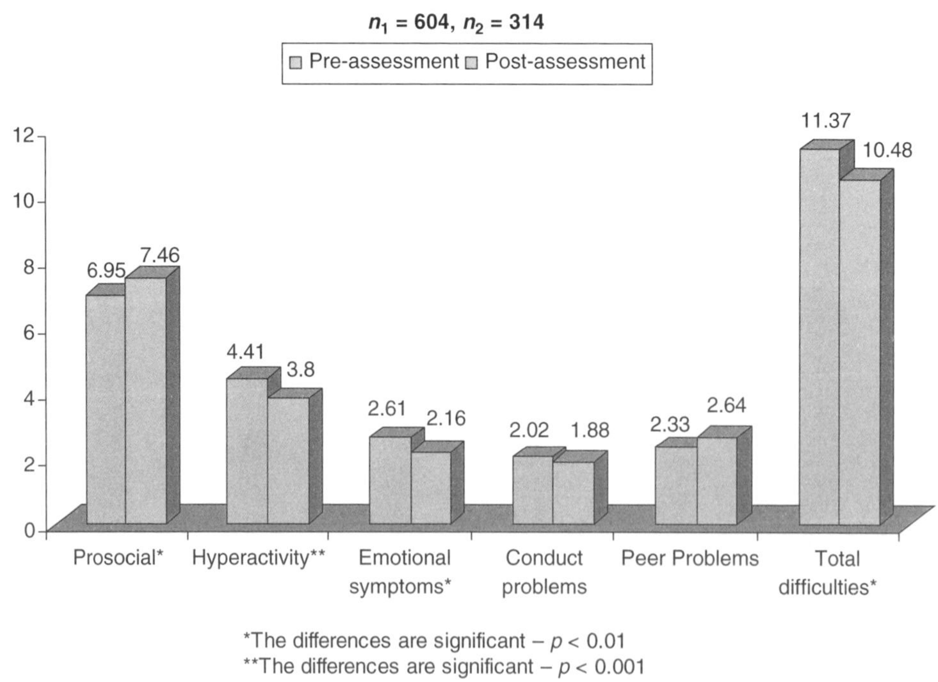

Figure 6.3.12 SDQ score experimental school (parents)

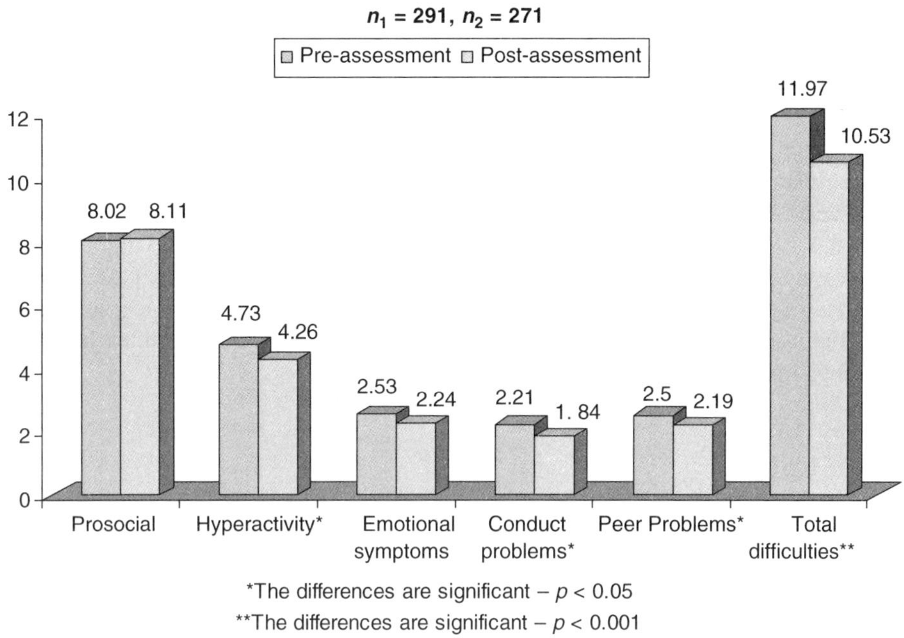

Figure 6.3.13 SDQ score control school (parents)

DISCUSSION

The prevention programme was associated with significant improvement in the rate of school absenteeism. The advantages of staying at school were extensively stressed to all students. The mobilization of the school community and the presence of the investigators in the school might have prepared the environment to accept that aspect of the intervention directed at at-risk students.

Because of the adverse school situation in both schools, especially relation to teachers, the experimental intervention aimed to improve the school environment. A more attractive school atmosphere could have helped to decrease the absenteeism rate in the experimental school. The significant improvement in SDQ ratings suggests that psychological adjustment of students in the experimental school improved in regard to peer relations, emotional symptoms, conduct problems, and prosocial behavior.

When the rate of potential dropouts in the control school is compared with that in the experimental school, a significant difference is found. Nevertheless, we found some improvements in absenteeism rates and SDQ scores in the control school during 2004/2005. It is possible that the presence of research team encouraged control school staff to pay more attention to at-risk students. However, the rate of absenteeism and dropout did not change, suggesting that the intervention did reach at-risk students in the experimental school. On the contrary, despite the intervention, almost half the students at risk continued to be absent from school. Clearly, a modification of the programme is required. Our suggestion is to investigate the family situation of absentees in more detail and to implement family-oriented components.

This intervention employed both universal and targeted strategies to address school dropout. It demonstrates the possibility of establishing an effective connection between the educational and mental health systems. The model could be replicated. Mental health professionals could work as consultants in schools with a high rate of student dropout, promoting the implementation of universal strategies at school and fostering links between families, school, mental health, and social facilities.

The acceptance of intervention by the school community was mixed. School staff readily reported cases of students who were out of school seven or more days, but at-risk families were less involved in the universal preventive strategies. In some cases, students induced to return after seven days out of school were not encouraged by teachers to stay. These findings suggest the need for more intensive preparatory work with teachers at the beginning of projects of this type.

CONCLUSION

A high rate of school absenteeism was found, together with high rates of psychological problems in absentee students. School-based prevention programmes should identify students at risk of dropping out of school by virtue of their regular absenteeism. The integrated preventive intervention in this study combined a universal strategy with a targeted, selective strategy for at-risk students. The overall intervention was successful in reducing the incidence of absenteeism and dropout but not the psychopathology of students. A future research aim could be to identify which components in the intervention are effective.

ACKNOWLEDGMENTS

We acknowledge Irina Burlakova (school psychologist) for her participation in the meetings with the parents and with the school staff; the staff from the City Department of Education and to the staffs of Schools N7 and N47 Nizhny Novgorod, especially to School Directors Nadezhda Smirnova and Olga Davidova, and social worker Lilia Siwokhina for their continuous support; and the members of the Taskforce on Prevention of the Presidential WPA Programme on Global Child Mental Health (Doctors Rohde, Seif El-Din, and Caffo; Professors Remschmidt, Flament, Nurcombe, and Rydelius).

REFERENCES

Achenbach, T. M., Howell, C. T., McConaughy, S. H., and Stanger, C. (1998) Six-year predictors of problems in a national sample: IV. Young adult signs of disturbance. *J Am Acad Child Adolesc Psychiatry*, **37**, 718–27.

Allen, J. P., Philliber, S., and Hoggson, N. (1990) School-based prevention of teen-age pregnancy and school dropout: Process evaluation of the national replication of the Teen Outreach Program. *Am J Community Psychol*, **18**(4), 505–24.

Astone, N. M. and McLanahan, S. S. (1994) Family structure, residential mobility, and school dropout: A research note. *Demography*, **31**, 575–84.

Barilnik, J. B., Pushkareva, L. N. (2003) The structure of conduct disorders in neglected under aged persons. *Materials of the Russian Congress "Medicine for children"*, Nizhny Novgorod, Remedium Publishers, p. 112.

Bechtold, D. W., Manson, S. M., and Shore, J. H. (1994) Psychosocial consequences of stress among Native American adolescents, in *Stress in Psychiatric Disorders. Springer series on psychiatry* (eds Liberman, Robert Paul and Yager Joel), Vol. 5, Springer Publishing Co. xv, 191 pp, New York, pp. 101–16.

Bryk, A. S. and Thum, Y. M. (1989) The effects of high school organization on dropping out: An exploratory investigation. *Am Educ Res J*, **26**, 353–83.

Center for Disease Control (CDC). (1994) Health risk behaviors among adolescents who do and do not attend school – United States, 1992. *JAMA*, **271**, 1068–70.

Dmitrieva, T., Seif El Din A. (2003) Questionnaire for Assessment of the Family and School Situation (QAFSS) for children and teachers, unpublished.

Eggert, L. L., Seyl, C. D., and Nicholas, L. J. (1990) Effects of a school-based prevention program for potential high school dropouts and drug abusers. *Int J Addic*, **25**(7), 773–801.

Ekstrom, R. B., Goertz, M. E., Pollack, J. M, and Rock, D. A. (1987) Who dropout of high school and why: Findings from a national study in *School Dropouts: Patterns and Policies* (ed C. Natriello), Teachers College Press, New York, pp. 52–69.

Fergusson, D. M. and Horwood, L. J. (1995) Validity of categorically and dimensionally scored measures of disruptive childhood behaviors. *J Am Acad Child Adolesc Psychiatry*, **34**, 477–87.

Fergusson, D. M. and Horwood, L. J. (1998) Early conduct problems and later life opportunities. *J Child Psychol Psychiatry*, **39**, 1097–108.

Gleason, P. and Dynarski, M. (2002) Do we know whom to serve? Issues in using risk factors to identify dropouts. *J Educ Students Placed at-Risk*, **7**(1), 25–41.

Goodman, R. (1997) Strengths and difficulties questionnaire: A research note. *J Child Psychol Psychiatry Allied Dis*, **38**, 581–86.

Hawkins, J. D., Catalano, R. F., Kosterman, R. *et al.* (1999) Preventing adolescent health-risk behaviors by strengthening protection during childhood. *Arch Pediatr Adolesc Med*, **153**(3), 226–34.

Hill, S., Locke, J., Lowers, L., and Connolly, J. (1999) Psychopathology and achievement in children at high risk for developing alcoholism. *J Am Acad Child Adolesc Psychiatry*, **38**, 883–91.

Jackson, M. H., Reddick, K. B., and Dubes, R. G. (1995) Self-concept correlates between at-risk and not-at-risk ninth-grade students. *Psychol Rep*, **76**, 683–87.

Kessler, R. C., Foster, C. L., Saunders, W. B., and Stang, P. E. (1995) Social consequences of psychiatric disorders, I: Educational attainment. *Am J Psychiatry*, **152**, 1026–32.

Kortering, L., Haring, N., and Klockars, A. (1992) The identification of high-school dropouts identified as learning disabled: Evaluating the utility of a discriminant analysis function. *Exceptional Children*, **58**, 422–35.

Mathai, J., Anderson, P., and Bourne, A. (2002) The Strengths and Difficulties Questionnaire (SDQ) as a screening measure prior to admission to a Child and Adolescent Mental Health Service (CAMHS). *Aus e-J Adv Ment Health (AeJAMH)*, **4**, Issue 3, ISSN, 1446–7984.

Maton, K. I. (1990) Meaningful involvement in instrumental activity and well-being: Studies of older adolescents and at risk urban teen-agers. *Am J Community Psychol*, **18**, 297–320.

Oakland, T. (1992) School dropouts: Characteristics and prevention. *Appl Preventive Psychol*, **1**(4), 201–08.

Reyes, O., Jason, L. A. (1991) An evaluation of high school dropout prevention program. *J Community Psychol*, **19**(3), 221–30.

Reynolds, A. J., Temple, J. A., Robertson, D. L., and Mann, E. A. (2001) Long-term effects of an early childhood intervention on educational achievement and juvenile arrest: A 15-year follow-up of low-income children in public schools. *JAMA*, **285**(18), 2339–46.

Ripple, C. H. (1996) Long-term predictors of academic achievement and high-school dropout among inner-city adolescents. *Dissertation Abstracts International: -Section B: The Sciences and Engineering*, **56**(8-B), 4608.

Srebnik, D. S. and Elias, M. J. (1993) An ecological, interpersonal skills approach to drop-out prevention. *Am J Orthopsychiatry*, **63**, 526–635.

Svec, H. (1987) Youth advocacy and high school dropout. *High School J*, **70**(4), 185–92.

Tramontina, S., Martins, S., Michalowski, M. B. *et al.* (2002) Estimated mental retardation and school dropout in a sample of students from state public schools in Porto Alegre, Brazil. *Rev Bras Psyquiatry*, **24**, 177–81.

Trusty, J. and Dooley-Dickey, K. (1993) Development of methods for identifying students with potential to drop out of school. *Special Servies in the Schools*, **7**(2), 21–33.

United Nations Children's Fund. (1999) *The Progress of Nations*, UNICEF publications, Brasília.

United Nation Children's Fund. (2005) *The State of the World's Children 2005*. Full text. Access on line at: www.unicef.org

Vitaro, F., Brendgen, M., and Tremblay, R. E. (1999) Prevention of school dropout through the reduction of disruptive behaviors and school failure in elementary school. *J School Psychol*, **37**(2), 205–26.

Index

Note: page numbers in **bold** refer to diagrams. Page numbers in *italics* refer to information contained in tables.